Pregnancy Disorders and Perinatal Outcomes

Edited By

Julie Lafond

Full Professor and Head, BioMed Research Centre
Department of Sciences Biologiques, Université du Québec à
Montréal, C.P. 8888, Succursale Centre-Ville, Montreal, QC
Canada

Cathy Vaillancourt

Associate Professor, INRS-Institut Armand-Frappier
Université du Québec, 531 blvd. des Prairies, Laval, QC, H7V 1B7
Canada

eBooks End User License Agreement

CONTENTS

FOREWORD

When Drs. Vaillancourt and Lafond asked me to write this foreword, I was honored to have the opportunity to introduce this eBook.

Despite the improvements in perinatal and neonatal outcomes with the progress in diagnostic, health care and service and treatment, the perinatal morbidity and mortality observed in conjunction with adverse pregnancy outcomes particularly in the developing countries remain an important health problem. A recent study of the American Health Institute suggests that half of all fetal deaths were caused by a complication during pregnancy. Specifically, a placental dysfunction was the cause in 26% of all fetal deaths, infections in the mother were the causes in 14-19% of cases, while in only 10% of cases, fetal malformations or umbilical cord dysfunctions were the cause. This study suggests that any disturbance during pregnancy including the state of the intrauterine environment during critical periods of organogenesis and fetal growth can permanently modify fetal programming; altering the organ structure and work in an epigenetic way.

In tracking healthy pregnancies through research, immense progress was made in understanding the types of disturbances and complications occur in pregnancy. This ongoing research helps to find innovative ways of minimizing these disturbances and complications, dealing with them when they do occur, ultimately leading to healthy pregnancies and healthier infants.

This eBook, while very comprehensive, remains simple in its approach. It aims at providing readers with an update on the current research on pregnancy disorders that affect fetal development and could lead to disability later in childhood and adulthood. The eBook is very well organized in eight chapters written by experts working in the burgeoning area of integrative physiology that attempts to unite nature and nurture.

In conclusion, I am excited about this eBook, not only because of its superbly organized, illustrated and presented content, but also because I anticipate that it will be useful to all those who have an interest in unraveling the mysteries of life. I believe that better management of pregnancy in the present will have long term wide-scale effects on the global health in our society.

Thierry Lacaze-Masmonteil, MD, PhD, FRCPC

Professor of Pediatrics, University of Ottawa
Regional Medical Lead-Newborn (Champlain Maternal Newborn Regional Program)
Neonatology, Division Head: CHEO-the Ottawa Hospital
Children's Hospital of Eastern Ontario
401 Smyth Road, Ottawa, ON, Canada, K1H 8L1

PREFACE

Adverse pregnancy outcomes are on the rise world-wide, leading to increased perinatal morbidity and mortality. Moreover, pregnancy disorders can lead to disruption in fetal programming. The fetal programming hypothesis suggests that the intrauterine environment during critical periods of organogenesis and tissue growth may permanently alter organ structure and function in an epigenetic manner. Accompanied with this are immense economic and emotional costs. In the course of its research on healthy pregnancy, scientists have made great progress in understanding features of disorders that may occur during pregnancy. These ongoing investigations are important to find ways to treat and prevent these disorders to support women in having healthy pregnancies and babies.

Since 1989, when David Barker showed an inverse relationship between birth weight and mortality due to adult ischemic heart disease, the role of prenatal programming, and by consequence pregnancy disorder, as a determinant of adult diseases has become increasingly clear. While epidemiological evidence for the role of early developmental growth patterns leading to specific adult disease outcomes has continued to strengthen, experimental evidence from animal models has brought new and compelling support for this important determinant of health throughout lifetime.

This eBook aims at providing readers with the latest research on the current state of knowledge related to pregnancy disorders that affect fetal development and possibly fetal programming. This eBook contains eight reviews by experts who are working in this burgeoning area of integrative physiology is an attempts to unite nature and nurture. We trust it to be useful to all of those who have an interest in unraveling the mysteries of life. We believe that better management of pregnancy today will have long term and wide-scale effects on the health of our society.

Cathy Vaillancourt
INRS-Institut Armand Frappier
Université du Québec
Canada

Julie Lafond
BioMed Research Centre
Department of Sciences Biologiques
Université du Québec à Montréal
Canada

List of Contributors

Eric Asselin

Research Group in Molecular Oncology and Endocrinology
Canada research chair in molecular gyneco-oncology
Department of Chemistry-Biology
University of Quebec at Trois-Rivières
Trois-Rivières, QC, Canada

Louiza Belkacemi

Perinatal Research Laboratories
Department of Obstetrics and Gynecology
David Geffen School of Medicine
University of California Los Angeles
Los Angeles Biomedical Research Institute
Harbor-UCLA Medical Center, Torrance, California, USA

Marc Charland

Reproduction, Perinatal Health and Child Health Research Axis
CHUQ Research Center
Québec City, QC, Canada

Parvesh Chaudhry

Research Group in Molecular Oncology and Endocrinology
Department of Chemistry-Biology
University of Quebec at Trois-Rivières
Trois-Rivières, QC, Canada

Jeffrey M. Craig

Early Life Epigenetics
Murdoch Childrens Research Institute
Royal Children's Hospital
Department of Paediatrics
University of Melbourne
Melbourne, Victoria, Australia

Maria del Pilar Vélez

Obstetrics and Gynecology Department
University of Montreal, Montreal, Quebec, Canada

Evemie Dubé

BioMed Research Centre
Department of Sciences Biologiques
Université du Québec à Montréal
Montreal, QC, Canada

Danièle Evain-Brion

Unité Mixte de Recherches-Santé UMR-S 767
Institut National de la Santé et de la Recherche Médicale (INSERM), Paris Descartes University
PremUP Foundation
Faculty of Pharmaceutical and Biological Sciences
Paris F-75006, France

Jean-Claude Forest

Reproduction, Perinatal Health and Child Health Research Axis
CHUQ Research Center
Department of Molecular Biology
Medical Biochemistry and Pathology
Faculty of Medicine, Université Laval
Québec City, QC, Canada

Thierry Forges

Department of Reproductive Medicine
Maternité Universitaire, 10 rue Dr Heydenreich
54042 Nancy, France

Thierry Fournier

Unité Mixte de Recherches-Santé UMR-S 767
Institut National de la Santé et de la Recherche Médicale (INSERM) and Paris Descartes University
PremUP Foundation
Faculty of Pharmaceutical and Biological Sciences
Paris F-75006, France

Yves Giguère

Reproduction, Perinatal Health and Child Health Research Axis
CHUQ Research Center
Department of Molecular Biology
Medical Biochemistry and Pathology
Faculty of Medicine, Université Laval
Québec City, QC, Canada

Joël Girouard

Reproduction, Perinatal Health and Child Health Research Axis
CHUQ Research Center
Québec City, QC, Canada

Dominique Guérette

Reproduction, Perinatal Health and Child Health Research Axis
CHUQ Research Center
Québec City, QC, Canada

Sophie Haché

BioMed Research Centre
Department of Sciences Biologiques
Université du Québec à Montréal
Montreal, QC, Canada

Ji-Hoon Eric Joo

Early Life Epigenetics
Murdoch Childrens Research Institute
Royal Children's Hospital
Department of Paediatrics
University of Melbourne
Melbourne, Victoria, Australia

Julie Lafond

BioMed Research Centre

Department of Sciences Biologiques
Université du Québec à Montréal
Montreal, QC, Canada

Dave Lanoix

INRS-Institut Armand-Frappier
Université du Québec
531 blvd. des Prairies, Laval, QC, Canada

André Malassiné

Unité Mixte de Recherches-Santé UMR-S 767
Institut National de la Santé et de la Recherche Médicale (INSERM) and Paris Descartes University
PremUP Foundation
Faculty of Pharmaceutical and Biological Sciences
Paris F-75006, France

Patricia Monnier

McGill Reproductive Centre
Department of Obstetrics and Gynecology
Division of Reproductive Endocrinology and Infertility
McGill University, Royal Victoria Hospital, Montreal, Quebec, Canada

Boris Novakovic

Cancer, Disease and Developmental Epigenetics
Murdoch Childrens Research Institute
Royal Children's Hospital
Department of Paediatrics
University of Melbourne
Melbourne, Victoria, Australia

François Rousseau

Reproduction, Perinatal Health and Child Health Research Axis
CHUQ Research Center
Department of Molecular Biology
Medical Biochemistry and Pathology
Faculty of Medicine, Université Laval
Québec City, QC, Canada

Richard Saffery

Cancer, Disease and Developmental Epigenetics
Murdoch Childrens Research Institute
Royal Children's Hospital
Department of Paediatrics
University of Melbourne
Melbourne, Victoria, Australia

Shigeru Saito

Department of Obstetrics and Gynecology
Toyama Medical and Pharmaceutical University
2630 Sugitani Toyama-shi, Toyama, Japan

Mohan Sran

Research Group in Molecular Oncology and Endocrinology
Department of Chemistry-Biology

University of Quebec at Trois-Rivières
Trois-Rivières, QC, Canada

Vassilis Tsatsaris

Assistance Publique-Hôpitaux de Paris
Centre Hospitalier Universitaire Cochin and Maternité Port-Royal
Paris F-75014, France

Cathy Vaillancourt

INRS-Institut Armand-Frappier
Université du Québec
531 blvd. des Prairies, Laval, QC, Canada

INTRODUCTION

The present eBook set of *Pregnancy disorders and perinatal outcomes* offers its readers a unique opportunity on the current status of knowledge related to maternal habits or disorders that could affect fetal development and lead to disability later in childhood and adulthood. It contains chapters on the role of placenta, hormones, nutrition, diabetes, hypertension, *in vitro* fertilization, immune systems and epigenetic in pregnancy well-being and perinatal outcomes. Importantly, the eBook integrates both fundamental and clinical medicine as well as molecular and cell biology. This eBook is written with the intent to allow multidisciplinary use and can be recommended to a wide spectrum of readers including students, clinicians (obstetricians, neonatologists, peadiatricians) and basic scientists in the field.

2

CHAPTER 1

Embryo Implantation Disorders

Mohan Singh, Parvesh Chaudhry and Eric Asselin*

Research Group in Molecular Oncology and Endocrinology, Canada Research Chair in Molecular Gyneco-Oncology, Department of Chemistry Biology, University of Quebec at Trois-Rivières, Trois-Rivières, Québec, Canada, G9A 5H7

Abstract: Embryo implantation is a complex process; primary step in implantation is the initiation of dialogue between free floating blastocyst and the receptive endometrium. This is followed by a stable adhesion of the blastocyst anchors to the endometrial basal lamina and stromal extracellular matrix. The last step is invasion of the embryo through the luminal epithelium and its basal lamina into the uterine stroma. Successful embryo implantation depends up on number of factors like steroid hormones (progesterone, estrogen), Cyclooxygenases, prostaglandins, cytokines, growth factors, transcription factors (HOXA-10 and HOXA-11), and adhesion molecules (integrins, selectins, cadherins, mucins) and receptive endometrium. Importantly, there is timely regulation of these factors and their cross talk which mediates the implantation process. Blastocyst is unable to implant successfully if there is deregulation in any of these factors leading to pregnancy loss. In this chapter we reviewed the information available till date to provide possible causes of implantation failure and its positive outcomes.

Keywords: Implantation, endometrial receptivity, growth factors, cytokines, hormones, adhesion molecules.

INTRODUCTION

Embryo implantation in the uterus is a critical and intricate event in the development of all mammals and its failure is widely considered to be a challenge to their furtherance. The process of blastocyst implantation requires synchronized interaction between trophoblast cells and the maternal endometrium [1]. Briefly, the events of implantation include: apposition of the blastocyst to the uterine luminal epithelium; adhesion to and penetration through the epithelium and basal lamina; and invasion into the stromal vasculature. This dynamic process involves a complex series of molecular and cellular events that are induced in the pregnant uterus by paracrine and autocrine regulators and also through cell–cell and cell–matrix interactions [2]. The success of implantation depends on achieving the appropriate embryo development to the blastocyst stage and at the same time, the development of an endometrium that is receptive to the embryo. However, embryonic loss in the first trimester occurs in 15–30% of all pregnancies [3], but the true figure is probably much higher because of the high incidence of pregnancy loss before the clinical detection of pregnancy. Although many losses are likely due to embryonic genetic anomalies, others are due to abnormalities in the uterine environment. In humans, little information is available about the genes whose expression in the endometrium is essential to its interaction with the blastocyst. Ethical and technical issues, such as restrictions in human blastocyst research, the lack of a reliable *in vitro* implantation model and limited availability of human placental tissue, limits the possibilities of human embryo implantation disorder studies. Thus, most of our current knowledge regarding expression/regulation of genes/proteins during the peri and implantation period has been derived from experimental animals. Rat and mouse models have provided valuable insights into the molecular mechanisms that occur during embryo implantation [4], however, these models do not necessarily translate to the human because the reproductive physiology of mice and humans is different at different levels [5].

A wide array of molecules participate in the embryo-uterine interaction, which includes cytokines, adhesion molecules, growth factors and various other molecules [6, 7]. Given the broad array of these molecules, special attention is given here to factors that are released at the implantation site, and particularly, on

*Address correspondence to Eric Asselin: Research Group in Molecular Oncology and Endocrinology, Canada Research Chair in Molecular Gyneco-Oncology, Department of Chemistry Biology, University of Quebec at Trois-Rivières, Trois-Rivières, Québec, Canada, G9A 5H7; Tel: 819-376-5011 ext. 3317; Fax: 819-376-5057; E-mail: eric.asselin@uqtr.ca

hormones, growth factors and cytokines which are likely to play an important role in regulating trophoblast differentiation and invasion. Discovery of indispensable molecules for successful embryo implantation has provided a great lead in the field of reproductive biology. Despite tremendous research in this field, molecular mechanisms responsible for the process of implantation still need a better understanding. There is a significant knowledge gap in the understanding of this embryo–uterine dialogue, and the *in vivo* events of implantation. Studies involving the molecular signalling pathways, which regulate uterine receptivity and successful implantation of blastocyst, are of paramount importance. These studies may provide a better understanding of the reasons for implantation failure, which could lead to an improvement in pregnancy rates in humans. In this chapter, we will examine the evidence that failure to develop a receptive endometrium contributes significantly to implantation failure. The purpose of this chapter is to describe the most important players of the embryo-uterine crosstalk in the apposition and adhesion phases which seem to be crucial for successful implantation. The current knowledge as to their expression, regulation, relationships and their involvement in physiological and pathological conditions will also be discussed. In addition, key areas in implantation research will be identified where efforts need to be focused in the future.

ENDOMETRIAL RECEPTIVITY AND IMPLANTATION

Endometrium is termed as receptive, when refractive endometrium is ready to receive blastocyst and allows its attachment with endometrium, which further induces morphological changes in the stromal region leading to decidualization and placentation. The phenomenon of endometrial receptivity was first established in the rat and later validated in other species [8]. Endometrium can exist in different stages like neutral, refractive and receptive. However, for successful implantation timely arrival of viable blastocyst along with receptive endometrium is a pre-requisite. Embryo transfer studies in rodent have established that the endometrium is receptive only for limited time period (for 24 hours) at day 4-5 of pregnancy [9]. However in humans, embryo implantation can only occur in the endometrium during limited period spanning days 20–24 of the menstrual cycle. After which the endometrium becomes refractory to implantation [8]. Embryos entering the uterine cavity before or after the window of receptivity do not attach and implant. This time period is called 'window of implantation', during which the uterine environment is conducive to blastocyst implantation.

Various morphological changes occur in the endometrial epithelial cells during implantation window. One of the changes is the appearance of membrane projections called pinopodes [10, 11]. Pinopodes develop in a progesterone dependent manner and become markedly visible between days 20-21 of the menstrual cycle [11, 12]. The mechanisms of action of pinopodes are still unclear, but their role as biomarkers of endometrial receptivity has been emphasized previously [13]. The presence of pinopodes at the embryo-endometrial interface during implantation has been demonstrated, where these pinopodes participate in the adhesion process of the human blastocyst. Furthermore, pinopodes may prevent sweeping off the blastocyst by cilia and helps the withdrawal of uterine fluid thus facilitating adhesion of the blastocyst to molecules of the pinopodes [14, 15].

Primary step in implantation is the initiation of dialogue between free floating blastocyst and the receptive endometrium (Fig. **1**). Presence of hormones and cytokines at this stage mediate synchronized endometrial maturation and embryo development [16]. Apposition is the next stage which is identified as an unstable adhesion of the blastocyst to the endometrial surface. During this stage, the trophoblast cells adhere to the receptive luminal epithelium. At this stage the pinopodes, which are micro protrusions from the apical uterine epithelium surface, inter-digitate with microvilli on the apical syncytiotrophoblast surface of the blastocyst [17] This is followed by a stable adhesion or attachment phase where blastocyst anchors to the endometrial basal lamina and stromal extracellular matrix. Paracrine signaling between the embryo and endometrium is responsible for stronger attachment of blastocyst. The first sign of the attachment reaction occurs on the evening of day 4 in mice/rats, or day 20 to 21 in humans, and it coincides with a localized increase in the stromal vascular permeability at the site of blastocyst attachment [18]. The last stage is the invasion process, which involves penetration of the embryo through the luminal epithelium and its basal lamina into the stroma thereby establishing a vascular relationship with the mother, and this activity is mainly controlled by trophoblasts; however the decidua also limits the extent of invasion [19]. In response to this invasion and the presence of constant progesterone stimulation, the endometrial stromal cells and endometrial extracellular matrix undergo decidualization. Which is an essential feature of normal implantation and pregnancy, during this process endometrial stroma transform into a dense cellular matrix known as deciduas [20]. In the process of decidualization, endometrial tissue remodulates, which includes secretory transformation of the uterine glands, influx of specialized uterine natural killer cells, and vascular remodelling [21]. Decidualization of stromal region impedes the movement of trophoblast by creating physical barrier and releasing cytokine in environment which promotes trophoblast attachment rather than invasion. [22, 23]. The timely completion of attachment and decidualization are essential for the viability of the pregnancy.

The establishment of the endometrial transition, which supports embryo implantation, is primarily coordinated by ovarian hormones, progesterone and estrogen, that modulate uterine events in a spatiotemporal manner and that prepare the endometrium to respond to blastocyst signals [24, 25]. In addition to the physical interaction of the embryonic tissue with the uterine cells, this process is undoubtedly influenced by maternal steroid hormones, growth factors and cytokines in paracrine manner thus playing a crucial role in embryonic signaling [7, 26]. The ovarian steroids have a major regulatory role by mobilizing several molecular modulators. Throughout this period, the human endometrium has been prepared to attach the blastocyst because it has acquired an appropriate morphological and functional state initiated by ovarian steroid hormones. Although numerous molecules involved in implantation have been identified in rodents [24, 25] and humans [27], microarray analysis of human endometrium from the receptive phase has given insight regarding involvement of certain molecules [28, 29] but the molecular mechanisms, regulation of genes, and signal cascades that govern this process of endometrium-blastocyst interaction remain poorly understood.

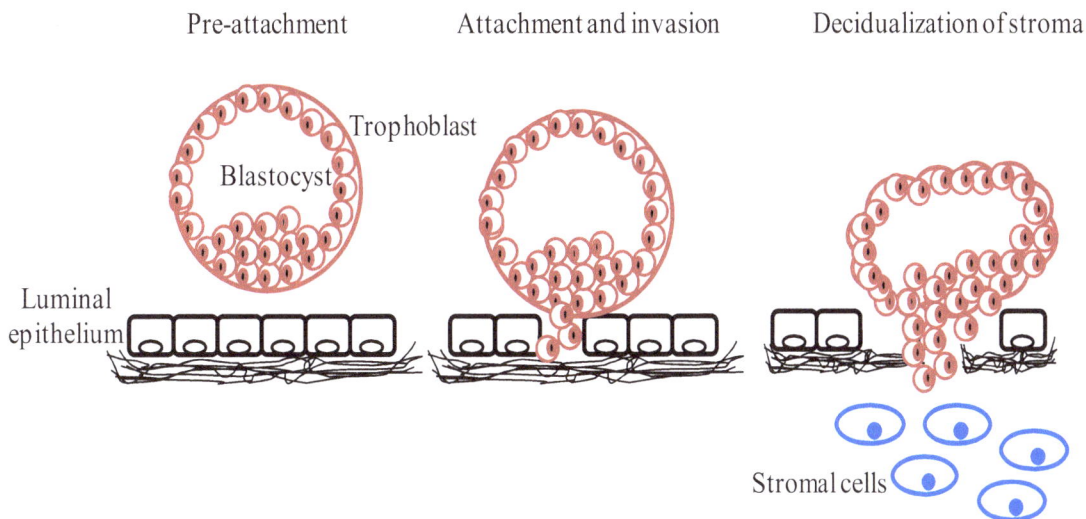

Figure 1: Cartoon representing the stages of implantation [Adapted from Sharkey, AM and Smith, SK (2003)].

Endocrinological Aspects

Progesterone and estrogen are the key hormones responsible for endometrial development. Progesterone is essential for implantation and pregnancy maintenance in all mammals, whereas the requirement for estrogen is species specific [30]. The preimplantation estrogen surge is essential in mice, whereas ovarian estrogen does not play an obligatory role in implantation of primates [31]. Both the epithelial and stromal compartments express progesterone and estrogen receptors and the response depend on the levels of these receptors as well as on the concentration of the hormones themselves. Synchronization between receptor expression and release of hormones is necessary for achieving endometrial receptivity and successful implantation [9, 32]. The uterine effects of estrogen and progesterone are primarily executed by nuclear estrogen and progesterone (ER and PR) receptors [33]. The discovery of ER (ERα and ERβ) and PR (PR-A and PR-B) isoforms and studies of the effects of their selective deletion provide evidence for their isoforms-specific functions in uterine biology and implantation. The uterus of ERα knockout (αERKO) mice develops normally but remains immature and hypoplastic, that is unable to support implantation [34]. Progesterone creates an immunologically conducive milieu for the developing fetus by mediating both the endocrine and immune systems [35]. Uterine natural killer (NK) cells accumulate in the endometrium during estrus and proestrus phases in rodents and during the luteal phase in humans. In addition, NK cells are also evidenced during early pregnancy at sites where fetal trophoblast infiltrates the decidua. Progesterone is the key player in uterine homing of NK cells by promoting NK cell interactions with the endothelium [36]. On the other hand, estradiol induces the expression of α_4 receptors for fibronectin, which is important component of uterine basement membrane [37]. During peri-implantation period, the increased release of estrogen over progesterone promotes proper distribution of integrins in the endometrium, which further facilitate attachment of blastocyst to the receptive endometrium. In future, these hormones and other factors may be used as predictors of endometrial receptivity or embryo quality for the improvement of implantation rates given a better understanding is achieved.

Plethora of other endocrinological factors is known to be involved in the process of pregnancy apart from progesterone and estrogen [38]. It is well documented in the literature that prostaglandins (PGs) play an important role in reproductive processes, including ovulation, implantation, and menstruation [39, 40]. The rate-limiting step in PG biosynthesis is catalyzed by cytosolic phospholipase A_2 (PLA_2) enzymes, which release arachidonic acid (AA) from membrane phospholipids [41] as shown in Fig. **2**. Cyclooxygenases (COX-1 and COX-2) mediate the conversion of arachidonic acid into prostaglandinH2 (PGH2), which is then converted into various PGs by specific synthase. Earlier study from our laboratory has shown that PGD synthase (PGDS) and prostacyclin synthase (PGIS) are present in the rat uterus during pregnancy and high levels could be seen at the early stage of pregnancy. The expression of various PG synthases could be regulated by steroids and that the endometrium could be a significant source of PGD_2 and PGI_2 at specific times during pregnancy [42].

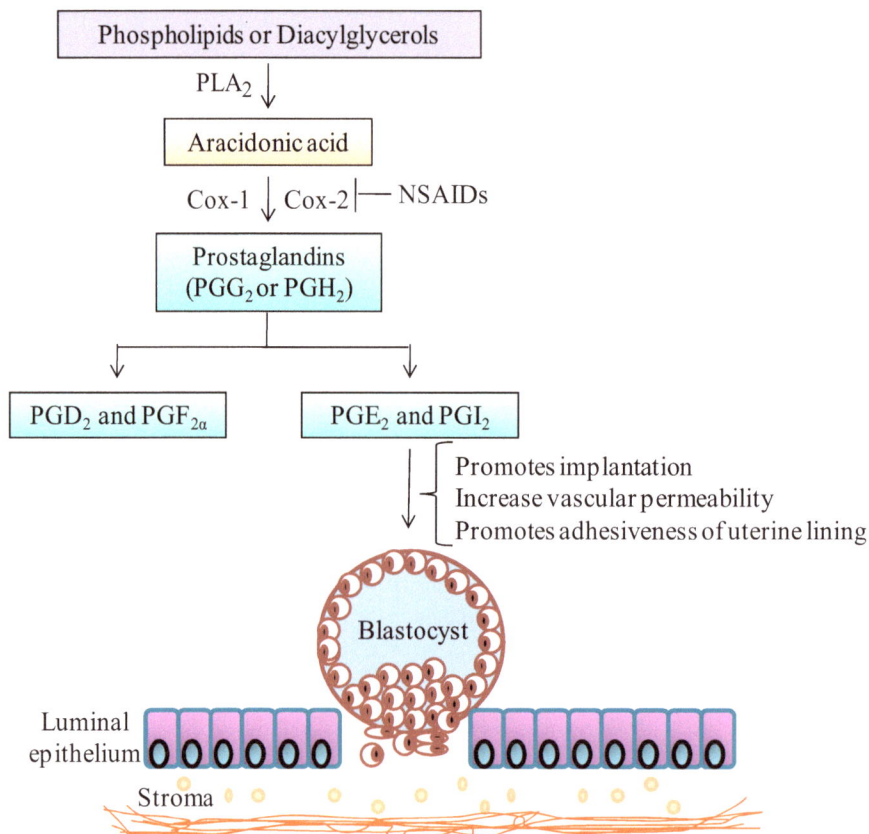

Figure 2: Role of prostaglandins in embryo implantation [Adapted from Shah, BH and Catt KJ (2005)].

Extensive research in the field of pregnancy highlighted and established the vital role of PGs in the implantation process. Achache *et al.* [43] have reported that patients with recurrent pregnancy failure were shown to have very low levels of $cPLA_{2\alpha}$ and COX-2, possibly reducing further PG synthesis, which could be responsible for implantation failure. Previous study by Song *et al.* [44] in female mice lacking $cPLA_2$ or COX-2 enzymes has also established the central role of PGs in implantation. Mice lacking either of these enzymes lead to absence of PG synthesis, which results in improper embryo implantation. Moreover, it had also been studied that $cPLA_2$ knockout mice experience pregnancy failure. Lysophosphatidic acid (LPA), a lipid-derived G-protein-coupled receptor (GPCR) agonist plays crucial roles in a wide array of processes, including cell proliferation, survival and differentiation, invasion and cell-cell interaction. LPA_3-deficient mice was markedly similar to those reported for rats and mice treated with the PG-synthesis inhibitor, indomethacin [45], and for mice deficient in $cPLA_{2\alpha}$ [44]. Modulation of PG synthesis before or during the time of implantation can be fatal for implantation by reducing the number of implantation sites with reduced decidual tissue, which can further lead to delayed implantation.

COX-1 is functions as a constitutive enzyme whereas COX-2 is highly inducible by diverse stimuli including mitogens, cytokines, growth factor and tumor promoters. COX-2 enzymes is known to regulate inflammation, differentiation and angiogenesis [46]. Recent study from our lab evidenced that COX-1 and COX-2 proteins are present during different stages of pregnancy in rat endometrium, indicating important role of these proteins in the process of pregnancy and expression of these cyclooxygenases are controlled by sex hormones [47]. The unique expression pattern of COX-1 and COX-2 genes in preimplantation mouse uterus suggests an important role for PGs in embryo implantation. This expression pattern suggests that COX-2 expression during the attachment reaction is critical for implantation [48]. COX-2 deficient mice were found to exhibit multiple reproductive failures, which were not observed in the case of COX-1 deficient mice. Furthermore, up regulation of COX-2 and prostacyclin (PGI_2) synthesis were found to be essential for implantation in the mouse [49]. Previous studies in rodents suggest that the enzymes responsible for prostaglandins (PGs) synthesis *i.e.*, COX-1 and COX-2 show cyclic changes in their expression pattern [47, 48, 50]. These PGs further affect the process of implantation by changing the vascular permeability of the uterus [51]. PGs are also speculated to play an important role in maintaining implantation window, as delayed implantation of blastocyst could generate ripple effect by crowding embryo near cervix, abnormal placentation and fetal resorption. However, PGs supplementation can partially restore a normal phenotype. There are concerns that non-steroidal anti-inflammatory drugs (NSAIDs) such as ibuprofen, aspirin, indomethacin and celecoxib may interfere with implantation of embryo. NSAIDs are considered to be the inhibitors of COX-2 and prostaglandin biosynthesis in most organ, including reproductive system, which could lead to abnormal implantation that predisposes an embryo to peri-implantation loss [52]. Previously, Sookvanichsilp and Pulbtur (2002) have also demonstrated that the administration of indomethacin and celecoxib to rats significantly reduced the uterine decidualization. The above mentioned studies suggest that COX-derived PGs are important factors at the critical time of implantation for subsequent post-implantation development.

Cell Adhesion Molecules

Integrins

The cell adhesion molecule (CAM) family is composed of four members known as integrins, cadherins, selectins and immunoglobulins. These surface ligands, usually glycoproteins, mediate cell-to-cell adhesion. Integrins are among the best characterized markers of endometrial receptivity [53].

Integrins are a family of transmembrane glycoproteins, formed by the association of two different, non-covalently linked, α and β subunits. Heterodimers of α and β integrins serve as receptors for extra cellular matrix (ECM) ligands such as collagen, laminin and fibronectin, as well as transducing signals from soluble ligands such as osteopontin [54]. To date, eighteen α and eight β chains have been identified in mammals. They can combine into 24 different integrin heterodimers having different functional significances [55]. A large variety of integrins have been described within the luminal and glandular endometrial epithelium [6,

56]. In spite of presence of various integrins during menstrual cycle differential expression pattern were observed for a few intergrin molecules. However, majority of the integrin molecules show constitutive expression throughout this period. [6]. Given their high expression during mid-luteal phase, some intergrins could play a crucial role as markers of the window of implantation [57]. α1β1, α4β1 and αVβ3 integrins are shown to be expressed in cyclic manner in human endometrium on days 20–24 of the human menstrual. According to a timed expression correlating with embryo attachment, the αVβ3 and the α4β1 integrins are considered markers of uterine receptivity [58, 59]. αVβ3 has been shown to be highly expressed at the time of embryo attachment, and aberrant expression of αVβ3 is associated with infertility [60, 61]. Women with recurrent miscarriages were found to have a lower concentration of α4β1 and α5β1 integrins in the stroma during the implantation window, than women with unexplained infertility [62]. In female mice lacking a functional integrin β1 gene, embryos develop normally to the blastocyst stage but fail to implant properly and die [63]. In knockout studies, no other integrins were found to be involved in implantation defects [7], except $α_V β3$, whose inactivation by echistatin significantly reduced implantation sites in mice [64]. All these reports indicates functional redundancy of several integrins in the process of implantation [65]. Moreover, $α_V β3$ integrin as well as its ligand osteopontin was positively detected by immunohistochemistry on the endometrial luminal epithelial surface, which first interacts with the trophoblast [66]. Therefore, αVβ3 has been proposed as a potential receptor for embryonic attachment [32].

Human trophoblast is known to express integrins at the time of implantation during implantation period [67]. Trophoblastic receptors for ECM (essentially, integrins α1β1 and α5β1) increase in concert with the differentiation of human cytotrophoblast cells to invasive extravillous phenotype [68]. The integrins present both on the uterine epithelium (osteopontin) and on trophoblast surface (oncofetal fibronectin) have affinity for specific ECM components. Incomplete maternal recognition of embryo was found in the absence of α4β1 integrin due to its inability to recognize fibronection on the surface of trophoblast [69]. This provides the possibility of a sandwich model of embryonic adhesion. Aberrant expression of integrins has been observed in the endometrium of women with reproductive failure [69].

Selectins

Selectins are glycoproteins which also belong to the CAM family. They include P-selectin, L-selectin and E-selectin [70]. Human L-selectin is a transmembrane protein with highly glycosylated extracellular domain and a small cytoplasmic tail [71]. The selectin adhesion system is well established at the maternal–fetal interface. At the time of endometrial receptivity, L-selectin has been found to be highly up regulated and present on the entire embryonic surface [72]. Previous studies in literature suggest that the interaction between L-selectin, expressed by trophoblast cells, and its oligosaccharide ligands, expressed by the endometrium, may constitute the initial step in the implantation process [73]. L-selectin has been found to initiate a signaling cascade that facilitates strong embryo attachment with the uterine epithelium which further helps the embryo in establishing contacts with maternal vasculature at the time of placenta formation [73]. In conclusion, very little is known about the involvement of selectins in embryo implantation.

Cadherins

Cadherins constitute a group of glycoproteins responsible for the calcium-dependent cell-to-cell adhesion mechanism. Amongst the various subclasses (E-, P-, and N-cadherins) of cadherins, E-cadherin represents the most studied subclass. E-cadherin is a cell surface transmembrane glycoprotein, which belongs to the family of calcium-dependent cell adhesion molecules (CAMs) that mediates cell–cell adhesion through homeotypic binding. E-cadherin is located in the adherents junctions that are specialized regions on the lateral side of the epithelial plasma membrane and is believed to be critical for the establishment and maintenance of these junctions in epithelial cells [74, 75]. Previous reports indicated that targeted mutations in the E-cadherin gene could result in defective pre-implantation development of the [76]. The role of E-cadherin in human embryo implantation is not known, but based on its expression pattern; it is suspected that might be of important during this process.

Mucins

Mucins are glycoylated molecules found on a great number of tissues, including the endometrial epithelial cells [77]. Enzymatic actions on the cellular surface are impeded by mucins, which also prevent cell–cell and cell–extracellular matrix adhesion. At least 19 human mucin genes have been distinguished by cDNA cloning but MUC-1 and MUC-4 are the two major mucins present in human endometrium both in proliferative and secretory phases [78, 79]. They are believed to be a barrier to trophoblast invasiveness, by controlling accessibility of integrin receptors to their ligands [80]. MUC1 increases from the proliferative to the secretory phase in endometrial tissue and then decreases in the late secretory phase [81]. It has been suggested that progesterone along with estrogen up-regulates MUC1 at the receptive endometrium [81]. This up regulation of MUC1 during apposition phase [82] prevents the attachment of blastocyst for first three days of blastocyst entry in uterus [83]. However, MUC1 was found to be down-regulated in the receptive endometrium before implantation suggesting anti-adhesive role during apposition [84, 85]. High levels of progesterone down-regulates MUC1 expression which further improves embryo–epithelial interactions by unmasking CAMs on the endometrial surface [86]. Hence, MUC1 inhibits implantation and its down-regulation could contribute to the achievement of endometrial receptivity. Unlike other species, human endometrial MUC1 was found to be up-regulated during the peri-implantation period [87, 88]. It was suggested that humans require a locally acting mechanism for the removal of the MUC1 barrier to the implanting embryo [89]. Reduced levels of endometrial MUC1 were reported in women with recurrent pregnancy loss. [90]. This suggests that primary infertility due to implantation failure might be associated with a polymorphism in the MUC1 variable number of tandem repeat (VNTR), resulting in a protein with a substantial reduction in the number of O-glycosylation sites. However, MUC4 VNTR polymorphism did not show any statistically significant difference between the spontaneous fertile and infertile population with or without unexplained embryo implantation failures.

Molecular Basis of Implantation

Transcription Factors

Implantation is governed by molecular mechanism mediated by homeobox (*HOX*) genes. The protein products of *HOX* genes belong to a class of proteins known as transcription factors, all of which are capable of binding to DNA, thereby regulating the transcription of genes [91]. The target of *HOX* genes promotes cell division, cell adhesion, apoptosis, and cell migration. *HOX* genes are arranged in four clusters (HOXA, HOXB, HOXC, HOXD) which are located on four separate chromosomes and each cluster houses between nine and 11 genes. The expression of *HOX* genes has been shown to regulate the growth and development of the human endometrium, which varies in response to hormones during the menstrual cycle, with significant up-regulation in the mid-secretory phase, coinciding with the implantation window [92]. Amongst all the homeobox genes, it has been suggested that HOXA-10 and HOXA-11, were shown to be important for implantation, because mice with mutations in these genes fail to achieve normal implantation [93, 94]. HOXA-10 and HOXA-11 are expressed in endometrial cells of mice and in the endometrial glands and stroma of the human uterus during the menstrual cycle [92, 95, 96]. Knock-down of HOXA-10 expression using siRNA mediated approach in mouse models prevents implantation. In addition, patients with endometriosis, fibroids, and polycystic ovary syndrome were found to have very low levels of HOXA-10 expression. Moreover, HOXA-10 has been demonstrated to regulate the expression of β3 integrin as well as several other genes involved in endometrial receptivity. Uterine stromal cells in HOXA-10 deficient female mice show reduced proliferation in response to progesterone, leading to decidualization defects [97, 98]. Furthermore, HOXA-10 expression plays an essential role in pinopod development. Indeed, blocking HOXA-10 expression dramatically decreases the number of pinopodes [99]. On the other hand, HOXA-11deficient mice are infertile due to endometrial implantation defects. HOXA11$^{-/-}$mice have reduced expression of leukemia inhibitory factor (LIF) [94]. The importance of LIF in embryo implantation will be discussed in the next section. In addition, HOXA-10 and HOXA-11 have been found to be essential for fertility in mice [94]. Previous studies evidenced that female mice that are homozygous mutants of either of these genes are infertile due to the endometrial factors [100, 101]. Thus, a gene therapy approach that may involve the manipulation of the expression of *HOX* genes could have a role in the enhancement of endometrial receptivity and implantation.

Cytokines

Cytokines and growth factors are cell-derived polypeptides and proteins which bind to specific cell surface receptor kinases leading to the activation of signaling cascades involved in the regulation of embryo-maternal interactions. By autocrine, paracrine and endocrine mechanisms, cytokines are believed to regulate various cellular functions like proliferation, differentiation and apoptosis [27, 102]. As regards of their role in implantation, cytokines secreted by uterus and the embryo promotes endometrial receptivity by regulating the levels of adhesion and anti-adhesion proteins [7]. Disturbances in the normal expression and action of these cytokines result in an absolute or partial failure of implantation and abnormal placental formation in mice and human [103].

Leukemia Inhibitory Factor (LIF)

LIF, which is a member of IL-6 type cytokine family, is a glycoprotein [104]. It is secreted from the uterus and is regarded as an important factor in embryo implantation. The pleiotropic effects of LIF are accomplished by binding to heterodimeric LIF receptor (LIFR), which consists of two transmembrane proteins, LIFR and gp130. The up-regulation of LIF also requires the action of the homeobox gene *Hmx3* [4]. The LIFR activates several signaling pathways in diverse cells types, including the Jak/STAT, MAPK, and PI3-kinase (PIPK) pathways [105]. Deletion of the genes for LIF, Hmx3 or a mutant gp130 deficient in STAT3 signalling all result in the failure of embryo attachment due to a failure of the epithelium to respond to the embryo [4, 106, 107]. In the endometrium of a fertile woman, LIF mRNA and protein are expressed throughout the menstrual cycle with a striking increase in the mid-and late secretory phase and during early pregnancy [108, 109]. LIF knockout female mice lacking a functional LIF gene are fertile, but the blastocysts fail to implant, even though they are viable and can implant when transferred to wild-type recipients. However, when LIF was injected into LIF knockout mice, they showed normal implantation [106, 110]. Previous studies showed that infertility could be associated with lower levels of LIF in endometrium [111, 112]. Furthermore, Giess *et al.* (1999) demonstrated that mutation in LIF genes might led to decreased activity of LIF in the endometrium and cause implantation failure. Embryos lacking either LIFR or gp130 develop to the blastocyst stage and implant normally but die during the perinatal period [113]. Thus LIF may signal to both embryonic and uterine cells during implantation [114]. Taken together, there is a strong evidence for an important role of LIF in both rodents and primate implantation. In view of the important role of LIF in implantation, administration of such r-hLIF could be valuable in future studies.

Interleukin-6 (IL-6)

IL-6, a multifunctional cytokine, controls diverse physiological processes including immune system. It shows functional redundancy with IL-11 and LIF [115]. In humans, the receptor for IL-6 is expressed throughout the menstrual cycle specifically localized in the glandular epithelium. Higher levels of IL-6 is found in the glandular and luminal epithelial cells during the mid-secretory phase, however, weak expression is evidenced in the proliferative phase [116, 117]. Therefore, a role in the human implantation could also be postulated for this cytokine. IL-6 is maximally expressed during the window of implantation and that its receptor is found both in the blastocyst and in the endometrium suggests a paracrine/autocrine role for IL-6 in the peri-implantation period. Deficiency of IL-6 leads to decrease in the number of viable implantation sites and thus affecting the outcome of pregnancy [118]. Experiments using mice with a targeted disruption in the IL-6 gene have shown that the development of blastocyst is compromised with no adverse effect on the blastocyst implantation [119, 120]. Based on the fact endometrial mRNA is suppressed in the mid-secretory phase of patients with recurrent abortions, the role of IL-6 during early pregnancy has been well established [121, 122].

Interleukin-11 (IL-11)

IL-11 is a cytokine with pleiotropic activities on range of cell types. It was initially described as growth factor acting on multiple stages during hematopoiesis, synergizing with other factors [123]. IL-11 and its receptor (IL-11Rα) have recently been demonstrated in human endometrium. All the major cell types in endometrium express IL-11 with cyclical variation. The most prominent immunoreactivity and mRNA expression was observed in the decidualized stromal cells late in the menstrual cycle [124-126]. Strong immunoreactivity for IL-11Rα and gp130 was observed in both luminal and glandular epithelium [126,

127]. Mice lacking the IL-11Rα have a fertility defect because of defective decidualization and in normal uterus maximal level of IL-11 was observed at the time of decidualization [128]. Furthermore, IL-11 signaling is required for maturation of natural killer (NK) cells at the time of decidualization in mice model [129]. As regards for human, increasing evidence indicates that IL-11 has an important function in implantation. A recent study on women with recurrent miscarriage reported decreased synthesis of IL-11 in the endometrial epithelium [130]. *In vitro* decidualization using progesterone or cAMP-induced was shown to induce IL-11 mRNA expression in the endometrial stromal cells [131, 132]. Taken together, all these evidences indicate that IL-11 may be important in the establishment of viable pregnancies.

Growth Factors

The expression of various growth factors such as transforming growth factor-β (TGF-β) and epidermal growth factor (EGF) and their receptors in the uterus is cell specific and temporal during the pre-implantation period, which implies the role of these factors in implantation process [133].

Transforming Growth Factor β

All three isoforms of transforming growth factor β (TGF-β1,-β2 and-β3) have been localized in rodent and human endometrial epithelium and stroma. Previously, our laboratory has shown that individual TGF-β isoforms (TGF-β1, TGF-β2 and TGF-β3) are differently expressed in the uterus during rat pregnancy [134] higher expression of TGF-β1 and TGF-β2 are present during implantation and decidua basalis regression, whereas TGF-β3 isoform is only present during DB regression and parturition. Recently, it has been demonstrated that TGF-β signaling pathway plays an important role in remodeling of rat endometrium by modulating the activity of PI3-K/Akt survival pathways, along with down regulating the XIAP levels thus inducing apoptosis in decidual cells [135]. Detection of TGF-β isoforms at the maternal–fetal interface, together with the known roles of TGF-β in the regulation of proliferation, differentiation, extracellular matrix production, invasion and in migration, suggests it potential role in implantation [136, 137].

In human endometrium, TGF-β protein and mRNA are localized in endometrial stromal, epithelial, and decidual cells [138]. Previously it has been demonstrated that TGF-β2 expression is more intense in stroma cells, while TGF-β1 and-β3 are equal in intensity in stromal and epithelial cells [139]. In late secretory phase of menstrual cycle, TGF-β3 expression was found to be expressed in glandular epithelium and secretion of TGF-β3 by the endometrial epithelial cells is indicative of its potential role in implantation process. Moreover, TGF-βs may play a role in human implantation *via* their stimulation of fibronectin or vascular endothelial growth factor production [140, 141] and by promotion of adhesion of trophoblast cells to the ECM [142]. Specifically, TGF-β1 increases ECM oncofetal fibronectin and stimulates trophoblast adhesion to the ECM; therefore, TGF-β1 is implicated in trophoblast attachment to the endometrium during the implantation [140, 143]. Therefore, disturbances of the normal expression and action of this major cytokine could result in absolute or partial failure of implantation in mice and humans.

Epidermal Growth Factors

The members of EGF family interact with receptor subtypes that belong to an ErbB gene family of tyrosine kinase receptors: ErbB1 (EGF-R), ErbB2, ErbB3, and ErbB4. They share common structural features but differ in their ligand specificity and kinase activity [30]. In human endometrium, EGF is moderately expressed in stromal cells during proliferative phase, however strong expression of EGF was observed at the time of secretory phase. EGF expression is also found in both decidual and trophoblastic cells [144]. Earlier studies have demonstrated that EGF plays a critical role in trophoblast invasion [145], differentiation, and proliferation [146] suggesting that EGF may affect implantation in several different ways thus suggesting that EGF is a significant regulator of the implantation process. Gene knockout studies for EGF receptor (ErbB1) in mice revealed impaired implantation and development of the embryos leading to their pre-implantation death [147]. Thereafter, several *in vitro* studies have demonstrated that EGF affects mouse embryo development and promotes trophoblast differentiation into the invasive type which is the most crucial cell type for implantation [148, 149]. EGF receptors were found to be present during peri-implantation period in the uterine epithelium of the mouse embryo [150, 151]. This timely expression of

EGFs and their receptors in the uterus during the peri-implantation period indicates the pivotal role of EGF-like growth in implantation process.

Heparin Binding-Epidermal Growth Factor

Heparin binding-epidermal growth factor (HB-EGF) shares a common receptor with EGF and TGF-α. HB-EGF is expressed in endometrial stromal and epithelial cells and has been demonstrated to regulate endometrial cell proliferation, glandular epithelial secretion, and decidual transformation [7]. HB-EGF was found to be expressed in human endometrium at the time of implantation [152, 153]. In an another study authors showed that HB-EGF mRNA expression is low in the proliferative endometrium and increases in the secretory phase, reaching its highest point of expression immediately prior to the implantation window [154]. Moreover, Leach *et al.* (1999) also demonstrated that HB-EGF expression is maximal in luminal and glandular epithelial cells during the implantation window, and during early pregnancy. HB-EGF expression was observed both in the decidualized and trophoblastic cells. It has been speculated that HB-EGF promotes implantation and trophoblast invasion through paracrine/autocrine signaling [155].

In mouse model, both the soluble and transmembrane forms of HB-EGF were detected as the earliest molecular marker of local endometrial receptivity just before the attachment of blastocyst. Based on these results the authors suggested that HB-EGF signaling occurs through paracrine and/or juxtacrine interactions with embryonic ErbBs as well as with ErbBs presents on the uterus during the peri-implantation period [86]. This process is followed by the induction in the expression of β-cellulin, amphiregulin, epiregulin, neuregulin-1, and COX-2 near the time of the blastocyst attachment [156, 157]. Targeted disruptions of EGF/TGF-α/amphiregulin in mice failed to have any adverse effect on the implantation process. This could be explained based on the fact that HB-EGF, betacellulin, epiregulin, neuregulin, and amphiregulin exhibit overlapping uterine expression during blastocyst attachment to the endometrium [156]. Previous reports suggest that HB-EGF acts as an inhibitor of apoptosis in human endometrium and promotes trophoblast invasion during embryonic implantation [158, 159]. Peak levels of HB-GF are observed in the luminal and glandular epithelium when fully developed pinopodes are present. Thus, establishing the potential role of HB-EGF in attachment and invasion processes during implantation [14]. Furthermore, these evidences suggest that HB-EGF is a critical signaling molecule for early pregnancy success by regulating the endometrial receptivity.

CONCLUSION AND FUTURE DIRECTION

Implantation, which involves the regulated interplay between the embryo and a receptive endometrium, is still incompletely understood intricate process. Despite extensive research in this field, the rates of pregnancy losses are still high. Progress towards improving early pregnancy success rates is one of the most challenging tasks of reproductive medicine. It is worth mentioning that ethical restrictions and limited availability of human tissues confined our studies on human implantation. Present knowledge is a result of the extrapolation of the events from primate and rodent models. It must be appreciated that most knowledge comes from *in vitro* experiments using human blastocysts co-cultured with polarized endometrial epithelial cells and *in vivo* studies from other species. Detailed understanding of the crosstalk between various growth factors, hormones, adhesion molecules, cytokines and transcription factors and downstream signaling cascades during endometrial receptivity and trophoblast attachment will improve the pregnancy outcomes. More insight will be gained by gene knockout studies which will help us to understand the action of each of these molecules during different stages of implantation process and to determine if these can be used in the treatment strategies of implantation failure. High throughput techniques such as microarray that allow the profiling of tissues at the genomic, transcriptomic and proteomic levels will allow the rapid assessment of many more potential markers of receptivity in a parallel manner. This will probably shed more light on the intricate dialogue between all the aforementioned molecular factors. The information gained will speed up the process of the identification of clinically useful markers which will enable to improve the diagnosis. This will help to identify the patients who suffer implantation failure due to problems of endometrial receptivity and will enable the gynecologists to use new clinical approaches against infertility related problems. Bridging the gap between endometrial receptivity and implantation will facilitate the treatment of fertility defects.

REFERENCES

[1]   Makrigiannakis A, Minas V, Kalantaridou SN, Nikas G, Chrousos GP. Hormonal and cytokine regulation of early implantation. Trends Endocrinol Metab 2006; 17(5): 178-85.

[2]   Krussel JS, Bielfeld P, Polan ML, Simon C. Regulation of embryonic implantation. Eur J Obstet Gynecol Reprod Biol 2003; 110(Suppl 1): S2-9.

[3]   Wilcox AJ, Weinberg CR, O'Connor JF, *et al.* Incidence of early loss of pregnancy. N Engl J Med 1988; 319(4): 189-94.

[4]   Wang W, Van De Water T, Lufkin T. Inner ear and maternal reproductive defects in mice lacking the Hmx3 homeobox gene. Development 1998; 125(4): 621-34.

[5]   Lee KY, DeMayo FJ. Animal models of implantation. Reproduction 2004; 128(6): 679-95.

[6]   Lessey BA, Damjanovich L, Coutifaris C, Castelbaum A, Albelda SM, Buck CA. Integrin adhesion molecules in the human endometrium. Correlation with the normal and abnormal menstrual cycle. J Clin Invest 1992; 90(1): 188-95.

[7]   Simon C, Martin JC, Pellicer A. Paracrine regulators of implantation. Baillieres Best Pract Res Clin Obstet Gynaecol 2000; 14(5): 815-26.

[8]   Psychoyos A. Uterine receptivity for nidation. Ann N Y Acad Sci 1986; 476: 36-42.

[9]   Ma WG, Song H, Das SK, Paria BC, Dey SK. Estrogen is a critical determinant that specifies the duration of the window of uterine receptivity for implantation. Proc Natl Acad Sci U S A 2003; 100(5): 2963-8.

[10]   Parr MB, Parr EL. Uterine luminal epithelium: protrusions mediate endocytosis, not apocrine secretion, in the rat. Biol Reprod 1974; 11(2): 220-33.

[11]   Nikas G, Drakakis P, Loutradis D, *et al.* Uterine pinopodes as markers of the 'nidation window' in cycling women receiving exogenous oestradiol and progesterone. Hum Reprod 1995; 10(5): 1208-13.

[12]   Nikas G, Aghajanova L. Endometrial pinopodes: some more understanding on human implantation? Reprod Biomed Online 2002; 4(Suppl 3): 18-23.

[13]   Bentin-Ley U, Sjogren A, Nilsson L, Hamberger L, Larsen JF, Horn T. Presence of uterine pinopodes at the embryo-endometrial interface during human implantation *in vitro*. Hum Reprod 1999; 14(2): 515-20.

[14]   Stavreus-Evers A, Aghajanova L, Brismar H, Eriksson H, Landgren BM, Hovatta O. Co-existence of heparin-binding epidermal growth factor-like growth factor and pinopodes in human endometrium at the time of implantation. Mol Hum Reprod 2002; 8(8): 765-9.

[15]   Stavreus-Evers A, Masironi B, Landgren BM, Holmgren A, Eriksson H, Sahlin L. Immunohistochemical localization of glutaredoxin and thioredoxin in human endometrium: a possible association with pinopodes. Mol Hum Reprod 2002; 8(6): 546-51.

[16]   Tabibzadeh S, Babaknia A. The signals and molecular pathways involved in implantation, a symbiotic interaction between blastocyst and endometrium involving adhesion and tissue invasion. Hum Reprod 1995; 10(6): 1579-602.

[17]   Lopata A, Bentin-Ley U, Enders A. "Pinopodes" and implantation. Rev Endocr Metab Disord 2002; 3(2): 77-86.

[18]   Sharkey AM, Smith SK. The endometrium as a cause of implantation failure. Best Pract Res Clin Obstet Gynaecol 2003; 17(2): 289-307.

[19]   Norwitz ER, Schust DJ, Fisher SJ. Implantation and the survival of early pregnancy. N Engl J Med 2001; 345(19): 1400-8.

[20]   Kearns M, Lala PK. Life history of decidual cells: a review. Am J Reprod Immunol 1983; 3(2): 78-82.

[21]   Gellersen B, Brosens IA, Brosens JJ. Decidualization of the human endometrium: mechanisms, functions, and clinical perspectives. Semin Reprod Med 2007; 25(6): 445-53.

[22]   Clark DA. Cytokines, decidua, and early pregnancy. Oxf Rev Reprod Biol 1993; 15: 83-111.

[23]   Graham CH, Lala PK. Mechanisms of placental invasion of the uterus and their control. Biochem Cell Biol 1992; 70(10-11): 867-74.

[24]   Carson DD, Bagchi I, Dey SK, *et al.* Embryo implantation. Dev Biol 2000; 223(2): 217-37.

[25]   Lim H, Song H, Paria BC, Reese J, Das SK, Dey SK. Molecules in blastocyst implantation: uterine and embryonic perspectives. Vitam Horm 2002; 64: 43-76.

[26]   Simon C, Valbuena D. Embryonic implantation. Ann Endocrinol (Paris) 1999; 60(2): 134-6.

[27]   Giudice LC. Potential biochemical markers of uterine receptivity. Hum Reprod 1999; 14(Suppl 2): 3-16.

[28]   Kao LC, Tulac S, Lobo S, *et al.* Global gene profiling in human endometrium during the window of implantation. Endocrinology 2002; 143(6): 2119-38.

[29]   Borthwick JM, Charnock-Jones DS, Tom BD, *et al.* Determination of the transcript profile of human endometrium. Mol Hum Reprod 2003; 9(1): 19-33.

[30]   Dey SK, Lim H, Das SK, *et al.* Molecular cues to implantation. Endocr Rev 2004; 25(3): 341-73.

[31]   Ghosh D, Sengupta J. Another look at the issue of peri-implantation oestrogen. Hum Reprod 1995; 10(1) :1-2.

[32]   Lessey BA. Two pathways of progesterone action in the human endometrium: implications for implantation and contraception. Steroids 2003; 68(10-13): 809-15.

[33]   Carpenter KD, Korach KS. Potential biological functions emerging from the different estrogen receptors. Ann N Y Acad Sci 2006; 1092: 361-73.

[34]   Curtis SW, Clark J, Myers P, Korach KS. Disruption of estrogen signaling does not prevent progesterone action in the estrogen receptor alpha knockout mouse uterus. Proc Natl Acad Sci U S A 1999; 96(7): 3646-51.

[35]   Szekeres-Bartho J, Halasz M, Palkovics T. Progesterone in pregnancy; receptor-ligand interaction and signaling pathways. J Reprod Immunol 2009; 83(1-2): 60-4.

[36]   van den Heuvel MJ, Chantakru S, Xuemei X, *et al.* Trafficking of circulating pro-NK cells to the decidualizing uterus: regulatory mechanisms in the mouse and human. Immunol Invest 2005; 34(3): 273-93.

[37]   Basak S, Dhar R, Das C. Steroids modulate the expression of alpha4 integrin in mouse blastocysts and uterus during implantation. Biol Reprod 2002; 66(6): 1784-9.

[38]   Kodaman PH, Taylor HS. Hormonal regulation of implantation. Obstet Gynecol Clin North Am 2004; 31(4): 745-66, ix.

[39]   Jabbour HN, Sales KJ. Prostaglandin receptor signalling and function in human endometrial pathology. Trends Endocrinol Metab 2004; 15(8): 398-404.

[40]   Kang J, Chapdelaine P, Parent J, Madore E, Laberge PY, Fortier MA. Expression of human prostaglandin transporter in the human endometrium across the menstrual cycle. J Clin Endocrinol Metab 2005; 90(4): 2308-13.

[41]   Capper EA, Marshall LA. Mammalian phospholipases A(2): mediators of inflammation, proliferation and apoptosis. Prog Lipid Res 2001; 40(3): 167-97.

[42]   Kengni JH, St-Louis I, Parent S, Leblanc V, Shooner C, Asselin E. Regulation of prostaglandin D synthase and prostacyclin synthase in the endometrium of cyclic, pregnant, and pseudopregnant rats and their regulation by sex steroids. J Endocrinol 2007; 195(2): 301-11.

[43]   Achache H, Tsafrir A, Prus D, Reich R, Revel A. Defective endometrial prostaglandin synthesis identified in patients with repeated implantation failure undergoing *in vitro* fertilization. Fertil Steril 2010; 94(4): 1271-1278.

[44]   Song H, Lim H, Paria BC, *et al.* Cytosolic phospholipase A2alpha is crucial [correction of A2alpha deficiency is crucial] for 'on-time' embryo implantation that directs subsequent development. Development 2002; 129(12): 2879-89.

[45]   Kennedy TG. Evidence for a role for prosaglandins in the initiation of blastocyst implantation in the rat. Biol Reprod 1977; 16(3): 286-91.

[46]   Smith WL, DeWitt DL, Garavito RM. Cyclooxygenases: structural, cellular, and molecular biology. Annu Rev Biochem 2000; 69: 145-82.

[47]   St-Louis I, Singh M, Brasseur K, Leblanc V, Parent S, Asselin E. Expression of COX-1 and COX-2 in the endometrium of cyclic, pregnant and in a model of pseudopregnant rats and their regulation by sex steroids. Reprod Biol Endocrinol 2010; 8: 103.

[48]   Chakraborty I, Das SK, Wang J, Dey SK. Developmental expression of the cyclo-oxygenase-1 and cyclo-oxygenase-2 genes in the peri-implantation mouse uterus and their differential regulation by the blastocyst and ovarian steroids. J Mol Endocrinol 1996; 16(2): 107-22.

[49]   Lim H, Gupta RA, Ma WG, *et al.* Cyclo-oxygenase-2-derived prostacyclin mediates embryo implantation in the mouse *via* PPARdelta. Genes Dev 1999; 13(12): 1561-74.

[50]   Das SK, Wang J, Dey SK, Mead RA. Spatiotemporal expression of cyclooxygenase 1 and cyclooxygenase 2 during delayed implantation and the periimplantation period in the Western spotted skunk. Biol Reprod 1999; 60(4): 893-9.

[51]   Kennedy TG. Prostaglandins and increased endometrial vascular permeabiltiy resulting from the application of artificial stimulus to the uterus of the rat sensitized for the decidual cell reaction. Biol Reprod 1979; 20(3): 560-6.

[52]   Li DK, Liu L, Odouli R. Exposure to non-steroidal anti-inflammatory drugs during pregnancy and risk of miscarriage: population based cohort study. BMJ 2003; 327(7411): 368.

[53]   Lessey BA, Castelbaum AJ. Integrins and implantation in the human. Rev Endocr Metab Disord 2002; 3(2): 107-17.

[54]   Humphries MJ. Integrin structure. Biochem Soc Trans 2000; 28(4): 311-39.

[55]   Hynes RO. Integrins: bidirectional, allosteric signaling machines. Cell 2002; 110(6): 673-87.

[56]   Klentzeris LD, Bulmer JN, Trejdosiewicz LK, Morrison L, Cooke ID. Beta-1 integrin cell adhesion molecules in the endometrium of fertile and infertile women. Hum Reprod 1993; 8(8): 1223-30.

[57]   Lessey BA, Castelbaum AJ, Wolf L, *et al.* Use of integrins to date the endometrium. Fertil Steril 2000; 73(4): 779-87.

[58]   Lessey BA, Castelbaum AJ, Buck CA, Lei Y, Yowell CW, Sun J. Further characterization of endometrial integrins during the menstrual cycle and in pregnancy. Fertil Steril 1994; 62(3): 497-506.

[59]   Nardo LG, Nikas G, Makrigiannakis A, Sinatra F, Nardo F. Synchronous expression of pinopodes and alpha v beta 3 and alpha 4 beta 1 integrins in the endometrial surface epithelium of normally menstruating women during the implantation window. J Reprod Med 2003; 48(5): 355-61.

[60]   Lessey BA, Castelbaum AJ, Sawin SW, Sun J. Integrins as markers of uterine receptivity in women with primary unexplained infertility. Fertil Steril 1995; 63(3): 535-42.

[61]   Lessey BA, Ilesanmi AO, Lessey MA, Riben M, Harris JE, Chwalisz K. Luminal and glandular endometrial epithelium express integrins differentially throughout the menstrual cycle: implications for implantation, contraception, and infertility. Am J Reprod Immunol 1996; 35(3): 195-204.

[62]   Skrzypczak J, Mikolajczyk M, Szymanowski K. Endometrial receptivity: expression of alpha3beta1, alpha4beta1 and alphaVbeta1 endometrial integrins in women with impaired fertility. Reprod Biol 2001; 1(2): 85-94.

[63]   Stephens LE, Sutherland AE, Klimanskaya IV, *et al.* Deletion of beta 1 integrins in mice results in inner cell mass failure and peri-implantation lethality. Genes Dev 1995; 9(15): 1883-95.

[64]   Illera MJ, Cullinan E, Gui Y, Yuan L, Beyler SA, Lessey BA. Blockade of the alpha(v)beta(3) integrin adversely affects implantation in the mouse. Biol Reprod 2000; 62(5): 1285-90.

[65]   Aplin JD, Kimber SJ. Trophoblast-uterine interactions at implantation. Reprod Biol Endocrinol 2004; 2: 48.

[66]   Apparao KB, Murray MJ, Fritz MA, *et al.* Osteopontin and its receptor alphavbeta(3) integrin are coexpressed in the human endometrium during the menstrual cycle but regulated differentially. J Clin Endocrinol Metab 2001; 86(10): 4991-5000.

[67]   Wang J, Armant DR. Integrin-mediated adhesion and signaling during blastocyst implantation. Cells Tissues Organs 2002; 172(3): 190-201.

[68]   Damsky CH, Librach C, Lim KH, *et al.* Integrin switching regulates normal trophoblast invasion. Development 1994; 120(12): 3657-66.

[69]   Klentzeris LD. The role of endometrium in implantation. Hum Reprod 1997; 12(11): 170-5.

[70]   Gallatin WM, Weissman IL, Butcher EC. A cell-surface molecule involved in organ-specific homing of lymphocytes. Nature 1983; 304(5921): 30-4.

[71]   Smalley DM, Ley K. L-selectin: mechanisms and physiological significance of ectodomain cleavage. J Cell Mol Med 2005; 9(2): 255-66.

[72]   Genbacev OD, Prakobphol A, Foulk RA, *et al.* Trophoblast L-selectin-mediated adhesion at the maternal-fetal interface. Science 2003; 299(5605): 405-8.

[73]   Fazleabas AT, Kim JJ. Development. What makes an embryo stick? Science 2003; 299(5605): 355-6.

[74]   Gumbiner BM. Cell adhesion: the molecular basis of tissue architecture and morphogenesis. Cell 1996; 84(3): 345-57.

[75]   Huber O, Bierkamp C, Kemler R. Cadherins and catenins in development. Curr Opin Cell Biol 1996; 8(5): 685-91.

[76]   Riethmacher D, Brinkmann V, Birchmeier C. A targeted mutation in the mouse E-cadherin gene results in defective preimplantation development. Proc Natl Acad Sci U S A 1995; 92(3): 855-9.

[77]   Lindhard A, Bentin-Ley U, Ravn V, *et al.* Biochemical evaluation of endometrial function at the time of implantation. Fertil Steril 2002; 78(2): 221-33.

[78]   Hey NA, Graham RA, Seif MW, Aplin JD. The polymorphic epithelial mucin MUC1 in human endometrium is regulated with maximal expression in the implantation phase. J Clin Endocrinol Metab 1994; 78(2): 337-42.

[79]   Audie JP, Tetaert D, Pigny P, *et al.* Mucin gene expression in the human endocervix. Hum Reprod 1995; 10(1): 98-102.

[80]   Burghardt RC, Johnson GA, Jaeger LA, *et al.* Integrins and extracellular matrix proteins at the maternal-fetal interface in domestic animals. Cells Tissues Organs 2002; 172(3): 202-17.

[81]   Dominguez F, Pellicer A, Simon C. Paracrine dialogue in implantation. Mol Cell Endocrinol 2002; 186(2): 175-81.

[82]   Meseguer M, Aplin JD, Caballero-Campo P, *et al.* Human endometrial mucin MUC1 is up-regulated by progesterone and down-regulated *in vitro* by the human blastocyst. Biol Reprod 2001; 64(2): 590-601.

[83]   Hill JA. Maternal-embryonic cross-talk. Ann N Y Acad Sci 2001; 943: 17-25.

[84] Braga VM, Gendler SJ. Modulation of Muc-1 mucin expression in the mouse uterus during the estrus cycle, early pregnancy and placentation. J Cell Sci 1993; 105(Pt 2): 397-405.

[85] DeSouza MM, Mani SK, Julian J, Carson DD. Reduction of mucin-1 expression during the receptive phase in the rat uterus. Biol Reprod 1998; 58(6): 1503-7.

[86] Surveyor GA, Gendler SJ, Pemberton L, et al. Expression and steroid hormonal control of Muc-1 in the mouse uterus. Endocrinology 1995; 136(8): 3639-47.

[87] Hey NA, Li TC, Devine PL, Graham RA, Saravelos H, Aplin JD. MUC1 in secretory phase endometrium: expression in precisely dated biopsies and flushings from normal and recurrent miscarriage patients. Hum Reprod 1995; 10(10): 2655-62.

[88] Aplin JD, Hey NA, Graham RA. Human endometrial MUC1 carries keratan sulfate: characteristic glycoforms in the luminal epithelium at receptivity. Glycobiology 1998; 8(3): 269-76.

[89] Thathiah A, Carson DD. MT1-MMP mediates MUC1 shedding independent of TACE/ADAM17. Biochem J 2004; 382(Pt 1): 363-73.

[90] Horne AW, White JO, Margara RA, Williams R, Winston RM, Lalani E. MUC 1: a genetic susceptibility to infertility? Lancet 2001; 357(9265): 1336-7.

[91] Vitiello D, Kodaman PH, Taylor HS. HOX genes in implantation. Semin Reprod Med 2007; 25(6): 431-6.

[92] Taylor HS, Igarashi P, Olive DL, Arici A. Sex steroids mediate HOXA11 expression in the human peri-implantation endometrium. J Clin Endocrinol Metab 1999; 84(3): 1129-35.

[93] Ma L, Benson GV, Lim H, Dey SK, Maas RL. Abdominal B (AbdB) Hoxa genes: regulation in adult uterus by estrogen and progesterone and repression in mullerian duct by the synthetic estrogen diethylstilbestrol (DES). Dev Biol 1998; 197(2): 141-54.

[94] Daftary GS, Taylor HS. Molecular markers of implantation: clinical implications. Curr Opin Obstet Gynecol 2001; 13(3): 269-74.

[95] Taylor HS, Vanden Heuvel GB, Igarashi P. A conserved Hox axis in the mouse and human female reproductive system: late establishment and persistent adult expression of the Hoxa cluster genes. Biol Reprod 1997; 57(6): 1338-45.

[96] Taylor HS, Arici A, Olive D, Igarashi P. HOXA10 is expressed in response to sex steroids at the time of implantation in the human endometrium. J Clin Invest 1998; 101(7): 1379-84.

[97] Benson GV, Lim H, Paria BC, Satokata I, Dey SK, Maas RL. Mechanisms of reduced fertility in Hoxa-10 mutant mice: uterine homeosis and loss of maternal Hoxa-10 expression. Development 1996; 122(9): 2687-96.

[98] Lim H, Ma L, Ma WG, Maas RL, Dey SK. Hoxa-10 regulates uterine stromal cell responsiveness to progesterone during implantation and decidualization in the mouse. Mol Endocrinol 1999; 13(6): 1005-17.

[99] Bagot CN, Kliman HJ, Taylor HS. Maternal Hoxa10 is required for pinopod formation in the development of mouse uterine receptivity to embryo implantation. Dev Dyn 2001; 222(3): 538-44.

[100] Satokata I, Benson G, Maas R. Sexually dimorphic sterility phenotypes in Hoxa10-deficient mice. Nature 1995; 374(6521): 460-3.

[101] Hsieh-Li HM, Witte DP, Weinstein M, et al. Hoxa 11 structure, extensive antisense transcription, and function in male and female fertility. Development 1995; 121(5): 1373-85.

[102] Beier HM, Beier-Hellwig K. Molecular and cellular aspects of endometrial receptivity. Hum Reprod Update 1998; 4(5): 448-58.

[103] Guzeloglu-Kayisli O, Kayisli UA, Taylor HS. The role of growth factors and cytokines during implantation: endocrine and paracrine interactions. Semin Reprod Med 2009; 27(1): 62-79.

[104] Hilton DJ. LIF: lots of interesting functions. Trends Biochem Sci 1992; 17(2): 72-6.

[105] Duval D, Reinhardt B, Kedinger C, Boeuf H. Role of suppressors of cytokine signaling (Socs) in leukemia inhibitory factor (LIF)-dependent embryonic stem cell survival. FASEB J 2000; 14(11): 1577-84.

[106] Stewart CL, Kaspar P, Brunet LJ, et al. Blastocyst implantation depends on maternal expression of leukaemia inhibitory factor. Nature 1992; 359(6390): 76-9.

[107] Ernst M, Inglese M, Waring P, et al. Defective gp130-mediated signal transducer and activator of transcription (STAT) signaling results in degenerative joint disease, gastrointestinal ulceration, and failure of uterine implantation. J Exp Med 2001; 194(2): 189-203.

[108] Arici A, Engin O, Attar E, Olive DL. Modulation of leukemia inhibitory factor gene expression and protein biosynthesis in human endometrium. J Clin Endocrinol Metab 1995; 80(6): 1908-15.

[109] Charnock-Jones DS, Sharkey AM, Fenwick P, Smith SK. Leukaemia inhibitory factor mRNA concentration peaks in human endometrium at the time of implantation and the blastocyst contains mRNA for the receptor at this time. J Reprod Fertil 1994; 101(2): 421-6.

[110] Chen JR, Cheng JG, Shatzer T, Sewell L, Hernandez L, Stewart CL. Leukemia inhibitory factor can substitute for nidatory estrogen and is essential to inducing a receptive uterus for implantation but is not essential for subsequent embryogenesis. Endocrinology 2000; 141(12): 4365-72.

[111] Hambartsoumian E. Endometrial leukemia inhibitory factor (LIF) as a possible cause of unexplained infertility and multiple failures of implantation. Am J Reprod Immunol 1998; 39(2): 137-43.

[112] Ledee-Bataille N, Lapree-Delage G, Taupin JL, Dubanchet S, Frydman R, Chaouat G. Concentration of leukaemia inhibitory factor (LIF) in uterine flushing fluid is highly predictive of embryo implantation. Hum Reprod 2002; 17(1): 213-8.

[113] Ware CB, Horowitz MC, Renshaw BR, *et al.* Targeted disruption of the low-affinity leukemia inhibitory factor receptor gene causes placental, skeletal, neural and metabolic defects and results in perinatal death. Development 1995; 121(5): 1283-99.

[114] Laird SM, Tuckerman EM, Dalton CF, Dunphy BC, Li TC, Zhang X. The production of leukaemia inhibitory factor by human endometrium: presence in uterine flushings and production by cells in culture. Hum Reprod 1997; 12(3): 569-74.

[115] Metcalf D. Hematopoietic regulators: redundancy or subtlety? Blood 1993; 82(12): 3515-23.

[116] Tabibzadeh S, Kong QF, Babaknia A, May LT. Progressive rise in the expression of interleukin-6 in human endometrium during menstrual cycle is initiated during the implantation window. Hum Reprod 1995; 10(10): 2793-9.

[117] Vandermolen DT, Gu Y. Human endometrial interleukin-6 (IL-6): *in vivo* messenger ribonucleic acid expression, *in vitro* protein production, and stimulation thereof by IL-1 beta. Fertil Steril 1996; 66(5): 741-7.

[118] Robertson SA OCAaRA. The effect of interleukin-6 deficiency on implantation, fetal development and parturition in mice. Proc Aust Soc Reprod Biol 2000; p. 97.

[119] Kopf M, Baumann H, Freer G, *et al.* Impaired immune and acute-phase responses in interleukin-6-deficient mice. Nature. 1994; 368(6469): 339-42.

[120] Salamonsen LA, Dimitriadis E, Robb L. Cytokines in implantation. Semin Reprod Med 2000; 18(3): 299-310.

[121] Lim KJ, Odukoya OA, Ajjan RA, Li TC, Weetman AP, Cooke ID. The role of T-helper cytokines in human reproduction. Fertil Steril 2000; 73(1): 136-42.

[122] von Wolff M, Thaler CJ, Strowitzki T, Broome J, Stolz W, Tabibzadeh S. Regulated expression of cytokines in human endometrium throughout the menstrual cycle: dysregulation in habitual abortion. Mol Hum Reprod 2000; 6(7): 627-34.

[123] Du XX, Williams DA. Interleukin-11: a multifunctional growth factor derived from the hematopoietic microenvironment. Blood 1994; 83(8): 2023-30.

[124] Cork BA, Li TC, Warren MA, Laird SM. Interleukin-11 (IL-11) in human endometrium: expression throughout the menstrual cycle and the effects of cytokines on endometrial IL-11 production *in vitro*. J Reprod Immunol 2001; 50(1): 3-17.

[125] Dimitriadis E, Salamonsen LA, Robb L. Expression of interleukin-11 during the human menstrual cycle: coincidence with stromal cell decidualization and relationship to leukaemia inhibitory factor and prolactin. Mol Hum Reprod 2000; 6(10): 907-14.

[126] von Rango U, Alfer J, Kertschanska S, *et al.* Interleukin-11 expression: its significance in eutopic and ectopic human implantation. Mol Hum Reprod 2004; 10(11): 783-92.

[127] Cullinan EB, Abbondanzo SJ, Anderson PS, Pollard JW, Lessey BA, Stewart CL. Leukemia inhibitory factor (LIF) and LIF receptor expression in human endometrium suggests a potential autocrine/paracrine function in regulating embryo implantation. Proc Natl Acad Sci U S A 1996; 93(7): 3115-20.

[128] Robb L, Li R, Hartley L, Nandurkar HH, Koentgen F, Begley CG. Infertility in female mice lacking the receptor for interleukin 11 is due to a defective uterine response to implantation. Nat Med 1998; 4(3): 303-8.

[129] Ain R, Trinh ML, Soares MJ. Interleukin-11 signaling is required for the differentiation of natural killer cells at the maternal-fetal interface. Dev Dyn 2004; 231(4): 700-8.

[130] Linjawi S, Li TC, Tuckerman EM, Blakemore AI, Laird SM. Expression of interleukin-11 receptor alpha and interleukin-11 protein in the endometrium of normal fertile women and women with recurrent miscarriage. J Reprod Immunol 2004; 64(1-2): 145-55.

[131] Popovici RM, Kao LC, Giudice LC. Discovery of new inducible genes in *in vitro* decidualized human endometrial stromal cells using microarray technology. Endocrinology 2000; 141(9): 3510-3.

[132] Tierney EP, Tulac S, Huang ST, Giudice LC. Activation of the protein kinase A pathway in human endometrial stromal cells reveals sequential categorical gene regulation. Physiol Genomics 2003; 16(1): 47-66.

[133] Tazuke SI, Giudice LC. Growth factors and cytokines in endometrium, embryonic development, and maternal: embryonic interactions. Semin Reprod Endocrinol 1996; 14(3): 231-45.

[134] Shooner C, Caron PL, Frechette-Frigon G, Leblanc V, Dery MC, Asselin E. TGF-beta expression during rat pregnancy and activity on decidual cell survival. Reprod Biol Endocrinol 2005; 3: 20.

[135] Caron PL, Frechette-Frigon G, Shooner C, Leblanc V, Asselin E. Transforming growth factor beta isoforms regulation of Akt activity and XIAP levels in rat endometrium during estrous cycle, in a model of pseudopregnancy and in cultured decidual cells. Reprod Biol Endocrinol 2009; 7: 80.

[136] Tabibzadeh S, Hemmati-Brivanlou A. Lefty at the crossroads of "stemness" and differentiative events. Stem Cells 2006; 24(9): 1998-2006.

[137] Lafontaine L, Chaudhry P, Lafleur MJ, Van Themsche C, Soares MJ, Asselin E. Transforming growth factor Beta regulates proliferation and invasion of rat placental cell lines. Biol Reprod 2011; 84(3): 553-9.

[138] Bischof P, Campana A. Molecular mediators of implantation. Baillieres Best Pract Res Clin Obstet Gynaecol 2000; 14(5): 801-14.

[139] Godkin JD, Dore JJ. Transforming growth factor beta and the endometrium. Rev Reprod 1998; 3(1): 1-6.

[140] Feinberg RF, Kliman HJ, Wang CL. Transforming growth factor-beta stimulates trophoblast oncofetal fibronectin synthesis *in vitro*: implications for trophoblast implantation *in vivo*. J Clin Endocrinol Metab 1994; 78(5): 1241-8.

[141] Chung IB, Yelian FD, Zaher FM, *et al.* Expression and regulation of vascular endothelial growth factor in a first trimester trophoblast cell line. Placenta 2000; 21(4): 320-4.

[142] Irving JA, Lala PK. Functional role of cell surface integrins on human trophoblast cell migration: regulation by TGF-beta, IGF-II, and IGFBP-1. Exp Cell Res 1995; 217(2): 419-27.

[143] Tamada H, McMaster MT, Flanders KC, Andrews GK, Dey SK. Cell type-specific expression of transforming growth factor-beta 1 in the mouse uterus during the periimplantation period. Mol Endocrinol 1990; 4(7): 965-72.

[144] Hofmann GE, Scott RT, Jr., Bergh PA, Deligdisch L. Immunohistochemical localization of epidermal growth factor in human endometrium, decidua, and placenta. J Clin Endocrinol Metab 1991; 73(4): 882-7.

[145] Bass KE, Morrish D, Roth I, *et al.* Human cytotrophoblast invasion is up-regulated by epidermal growth factor: evidence that paracrine factors modify this process. Dev Biol 1994 Aug; 164(2): 550-61.

[146] Li RH, Zhuang LZ. The effects of growth factors on human normal placental cytotrophoblast cell proliferation. Hum Reprod 1997; 12(4): 830-4.

[147] Threadgill DW, Dlugosz AA, Hansen LA, *et al.* Targeted disruption of mouse EGF receptor: effect of genetic background on mutant phenotype. Science 1995; 269(5221): 230-4.

[148] Harvey MB, Leco KJ, Arcellana-Panlilio MY, Zhang X, Edwards DR, Schultz GA. Proteinase expression in early mouse embryos is regulated by leukaemia inhibitory factor and epidermal growth factor. Development 1995; 121(4): 1005-14.

[149] Khamsi F, Armstrong DT, Zhang X. Expression of urokinase-type plasminogen activator in human preimplantation embryos. Mol Hum Reprod 1996; 2(4): 273-6.

[150] Wiley LM, Wu JX, Harari I, Adamson ED. Epidermal growth factor receptor mRNA and protein increase after the four-cell preimplantation stage in murine development. Dev Biol 1992; 149(2): 247-60.

[151] Lim H, Das SK, Dey SK. erbB genes in the mouse uterus: cell-specific signaling by epidermal growth factor (EGF) family of growth factors during implantation. Dev Biol 1998; 204(1): 97-110.

[152] Birdsall MA, Hopkisson JF, Grant KE, Barlow DH, Mardon HJ. Expression of heparin-binding epidermal growth factor messenger RNA in the human endometrium. Mol Hum Reprod 1996; 2(1): 31-4.

[153] Lessey BA, Gui Y, Apparao KB, Young SL, Mulholland J. Regulated expression of heparin-binding EGF-like growth factor (HB-EGF) in the human endometrium: a potential paracrine role during implantation. Mol Reprod Dev 2002; 62(4): 446-55.

[154] Yoo HJ, Barlow DH, Mardon HJ. Temporal and spatial regulation of expression of heparin-binding epidermal growth factor-like growth factor in the human endometrium: a possible role in blastocyst implantation. Dev Genet 1997; 21(1): 102-8.

[155] Leach RE, Khalifa R, Ramirez ND, *et al.* Multiple roles for heparin-binding epidermal growth factor-like growth factor are suggested by its cell-specific expression during the human endometrial cycle and early placentation. J Clin Endocrinol Metab 1999; 84(9): 3355-63.

[156] Das SK, Chakraborty I, Paria BC, Wang XN, Plowman G, Dey SK. Amphiregulin is an implantation-specific and progesterone-regulated gene in the mouse uterus. Mol Endocrinol 1995; 9(6): 691-705.

[157] Das SK, Das N, Wang J, *et al.* Expression of betacellulin and epiregulin genes in the mouse uterus temporally by the blastocyst solely at the site of its apposition is coincident with the "window" of implantation. Dev Biol 1997; 190(2): 178-90.

[158] Martin KL, Barlow DH, Sargent IL. Heparin-binding epidermal growth factor significantly improves human blastocyst development and hatching in serum-free medium. Hum Reprod 1998; 13(6): 1645-52.

[159] Michalsky MP, Kuhn A, Mehta V, Besner GE. Heparin-binding EGF-like growth factor decreases apoptosis in intestinal epithelial cells *in vitro*. J Pediatr Surg 2001; 36(8): 1130-5.

CHAPTER 2

The Impact of Assisted Reproductive Technologies on Perinatal Outcomes

Patricia Monnier[1,*], Maria del Pilar Vélez[2] and Thierry Forges[3]

[1]*McGill Reproductive Centre, Department of Obstetrics and Gynecology, Division of Reproductive Endocrinology and Infertility, McGill University, Royal Victoria Hospital, Montreal, QC, Canada, H3A 1A1;* [2]*Obstetrics and Gynecology department, University of Montreal, Montreal, QC, Canada;* [3]*Department of Reproductive Medicine, Maternité Universitaire, 10 rue Dr Heydenreich, 54042 Nancy, France*

Abstract: The success of Assisted Reproductive Technologies (ART) during the last decades has transformed the evaluation and treatment of infertility. Nonetheless, there are concerns about the risk for adverse pregnancy outcomes. Research on ART and perinatal outcomes faces several methodological challenges that need to be considered to allow reliable interpretation of results. Major perinatal risks are consequence of the high rate of multiple gestations associated with ART treatment. The improvement of embryo cryopreservation programmes and the development of elective Single Embryo Transfer policies will reduce significantly the number of multiple pregnancies while maintaining acceptable overall pregnancy rates. Although the great majority of singleton ART pregnancies are uncomplicated, numerous studies have raised questions concerning a range of adverse pregnancy outcomes in singleton ART pregnancies. Spontaneous abortion, first trimester vaginal bleeding, ectopic pregnancies, adnexal torsion, chromosomal abnormalities, imprinting disorders, preterm birth, low birth weight and small for gestational age infants, birth defects, preeclampsia, placenta praevia and placental abruption have been associated with ART. Nonetheless, questions remain about the underlying mechanisms. Maternal age is an important confounder, as well as the role of the underlying infertility in the observed adverse perinatal outcomes. There are many data gaps to date. Future research initiatives are emergently needed, with enhancing transdisciplinary collaboration.

Keywords: Assisted reproductive technologies, *in vitro* fertilization, intracytoplasmic sperm injection, obstetric outcomes, perinatal outcomes.

INTRODUCTION

Because of the growing proportion of children born after Assisted Reproductive Technologies (ART) throughout the world, the assessment of the health impact of these techniques constitutes a stake mattering in our society.

The American Society for Reproductive Medicine (ASRM)/Society for Assisted reproductive technology (SART) registry reported 138,198 ART procedures conducted in 2006 in 88% of the medical centers providing ART treatments in the United States, thus their number has more than doubled over the past ten years. As a result, 1.2% of US infants born in 2006 were declared to be conceived through ART [1]. The European Society of Human Reproduction and Embryology (ESHRE) registry in 2005 reported 418,111 treatment cycles in 81% of centers in the 30 countries providing information to ESHRE [2]. Within Europe, the largest number of ART cycles was reported in France where ART is re-imbursed by the public health insurance, with 2.5% of French infants born after ART [3]. In Canada, 13,482 ART cycles were reported in 2007, which corresponds to a 12% increase when compared to 2006 data [4]. According to the European experience, the public re-imbursement policy of ART in Quebec that started in August 2010 will probably result in a dramatic increase of the number of ART treatments in this province.

Despite the increasing use of ART over the last decades, there are concerns about the risk for adverse pregnancy outcomes. Nonetheless, numerous epidemiological considerations should be taken into account

*Address correspondence to Patricia Monnier: McGill Reproductive Centre, Department of Obstetrics and Gynecology, Division of Reproductive Endocrinology and Infertility, McGill University, Royal Victoria Hospital, Montreal, Quebec, Canada, H3A 1A1; Tel 514 934-1934 ext. 34373, Fax: 514 843-1496; E-mail: monnier.patricia@muhc.mcgill.ca

Julie Lafond and Cathy Vaillancourt (Eds)

to analyse the literature in a balanced manner. Especially, it is recognized that major risks are associated with an increased prevalence of multiple gestations. However, even ART singletons seem to have higher rates of adverse pregnancy outcome than spontaneously conceived singletons. On the other hand, publications concerning developmental outcomes are still scarce. Finally, the impact of the underlying infertility remains a long-standing question.

OVERVIEW OF ART TECHNOLOGIES (FIG. 1)

Many definitions of ART exist. For this chapter we adopted the definition of the Centers for Disease Control and Prevention: "all fertility treatments in which both eggs and sperm are handled. In general, ART procedures involve surgically removing eggs from a woman's ovaries, combining them with sperm in the laboratory, and returning them to the woman's body or donating them to another woman" [5]. This definition excludes artificial insemination as well as ovarian stimulation alone, without oocyte retrieval.

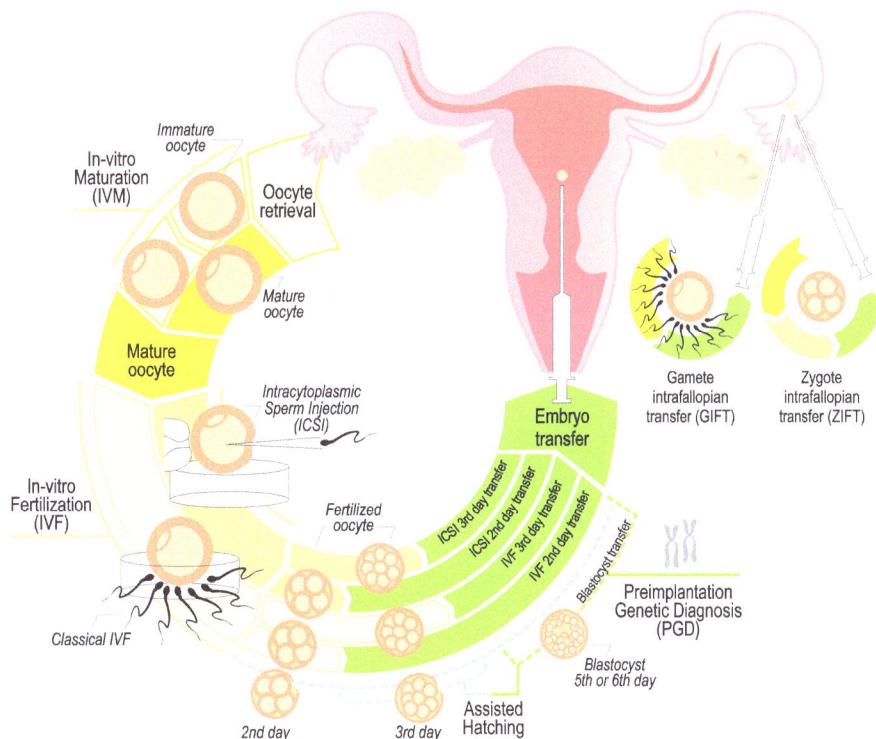

Figure 1: Assisted reproductive technologies.

In Vitro Fertilization (IVF or classical IVF) is a major part of ART. Briefly, after controlled ovarian stimulation, mature eggs are brought together with sperm in culture medium, attending for a spontaneous fertilization. Several embryos are often obtained. One or more of these embryos are placed into the uterus of the woman with the goal to establish a pregnancy.

Since the birth of the first human baby conceived by IVF in 1978 [6], the indications of these treatments have diversified dramatically. Used primarily in case of fallopian tube obstruction, the technique was then proposed in various conditions such as sperm abnormalities, anovulation or severe dysovulation as well as in idiopathic infertility. With the multiplication of indications, several modified techniques appeared: in Zygote intrafallopian transfer (ZIFT) fertilized eggs are placed into the fallopian tube while in Gamete intrafallopian tranfer (GIFT) a mixture of sperm and eggs is placed directly into a woman's fallopian tubes using laparoscopy following transvaginal oocyte retrieval.

However, IVF results were poor in case of male factor infertility and subzonal injection (SUZI) was developed. In this technique, a few spermatozoa were inserted into the perivitelline space after breaching of the zona pellucida by mechanical or chemical means. A Belgian team went farther and injected a single spermatozoon into the ooplasm of a mature oocyte: Intra-Cytoplasmic Sperm Injection (ICSI) was born [7] and SUZI was given up. Since the first babies conceived by ICSI in 1992 [7], the proportion of ICSI attempts has been raising incredibly and has now become higher than that of IVF. In the 2005 ESHRE report, the proportion of IVF was 36.7% *versus* 63.3% for ICSI [2]. In the USA, in 2006, a similar evolution has been reported with a percentage of 71% of ICSI cycles, which had increased by a factor of seven since 1995 [1].

Technical assistance is not limited to the entry of the sperm into the oocyte, as it can also be applied to the hatching of the embryo out of the zona pellucida. This glycoprotein coat is surrounding the oocyte and early cleaving embryo until it arrives in the uterine cavity. When the embryo has reached the so-called blastocyst stage, it will eventually hatch out of its coat and come into contact with the endometrium. This phenomenon may be impaired in case of an abnormal zona thickness or in various clinical subgroups of patients. Artificially disrupting the zona by mechanical, chemical, or laser-assisted techniques can be performed in order to facilitate implantation (Assisted Zona Hatchnig, AZH), but the benefit of this approach has not yet been clearly demonstrated [8]. Nevertheless, it has to be taken into account when analyzing ART impact on human health.

Besides these laboratory techniques, the pharmacopoeia has also considerably evolved. Since the first births performed during a natural cycle, where the body itself selects its own dominant egg, today, various ovarian stimulation protocols have been introduced in order to collect more eggs while controlling the LH surge. With the retrieval of a larger number of oocytes, more embryos than are actually needed for transfer often develop. As a consequence, supernumerary embryos can be cryopreserved in liquid nitrogen or nitrogen vapours, for future intraconjugal use or for a donation programme. Classically, embryos are frozen according to a slow cooling protocol in a programmable freezer, before their final storage. More recently, vitrification, has emerged as a simple and safe procedure by which embryos are directly plunged into liquid nitrogen [9, 10].

Dealing with large numbers of embryos also raises the question how to select the best of them for transfer. A lot of criteria have been put forward to assess their morphological quality and the dynamics of early development. Alternatively, embryos can be kept *in vitro* beyond the 2nd or 3rd day after egg collection, where transfer is usually performed. Under adequate culture conditions, they can be grown until day 5 or 6, up to the blastocyst stage. The procedure is quite selective, but blastocyst implantation rates are higher than those of cleaved embryos. However, while human blastocyst culture at the beginning was performed with co-culture (culture in the presence of various human or non-human epithelial cells), the development of standardized commercially available culture media systems has now lead to a high rate of viable blastocysts [11]. One issue that must be recognized is that we cannot compare old technology with a new one. Nowadays, in order to lower the risks of ovarian hyperstimulation, a growing number of ART providers offer modified natural IVF cycles or mild stimulation protocols, so called "patient-friendly IVF" [12-14]. Another option, when gonadotrophin stimulation has to be avoided, is oocyte *in vitro* maturation (IVM). In 1994, the first report of a successful pregnancy following this technique was published [15]. Egg retrieval is performed without previous ovarian stimulation, and immature eggs are cultured in maturation medium for 24 to 48 hours. *In vitro* matured eggs are then fertilized using IVF or more frequently ICSI. Despite of the fact that the effects of human immature oocyte culture on the subsequent development are not well known, hundreds of children have been born worldwide after IVM.

With the development and the optimization of techniques, the indications also diversified. Some forms of ART, such as pre-implantation genetic diagnosis (PGD), are used also in fertile couples presenting with genetic disease, to reduce the risk of transmission to the baby when a pregnancy is desired. The most common approach is to biopsy one or two blastomeres from day 3 embryos, and to select those who are not carrying the genetic risk. ART may also be offered to young patients with a high risk of infertility (*e.g.* cancer diagnosis, autoimmune disease, and other risks of premature ovarian failure), who underwent cryopreservation of eggs, sperm or gonadal tissue for later use. The fertility preservation strategy depends on the hormonal status (prepubertal/pubertal), the nature of the disease and the marital status. In case of various infectious diseases, serodiscordant couples can also ask for ART. This approach will minimize the risk of infection for the seronegative partner and for the baby. Finally, some countries allow assisted reproduction for personal reasons (same-sex couples, women without partner, preservation of fertility for social reasons).

METHODOLOGICAL CONSIDERATIONS WHEN ASSESSING THE EFFECT OF INFERTILITY TREATMENT AND PERINATAL OUTCOMES

Research on ART and perinatal outcomes faces several methodological challenges that need to be considered to allow reliable interpretation of results. Three possible categories might represent the factors involved in the association between ART and pregnancy outcomes: 1) ART treatment; 2) pharmacologic agents for ovulation induction or pregnancy maintenance; and 3) underlying infertility [16]. The diversity of aetiological factors implicated in the origin of infertility as well as the diversity of techniques and pharmacological agents hampers the assessment of the effect of ART on perinatal outcomes. Moreover, since different complementary techniques can be used at the same time, it is difficult to analyse the individual contribution of each technique to the perinatal outcome. Other methodological considerations are the study design, inadequate or inappropriate comparison groups, selection bias, and limited statistical power.

Concerning the study design, randomized clinical trials are not suitable from a practical and ethical point of view [17]. Prospective pregnancy-cohort studies following consecutively ART treatment and naturally conceived control pregnancies are desirable and feasible due to the relatively short interval between ART treatment and pregnancy outcome [18]. In the case of uncommon events such as birth defects or the long-term intergenerational effect of ART treatment, retrospective observational studies might be more efficient. However care must be taken as to potential bias, lack of temporal precision, and correlation of exposure patterns [17].

The unfeasibility of randomized clinical trials results in a lack of appropriate control groups, which impedes the differentiation between the effect of ART and the underlying infertility. Nonetheless, it has been proposed that some subgroups of women may be analyzed [16]: 1) infertile women who become pregnant spontaneously compared with infertile treated women; 2) fertile women who become pregnant with ART compared with fertile women who conceive spontaneously; and 3) infertile women treated with different types of infertility treatment. However, the implementation of studies including the first two subgroups of women might be more complicated. In the first subgroup, there are no population estimates for infertile women who achieved pregnancy without ART, making these studies difficult to carry out. Additionally, couples who do eventually conceive without assistance have probably different characteristics than those who conceive following ART [17]. Studies included into the second subgroup are practically impossible to be conducted at the population level since the circumstances under which ART treatment is provided to this group of patients are very limited. Moreover, national-wide registries do not identify fertile women who become pregnant with ART [17]. Thus, the third subgroup, which evaluates the compound effect of infertility and treatment, is the most realistic study design [16].

The scarcity of sampling frameworks for ascertaining populations at risk for fertility impairments, has led to the use of populations seeking treatment at fertility clinics [17]. However, for the purpose of epidemiological studies this sampling strategy is inappropriate because a large percentage of infecund couples do not seek medical care. Woman's age, education, income, duration of marriage and nulliparity, are associated with care-seeking behaviour, raising concern about potential selection bias [19]. On the other hand, nation-wide ART registries that are available in a few countries have provided useful information at the population-level allowing for control of possible confounding variables; however, this source of data might be also suffer from selection bias in countries where ART treatment is not accessible to the all population. Additionally, the methods used for data collection, the definitions of exposures and outcomes, the data validation, and the fact of voluntary compared with compulsory reporting may impact the interpretation of results of registry based research.

In addition, sufficient sample size is needed to minimize erroneous interpretation of the study results such as the absence of an ART treatment effect. This situation is frequently evoked in studies of ART and birth defects, where the low frequency of both, ART and birth defects, makes large sample sizes necessary [17].

Considering these challenges when evaluating the effect of ART on perinatal outcomes is essential. Although it is not possible to evaluate the independent effect of the underlying infertility diagnosis compared to the ART treatment or medication in the setting of a randomized clinical trial, other alternatives exist. Caution is needed regarding the choice of control groups, the ascertainment of the population to avoid selection bias, the standardization of protocols to precisely define the exposures and outcomes, and the estimate of an adequate sample size to guarantee sufficient statistical power.

PERINATAL OUTCOMES IN ART MULTIPLE PREGNANCIES

Major perinatal risks are consequence of the high rate of multiple gestations associated with ART treatment. Even in recent years, when the transfer of fewer embryos has been advocated, the reported prevalence of multiple pregnancies is still elevated. In Europe the reported average risk of multiple pregnancies as consequence of ART for 2005 was 21.8% [2]; while it was 31% in USA for 2006 when using fresh embryos and patient's eggs [1]. The prevalence may differ according to women's age and the use of frozen-thawed embryos.

Most of the ART twin pregnancies are dizygotic as result of multiple embryo transfer. However, some studies have documented a higher prevalence of monozygotic pregnancies among ART twins than in the general population. Monozygotic (MZ) twin occurrence is universally about 0.4–0.45% following non-stimulated *in vivo* conception [20], while the prevalence of MZ twinning following ART procedures has been reported to be between two and twelve times higher [21]. The increased prevalence of MZ twins is of clinical importance because of the higher risk of complications associated with these pregnancies, particularly the twin-twin transfusion syndrome. Various aetiological factors have been proposed but the debate is still open. Manipulation of the zona pellucida (ICSI, AZH) and blastocyst transfer appear to be of particular risk [21, 22].

Several studies conclude that ART twins have similar outcomes than spontaneous twins as illustrated by a systematic review of controlled studies [23], even after controlling for socioeconomic status [24]. Moreover, some adverse outcomes seem to be lower in ART twins, particularly as far as the risk of low and very low birth weight is concerned [24]. Although some studies have reported lower incidence of infant mortality among ART twins [23-25], a meta-analysis did not find any difference in perinatal death among ART and non-ART twins [26] Concerning the delivery route, an increased rate of caesarean section among ART twins has been reported in various publications [24, 27, 28].

However, it is important to remind that adverse perinatal outcomes are more frequent in ART twins than in singletons conceived with ART. The development of elective single embryo transfer (eSET) strategies aiming at reduce ART multiple births while maintaining acceptable overall pregnancy rates in good prognosis patients is the best approach [29, 30].

PERINATAL OUTCOMES IN ART SINGLETON PREGNANCIES

Although the great majority of singleton ART pregnancies are uncomplicated, numerous studies have raised questions concerning a range of adverse pregnancy outcomes in singleton ART pregnancies compared with spontaneously conceived singleton gestations.

First Half of Pregnancy

Spontaneous Abortion

Spontaneous abortion is defined by the World Health Organization (WHO) as the expulsion or extraction from its mother of an embryo or fetus weighing 500 g or less [31]. Additionally, in the field of assisted reproduction, a clinical pregnancy is defined by the ultrasound confirmation of a gestational sac. Thus, while in the general population the incidence of spontaneous abortion is around 11-16% [32], it increases to 31% if early clinical pregnancy losses are considered [33]. In clinical practice, two important factors should be taken into account when interpreting the literature. First, ART pregnancies are diagnosed earlier and followed more closely than pregnancies conceived naturally, and second, confounding factors such as maternal age or the rate of multiple pregnancies need to be considered. Indeed, a U.S. population-based study concluded that spontaneous abortion rates for ART patients conceived with the patient's oocytes and freshly transferred embryos were not different from the rates calculated from a representative sample of U.S. spontaneous conceptions [34]. Nonetheless, even when only clinically recognized pregnancies are considered, there are sub-groups of patients that seem to have an increased risk of spontaneous abortion, such as those who use clomiphene citrate for ovarian stimulation [34, 35]. Recently, the McGill assisted reproductive center group reported a high miscarriage rate after the introduction of IVM [36]. However, because 80% of these patients suffered from Polycystic Ovary Syndrome (PCOS), a debate is still open about the underlying mechanism: the disease itself and/or a treatment-mediated effect.

Vaginal Bleeding

In ART pregnancies, vaginal bleeding during the first trimester is not always a sign of spontaneous abortion. However, it is an independent risk factor for adverse obstetrical and perinatal outcomes during gestation [37]. The underlying mechanisms are unclear, but a vanishing twin effect following an embryo transfer of more than one embryo is probable [38]. Indeed, some studies concluded that pregnancy outcomes in ART singletons are more favorable after single-than after double-embryo transfer [39-41].

Ectopic Pregnancies

In developed countries, the estimated prevalence of ectopic pregnancy in the general population is 2% [42, 43]. Although, it is classical to consider that the rate of ectopic pregnancy is higher in pregnancies resulting from ART than in spontaneous pregnancies, this could be attributed to coexisting maternal pathologies. A recent review supported that distorted tubal anatomy is a strong predisposing factor for ectopic pregnancy after ART [44]. Indeed, the female status highly influences this risk explaining why the incidence of ectopic pregnancy has been shown to be as high as 11.1% in tubal infertility [45]. Nonetheless, data from the 2001 SART registry reported a rate of ectopic pregnancy among ICSI patients of 1.7% per pregnancy, compared with 2% among non-ICSI patients [46]. These percentages are similar to the estimated overall incidence of ectopic pregnancy in the USA of 2% per reported pregnancy [43]. In total, the prevalence of ectopic pregnancy after ART and after spontaneous conceptions is now comparable. This evolution is attributable to the decrease in the proportion of couples with tubal factor infertility undergoing classical IVF and a concomitant increase in couples with male factor infertility undergoing ICSI as described before (see "Overview of IVF technologies"). Besides, to study the effect of other risk factors such as ZIFT, assisted hatching, high embryo transfer volume, deep fundal transfer, and frozen embryo transfer larger multicentre series are required to attain enough statistical power.

Ectopic pregnancy may also be associated with a simultaneous intrauterine pregnancy. The incidence of this particular form, called heterotopic pregnancy, has increased dramatically with the development of ART procedures. While the incidence of heterotopic pregnancy in spontaneous cycles is 1 in 30,000 pregnancies [47], its incidence is about 1 in 100 pregnancies in women treated with IVF [48, 49]. The clinical diagnosis of this entity is difficult as the major symptom is abdominal pain, a common symptom of ovarian hyperstimulation. Different treatment options are available: surgical intervention, selective fetal reduction by embryo aspiration under ultrasound guidance, or expectant management of the extra-uterine gestation ensuring minimal distress of the intrauterine pregnancy. In a review of the literature, the overall live birth rate for the intrauterine pregnancy was 56.7% [50]. These data are supported by a recent case report of 12 heterotopic pregnancies with a live birth rate of 66.7% [51].

Adnexal Torsion

Another well-known complication in ART pregnancies, although less frequent than vaginal bleeding, is adnexal torsion. A 10-fold increase in the likelihood of ovarian torsion during ART pregnancies was seen on a large population-based study [52]. Of interest, even if ovarian hyperstimulation syndrome is associated with an increased risk of adnexal torsion related to enlarge cystic ovaries, the pregnancy itself increases the likelihood of ovarian torsion [53, 54]. This true gynecologic emergency is difficult to recognize clinically after ovarian stimulation, because lower abdominal pain, distended abdomen, nausea and emesis are not specific. Pelvic ultrasonography with Doppler evaluation is helpful for diagnosis because Doppler's sensitivity is improved in this context (75% for Pena *et al.* [55]). When possible, a laparoscopic conservative treatment (detorsion) must be proposed during the first and second trimester of pregnancy despite an unfavorable appearance of the ovary [56]. For technical reasons, laparotomy remains a traditional approach in advanced gestation [57].

Prenatal Screening of-Chromosomal Abnormalities

There is concern about the validity of maternal serum screening for chromosomal abnormalities. Higher false-positive rates of screening tests than in spontaneously conceived pregnancies after adjusting for maternal age are described. Therefore, ART pregnant patients are at increased risk of having an invasive prenatal diagnosis test, which may generate unnecessary anxiety and increase the risk of miscarriage on a healthy pregnancy. Biomarkers are modified in singleton ART pregnancies during the first [58] and second trimester [59]. Over the last 10 years, second trimester serum screening has been progressively replaced by first trimester combined screening. The first trimester combined screen measures maternal serum levels of free beta-human chorionic gonadotrophin (fb-hCG) and pregnancy-associated plasma protein-A (PAPP-A) at 9–12 weeks gestation as well as nuchal translucency by ultrasound at 11–13 weeks gestation. These measurements are combined with maternal age, weight and gestational age to produce a risk estimate of chromosomal abnormalities [60]. In the first trimester of ART pregnancies, several studies have reported lower levels of PAPP-A following fresh embryo transfer, even in pregnancies without later obstetrical complication [58, 61, 62] explaining the high false-positive rate described as fb-hCG was not significantly altered. However, one study reported that in pregnancies following the transfer of frozen-thawed embryo, PAPP-A levels were not modified, except when the mother received hormonal treatment around the time of embryo transfer [58]. Among the mechanisms proposed to explain these results are a delay in placental maturation [63] and abnormal interactions between the corpus luteum, endometrium, embryo and placenta [58, 64]. Concerning nuchal translucency thickness, an ultrasound marker of chromosomal abnormalities, a marginal increase, was noted in the largest study to date on the influence of ART conception on first trimester combined screening (1,739 ART pregnancies and 50,253 non-ART pregnancies). However the authors suggested that it was due to operator effects [58]. Moreover, two recent studies on smaller groups reported a decrease in nuchal tranlucency thickness in ART pregnancies [61, 62]. The future is perhaps in measuring circulating cell-free fetal DNA in maternal serum which does not appear to be affected by IVF conception [65].

Second Half of Pregnancy and Neonate

Preterm Birth

The WHO defines preterm birth as the delivery of an infant between 20 and 37 weeks' gestation [66]. Preterm birth is the major cause of perinatal mortality and morbidity worldwide [67]. It is associated with 70% of neonatal deaths [68] and many who survive suffer from major long-term neurocognitive, respiratory, and ophthalmologic morbidity [69]. Several studies have evaluated the association between ART and preterm birth [70-79]. Consistently, women pregnant after ART had an increased risk of delivery prior to 37 weeks. In one meta-analysis of 14 studies which were controlled at least for age and parity, and included 12,114 IVF pregnancies, the reported risk of preterm birth after ART was increased by 1.95 (95% CI 1.73, 2.20), when compared with the risk in spontaneous singleton pregnancies [80]. Another meta-analysis confirmed these results in maternal age-matched studies (OR 1.93; 95% CI 1.36-2.74), with an even higher risk for preterm birth at less than 33 weeks' gestation (OR 2.99; 95% CI 1.54-5.80) [26]. Thus, preterm birth in singletons is approximately twice as likely after ART treatment compared to spontaneous pregnancies. Nonetheless, from the existing literature, it is not possible to ascertain the proportion of preterm induced deliveries (as consequence of maternal or fetal complications) *versus* preterm birth secondary to spontaneous preterm labor [81].

Low Birth Weight, Very Low Birth Weight and Small for Gestational Age

Weight at birth is directly correlated to gestational age. Thus, if ART pregnancies have an increased risk of preterm birth, it is expected that these pregnancies have also a higher prevalence of low birth weight (LBW) defined as weight at birth less than 2500 g or very low birth weight (VLBW) defined as weight at birth less than 1500 g. Indeed, several meta-analyses have consistently reported significantly increased risks of LBW and VLBW among singletons born after ART [23, 80, 82]. Nevertheless, to determine the independent effect of ART on fetal growth during pregnancy the ultimate goal would be to know if, for a given gestational age, infants born after ART are smaller than infants born after spontaneous conception. Therefore, studies evaluating the gestational age-specific relative weight, generally expressed as the proportion below the 10th percentile ("small for gestational age" SGA), are of valuable importance [81]. In Finland, no differences in SGA rates were detected among singleton pregnancies after ART in women with unexplained infertility [83], while a Dutch study reported a significant increased risk of SGA in ART singleton pregnancies (RR 2.08; 95% CI 1.21, 3.70) [70]; these results are supported also by a Danish population-based study (RR 1.38; 95% CI 1.22, 1.56) [84]. Moreover, analyses conducted in the SART registry in the United States showed that the standardized risk ratio for term low birth weight after ART was increased (RR 2.6; 95% CI 2.4,2.7) [85]. In summary, besides the expected increased risk of LBW and VLBW associated with the increased risk of preterm birth, there is some evidence that singleton infants born after ART are more likely to be SGA than infants born after spontaneous conception. However, the mechanisms involved are still to be determined.

Mis-Implantation-Related Complications

The risk of preeclampsia is significantly increased in ART pregnancies compared to spontaneous pregnancies, even after adjustment for confounding factors [52, 80, 86]. This increased risk was described after both standard IVF and ICSI. Other complications associated with implantation such as placental abruption and placenta *praevia* are also increased in women undergoing ART [80, 86-88].

Other Obstetrical Complications

The association between ART singleton pregnancies and gestational diabetes is less clear since some risk factors for gestational diabetes are also related to infertility, such as anovulation and previous insulin resistance. Among other pregnancy complications, a Swedish register study reported a statistically significant increased risk of premature rupture of membranes in IVF singleton pregnancies [52].

Perinatal Mortality

Perinatal mortality differed widely among studies with some [27, 89, 90] but not all [70, 90-93] reporting an increased risk. However, different meta-analyses have consistently supported an elevated risk of perinatal mortality in IVF singletons [23, 26, 80]. Nonetheless, it is unclear to what extent this was due to the observed differences in preterm birth and low birth weight [81].

Delivery

The ART pregnancies are more prone to medical intervention. Several publications report an increased rate of obstetrical interventions such as induced labor, elective and emergent caesarean delivery [23, 80, 94-97], even when matched for age and duration of gestation [98]. This trend reflects in part the increased anxiety that surrounds the management of ART-pregnancies for both the patient and the physician.

Birth Defects

Since the 1980s, concerns were raised regarding the risk of congenital malformations following IVF, and later following ICSI. In this particular context, major methodological difficulties exist [99]. Besides the low frequency of certain events or the non-standard definition and classification of congenital malformations, the proportion of affected children depends on whether or not abortions and stillbirths are included; on the differences of methods used to assess the malformations; on the length of follow-up and on the consideration of potential confounding factors. Nonetheless, meta-analyses, case-control studies and population-based registry studies, as recently reviewed by Basatemur and Sutcliffe, have reported an increased risk of major malformations between 29 and 41% in children born following ART when compared with non-assisted conceived children [100]. No significant differences in malformation rates between IVF and ICSI groups were found.

Even if an insufficient statistical power limits the association between ART and specific defects, some malformations are pointed [101]: genitourinary defects and particularly hypospadias, neural tubes defects, gastrointestinal defects, musculoskeletal defects, chromosomal defects and cardiovascular defects.

Imprinting Disorders

Despite Mendelian principles, maternal and paternal genomes are not functionally equivalent; a number of genes may have modifications, specific to their maternal or paternal origin, and are said to be imprinted. About 50 genes are currently known to be differentially expressed according to their origin in either the oocyte or the sperm [102].

Recently, several authors have reported correlations between certain genomic imprinting disorders and ART: Beckwith–Wiedemann syndrome, Angelman syndrome, Silver-Russel syndrome and retinoblastoma. Other studies however found discordant results. Again, major methodological difficulties must be highlighted [101, 103-105] such as small sample sizes, the absence of correction for confounding factors (*e.g.* paternal or maternal age, infertility diagnoses), possible biases (*e.g.* socioeconomic status and participation in genetic disease registries) and statistical misinterpretation. However, various steps occurring during ART treatment could lead to imprinting defects, altering either gametes or embryos [103, 104]. Animal studies have suggested that the impact can occur 1) during superovulation for both IVF and ICSI; 2) at some stage of ICSI itself, during removal of cumulus cells prior to micromanipulation, and/or during the injection of spermatozoon into the ooplasm; and 3) during the oocyte and embryo culture period (culture media, length of exposure), with special concern in case of oocyte *in vitro* maturation since imprint establishment may not be complete in immature human germinal vesicle oocytes.

Prospective longitudinal studies of children conceived by ART at multiple centres are emergently needed, particularly in case of such rare events like imprinting disorders.

DIFFERENTIATING MATERNAL FACTORS *VERSUS* ART EFFECT ON PREGNANCY OUTCOMES

ART pregnancies have been associated with higher health risks than naturally-conceived singletons. Nonetheless, questions remain about the underlying mechanisms.

Two common risk factors are evoked: maternal age and parity. A US population-based study of ART and maternal and perinatal outcomes reported that among singletons, the risk of maternal and perinatal adverse outcomes was independent of demographic differences between ART and non-ART births such as advanced maternal age or primiparity [94]. An higher frequency of pre-existent maternal chronic conditions is also evoked in older women who suffer from infertility. In the above mentioned American study [94], associations between ART and both preterm and low birth weight remained significant in a subset of births for which no maternal chronic conditions, pregnancy complications, or labor and delivery complications were reported.

On the other hand, a recurrent question is about the role of the underlying infertility and/or ART treatment in the observed adverse perinatal outcomes. Thus, in a Swedish register-based study on large numbers of patients, the increase in likelihood of many complications was greater after standard IVF than after ICSI. The authors suggest that women receiving standard IVF treatment and women receiving ICSI have differences in clinical characteristics, such as a lower rate of fertility problems among the latter [52]. Furthermore, even in singletons, several studies have found a higher prevalence of adverse perinatal outcomes in subfertile/infertile couples who conceived spontaneously. In a Danish national birth cohort, the prevalence of congenital malformations increased with increasing time to pregnancy [106] as well as the risk for low birth weight, preterm birth, caesarean section [107], preeclampsia [108], small-for-gestational age [109] and neonatal mortality [110]. An increased risk of low birth weight and preterm birth has been also reported by other authors [111-113].

Additionally, in a population-based cohort study in Norway, two different approaches of analyses where conducted: the usual comparison of perinatal outcomes among spontaneous conception and ART singletons, and a sibling-relationship analysis. The sibling-relationship analysis compared women who had given birth to a singleton infant after assisted fertilization and who previously delivered a singleton infant after spontaneous conception or *vice versa*. The usual comparison reported similar results as in the existent literature, supporting an increased risk of adverse perinatal outcomes after ART treatment. However, when sibling-relationship analyses were conducted, no association was found between assisted fertilization and the risk of low birth weight, preterm delivery, and small for gestational age infants, even when controlling for birth order effect [114]. The authors concluded that previous studies that have assessed effects of ART on pregnancy outcomes could be biased. Thus, outcomes might differ between pregnancies conceived spontaneously and after assisted fertilization because of factors attributable to the underlying infertility, and not to the reproductive technology itself.

Finally, some unexplained infertility may be due to so far unrecognized epigenetic disorders increasing the risk of affected offspring, with or without ART. A recent report on 79 Angelman syndrome children revealed that children of subfertile couples, whether they were conceived naturally, by ICSI, or after superovulation, had a greater risk of Angelman syndrome compared to children who were born to normal fertile couples [115]. Because early embryonic development is critically dependent on the normal function of imprinted genes [116], the underlying infertility could be implicated in various adverse pregnancy outcomes including intra-uterine growth retardation and some congenital anomalies.

The debate is still open. However, the Norway population-based study illustrates the importance of the control group. Thus, when nation-wide registries of good quality are available these can be used to compare perinatal outcomes of ART patients with those of infertile couples who achieve pregnancy spontaneously.

CONCLUSION

As the number of ART pregnancies increases, it becomes fundamental to better identify health outcomes specific to these pregnancies. The main risk associated with ART is related to multiple pregnancies. The improvement of embryo cryopreservation programmes and the development of eSET policies will reduce significantly the number of multiple pregnancies while maintaining acceptable overall pregnancy rates. Publication of cumulative live birth rates per attempt of IVF or ICSI using fresh and frozen-thawed embryos will promote the acceptance of such policies. On the other hand, the available weight of evidence suggests an association between ART treatment and adverse outcomes in singleton pregnancies. However, the underlying infertility might be in the causal pathway. It is important to note that there are many data gaps to date. Future research initiatives are emergently needed, with enhancing transdisciplinary collaboration. The knowledge acquired will impact on infertility specialists, obstetricians, urologists, and geneticists when counselling patients requesting fertility treatment.

ACKNOWLEDGEMENTS

Particular thanks to Gabriel Abad for his technical support with the graphic design. M.P. Vélez is supported by a doctoral fellowship from the Strategic Training Initiative in Research in Reproductive Health Sciences (STIRRHS-CIHR).

REFERENCES

[1]   Sunderam S, Chang J, Flowers L, *et al.* Assisted reproductive technology surveillance--United States, 2006. MMWR Surveill Summ 2009; 58(5): 1-25.

[2]   Nyboe Andersen A, Goossens V, Bhattacharya S, *et al.* Assisted reproductive technology and intrauterine inseminations in Europe, 2005: results generated from European registers by ESHRE: ESHRE. The European IVF Monitoring Programme (EIM), for the European Society of Human Reproduction and Embryology (ESHRE). Human Reprod 2009; 24(6): 1267-87.

[3]   Agence de la biomédecine. Bilan des activités de procréation et génétique humaines en France 2007. 2010 [Accessed May 17, 2010]; Available from: http://www.agence-biomedecine.fr/annexes/bilan2008/som/som_general_proc.htm.

[4]   Gunby J, Bissonnette F, Librach C, Cowan L. Assisted reproductive technologies (ART) in Canada: 2007 results from the Canadian ART Register. Fertil Steril 2011; 95(2): 542-7 e1-10.

[5]   Centres for Disease Control and Prevention. Assisted Reproductive Technology: Home. 2010 [updated November 11, 2009. Accessed May 11, 2010]; Available from: http://www.cdc.gov/art/.

[6]   Steptoe PC, Edwards RG. Birth after the reimplantation of a human embryo. Lancet 1978; 2(8085): 366.

[7]   Palermo G, Joris H, Devroey P, Van Steirteghem AC. Pregnancies after intracytoplasmic injection of single spermatozoon into an oocyte. Lancet 1992; 340 (8810): 17-8.

[8]   Das S, Blake D, Farquhar C, Seif MM. Assisted hatching on assisted conception (IVF and ICSI). Cochrane Database Syst Rev 2009; (2): CD001894.

[9]   Kuwayama M. Highly efficient vitrification for cryopreservation of human oocytes and embryos: the Cryotop method. Theriogenology 2007; 67(1): 73-80.

[10]   Vajta G, Nagy ZP, Cobo A, Conceicao J, Yovich J. Vitrification in assisted reproduction: myths, mistakes, disbeliefs and confusion. Reprod Biomed Online 2009; 19(Suppl 3): 1-7.

[11]   Gardner DK, Lane M, Schoolcraft WB. Physiology and culture of the human blastocyst. J Reprod Immunol 2002; 55(1-2): 85-100.

[12]   Pelinck MJ, Hoek A, Simons AH, Heineman MJ. Efficacy of natural cycle IVF: a review of the literature. Hum Reprod Update 2002; 8(2): 129-39.

[13]   Pelinck MJ, Vogel NE, Arts EG, Simons AH, Heineman MJ, Hoek A. Cumulative pregnancy rates after a maximum of nine cycles of modified natural cycle IVF and analysis of patient drop-out: a cohort study. Human reproduction 2007; 22(9): 2463-70.

[14]   Verberg MF, Eijkemans MJ, Macklon NS, *et al.* The clinical significance of the retrieval of a low number of oocytes following mild ovarian stimulation for IVF: a meta-analysis. Hum Reprod Update 2009; 15(1): 5-12.

[15]   Trounson A, Wood C, Kausche A. *In vitro* maturation and the fertilization and developmental competence of oocytes recovered from untreated polycystic ovarian patients. Fertil Steril 1994; 62(2): 353-62.

[16]   Reddy UM, Wapner RJ, Rebar RW, Tasca RJ. Infertility, assisted reproductive technology, and adverse pregnancy outcomes: executive summary of a National Institute of Child Health and Human Development workshop. Obstet Gynecol 2007; 109(4): 967-77.

[17]   Buck Louis GM, Schisterman EF, Dukic VM, Schieve LA. Research hurdles complicating the analysis of infertility treatment and child health. Hum Reprod 2005; 20(1): 12-8.

[18]   Olsen J, Skov T. Design options and methodological fallacies in the studies of reproductive failures. Environ Health Perspect 1993; 101(Suppl 2): 145-52.

[19]   Rachootin P, Olsen J. Social selection in seeking medical care for reduced fecundity among women in Denmark. J Epidemiol Community Health 1981; 35(4): 262-4.

[20]   Derom C, Vlietinck R, Derom R, Van den Berghe H, Thiery M. Increased monozygotic twinning rate after ovulation induction. Lancet 1987; 1(8544): 1236-8.

[21]   Aston KI, Peterson CM, Carrell DT. Monozygotic twinning associated with assisted reproductive technologies: a review. Reproduction 2008; 136(4): 377-86.

[22]   Chang HJ, Lee JR, Jee BC, Suh CS, Kim SH. Impact of blastocyst transfer on offspring sex ratio and the monozygotic twinning rate: a systematic review and meta-analysis. Fertil Steril 2009; 91(6): 2381-90.

[23]   Helmerhorst FM, Perquin DA, Donker D, Keirse MJ. Perinatal outcome of singletons and twins after assisted conception: a systematic review of controlled studies. BMJ 2004; 328(7434): 261.

[24]   Boulet SL, Schieve LA, Nannini A, *et al.* Perinatal outcomes of twin births conceived using assisted reproduction technology: a population-based study. Human Reprod 2008; 23(8): 1941-8.

[25]   Fitzsimmons BP, Bebbington MW, Fluker MR. Perinatal and neonatal outcomes in multiple gestations: assisted reproduction versus spontaneous conception. Am J Obstet Gynecol 1998; 179(5): 1162-7.

[26]   McDonald S, Murphy K, Beyene J, Ohlsson A. Perinatal outcomes of *in vitro* fertilization twins: a systematic review and meta-analyses. Am J Obstet Gynecol 2005; 193(1): 141-52.

[27]   Dhont M, De Sutter P, Ruyssinck G, Martens G, Bekaert A. Perinatal outcome of pregnancies after assisted reproduction: a case-control study. Am J Obstet Gynecol 1999; 181(3): 688-95.

[28]   Shebl O, Ebner T, Sir A, Sommergruber M, Tews G. The role of mode of conception in the outcome of twin pregnancies. Minerva Ginecol 2009; 61(2): 141-52.

[29]   Gerris JM. Single embryo transfer and IVF/ICSI outcome: a balanced appraisal. Hum Reprod Update 2005; 11(2): 105-21.

[30]   Pandian Z, Bhattacharya S, Ozturk O, Serour G, Templeton A. Number of embryos for transfer following *in-vitro* fertilisation or intra-cytoplasmic sperm injection. Cochrane Database Syst Rev 2009; (2): CD003416.

[31]   WHO: recommended definitions, terminology and format for statistical tables related to the perinatal period and use of a new certificate for cause of perinatal deaths. Modifications recommended by FIGO as amended October 14, 1976. Acta Obstet Gynecol Scand 1977; 56(3): 247-53.

[32]   Everett C. Incidence and outcome of bleeding before the 20th week of pregnancy: prospective study from general practice. BMJ 1997; 315(7099): 32-4.

[33]   Wilcox AJ, Weinberg CR, O'Connor JF, *et al.* Incidence of early loss of pregnancy. N Engl J Med 1988; 319(4): 189-94.

[34]   Schieve LA, Tatham L, Peterson HB, Toner J, Jeng G. Spontaneous abortion among pregnancies conceived using assisted reproductive technology in the United States. Obstet Gynecol 2003; 101(5 Pt 1): 959-67.

[35]   Dickey RP, Taylor SN, Curole DN, Rye PH, Pyrzak R. Incidence of spontaneous abortion in clomiphene pregnancies. Human Reprod 1996; 11(12): 2623-8.

[36]   Buckett WM, Chian RC, Dean NL, Sylvestre C, Holzer HE, Tan SL. Pregnancy loss in pregnancies conceived after *in vitro* oocyte maturation, conventional *in vitro* fertilization, and intracytoplasmic sperm injection. Fertil Steril 2008; 90(3): 546-50.

[37]   Weiss JL, Malone FD, Vidaver J, *et al.* Threatened abortion: A risk factor for poor pregnancy outcome, a population-based screening study. Am J Obstet Gynecol 2004; 190(3): 745-50.

[38]   De Sutter P, Bontinck J, Schutysers V, Van der Elst J, Gerris J, Dhont M. First-trimester bleeding and pregnancy outcome in singletons after assisted reproduction. Human Reprod 2006; 21(7): 1907-11.

[39]   Pinborg A, Lidegaard O, la Cour Freiesleben N, Andersen AN. Consequences of vanishing twins in IVF/ICSI pregnancies. Human Reprod 2005; 20(10): 2821-9.

[40]   Pinborg A, Lidegaard O, Freiesleben NC, Andersen AN. Vanishing twins: a predictor of small-for-gestational age in IVF singletons. Human Reprod 2007; 22(10): 2707-14.

[41]   De Sutter P, Van der Elst J, Coetsier T, Dhont M. Single embryo transfer and multiple pregnancy rate reduction in IVF/ICSI: a 5-year appraisal. Reprod Biomed Online 2003; 6(4): 464-9.

[42]   Bouyer J. [Epidemiology of ectopic pregnancy: incidence, risk factors and outcomes] J Gynecol Obstet Biol Reprod 2003; 32(Suppl 7): S8-17.

[43]   Ectopic pregnancy--United States, 1990-1992. MMWR Morb Mortal Wkly Rep 1995; 44(3): 46-8.

[44]   Chang HJ, Suh CS. Ectopic pregnancy after assisted reproductive technology: what are the risk factors? Curr Opin Obstet Gynecol 2010; 22(3): 202-7.

[45]   Dubuisson JB, Aubriot FX, Mathieu L, Foulot H, Mandelbrot L, de Joliere JB. Risk factors for ectopic pregnancy in 556 pregnancies after *in vitro* fertilization: implications for preventive management. Fertil Steril 1991; 56(4): 686-90.

[46]   Assisted reproductive technology in the United States: 2001 results generated from the American Society for Reproductive Medicine/Society for Assisted Reproductive Technology registry. Fertil Steril 2007; 87(6): 1253-66.

[47]   Reece EA, Petrie RH, Sirmans MF, Finster M, Todd WD. Combined intrauterine and extrauterine gestations: a review. Am J Obstet Gynecol 1983; 146(3): 323-30.

[48]   Marcus SF, Macnamee M, Brinsden P. Heterotopic pregnancies after *in-vitro* fertilization and embryo transfer. Human Reprod 1995; 10(5): 1232-6.

[49]   Svare J, Norup P, Grove Thomsen S, *et al.* Heterotopic pregnancies after *in-vitro* fertilization and embryo transfer--a Danish survey. Human Reprod 1993; 8(1): 116-8.

[50]   Chin HY, Chen FP, Wang CJ, Shui LT, Liu YH, Soong YK. Heterotopic pregnancy after *in vitro* fertilization-embryo transfer. Int J Gynaecol Obstet 2004; 86(3): 411-6.

[51]   Luo X, Lim CE, Huang C, Wu J, Wong WS, Cheng NC. Heterotopic pregnancy following *in vitro* fertilization and embryo transfer: 12 cases report. Arch Gynecol Obstet 2009; 280(2): 325-9.

[52]   Kallen B, Finnstrom O, Nygren KG, Otterblad Olausson P, Wennerholm UB. *In vitro* fertilisation in Sweden: obstetric characteristics, maternal morbidity and mortality. BJOG 2005; 112(11): 1529-35.

[53]   Mashiach S, Bider D, Moran O, Goldenberg M, Ben-Rafael Z. Adnexal torsion of hyperstimulated ovaries in pregnancies after gonadotropin therapy. Fertil Steril 1990; 53(1): 76-80.

[54]   Wiser A, Levron J, Kreizer D, *et al.* Outcome of pregnancies complicated by severe ovarian hyperstimulation syndrome (OHSS): a follow-up beyond the second trimester. Human Reprod 2005; 20(4): 910-4.

[55]   Pena JE, Ufberg D, Cooney N, Denis AL. Usefulness of Doppler sonography in the diagnosis of ovarian torsion. Fertil Steril 2000; 73(5): 1047-50.

[56]   Rackow BW, Patrizio P. Successful pregnancy complicated by early and late adnexal torsion after *in vitro* fertilization. Fertil Steril 2007; 87(3): 697 e9-12.

[57]   Hasiakos D, Papakonstantinou K, Kontoravdis A, Gogas L, Aravantinos L, Vitoratos N. Adnexal torsion during pregnancy: report of four cases and review of the literature. J Obstet Gynaecol Res 2008; 34(4 Pt 2): 683-7.

[58]   Amor DJ, Xu JX, Halliday JL, *et al.* Pregnancies conceived using assisted reproductive technologies (ART) have low levels of pregnancy-associated plasma protein-A (PAPP-A) leading to a high rate of false-positive results in first trimester screening for Down syndrome. Human Reprod 2009; 24(6): 1330-8.

[59]   Lambert-Messerlian G, Dugoff L, Vidaver J, *et al.* First-and second-trimester Down syndrome screening markers in pregnancies achieved through assisted reproductive technologies (ART): a FASTER trial study. Prenat Diagn 2006; 26(8): 672-8.

[60]   Wald NJ, Rodeck C, Hackshaw AK, Walters J, Chitty L, Mackinson AM. First and second trimester antenatal screening for Down's syndrome: the results of the Serum, Urine and Ultrasound Screening Study (SURUSS). Health Technol Assess 2003; 7(11): 1-77.

[61]   Engels MA, Kooij M, Schats R, Twisk JW, Blankenstein MA, van Vugt JM. First-trimester serum marker distribution in singleton pregnancies conceived with assisted reproduction. Prenat Diagn 2010; 30(4): 372-7.

[62]   Gjerris AC, Loft A, Pinborg A, Christiansen M, Tabor A. First-trimester screening markers are altered in pregnancies conceived after IVF/ICSI. Ultrasound Obstet Gynecol 2009; 33(1): 8-17.

[63]   Bersinger NA, Wunder D, Vanderlick F, *et al.* Maternal serum levels of placental proteins after *in vitro* fertilisation and their implications for prenatal screening. Prenat Diagn 2004; 24(6): 471-7.

[64]   Tul N, Novak-Antolic Z. Serum PAPP-A levels at 10-14 weeks of gestation are altered in women after assisted conception. Prenat Diagn 2006; 26(13): 1206-11.

[65]   Pan PD, Peter I, Lambert-Messerlian GM, Canick JA, Bianchi DW, Johnson KL. Cell-free fetal DNA levels in pregnancies conceived by IVF. Human Reprod 2005; 20(11): 3152-6.

[66]   World Health Organization. The prevention of perinatal mortality and morbidity. Report No.: 457. Geneva, Switzerland 1970.

[67]   Ananth CV, Vintzileos AM. Epidemiology of preterm birth and its clinical subtypes. J Matern Fetal Neonatal Med 2006; 19(12): 773-82.

[68]   Challis JR, Lye SJ, Gibb W, Whittle W, Patel F, Alfaidy N. Understanding preterm labor. Ann N Y Acad Sci 2001; 943: 225-34.

[69]   Saigal S, Doyle LW. An overview of mortality and sequelae of preterm birth from infancy to adulthood. Lancet 2008; 371(9608): 261-9.

[70]   Koudstaal J, Braat DD, Bruinse HW, Naaktgeboren N, Vermeiden JP, Visser GH. Obstetric outcome of singleton pregnancies after IVF: a matched control study in four Dutch university hospitals. Hum Reprod 2000; 15(8): 1819-25.

[71]   Perri T, Chen R, Yoeli R, *et al.* Are singleton assisted reproductive technology pregnancies at risk of prematurity? J Assist Reprod Genet 2001; 18(5): 245-9.

[72]   Poikkeus P, Unkila-Kallio L, Vilska S, *et al.* Impact of infertility characteristics and treatment modalities on singleton pregnancies after assisted reproduction. Reprod Biomed Online 2006; 13(1): 135-44.

[73]   Klemetti R, Gissler M, Hemminki E. Comparison of perinatal health of children born from IVF in Finland in the early and late 1990s. Hum Reprod 2002; 17(8): 2192-8.

[74]   Wang JX, Norman RJ, Kristiansson P. The effect of various infertility treatments on the risk of preterm birth. Hum Reprod 2002; 17(4): 945-9.

[75]   De Sutter P, Delbaere I, Gerris J, *et al.* Birthweight of singletons after assisted reproduction is higher after single-than after double-embryo transfer. Hum Reprod 2006; 21(10): 2633-7.

[76]   De Neubourg D, Gerris J, Van Royen E, Mangelschots K, Vercruyssen M. Impact of a restriction in the number of embryos transferred on the multiple pregnancy rate. Eur J Obstet Gynecol Reprod Biol 2006; 124(2): 212-5.

[77]   Rajesh H, Yap HA, Wu YJ. Pregnancy outcomes from *in-vitro* fertilisation and intracytoplasmic sperm injection: a comparison. Singapore Med J 2006; 47(4): 309-14.

[78] Poikkeus P, Gissler M, Unkila-Kallio L, Hyden-Granskog C, Tiitinen A. Obstetric and neonatal outcome after single embryo transfer. Hum Reprod 2007; 22(4): 1073-9.

[79] Bonduelle M, Liebaers I, Deketelaere V, *et al.* Neonatal data on a cohort of 2889 infants born after ICSI (1991-1999) and of 2995 infants born after IVF (1983-1999). Hum Reprod 2002; 17(3): 671-94.

[80] Jackson RA, Gibson KA, Wu YW, Croughan MS. Perinatal outcomes in singletons following *in vitro* fertilization: a meta-analysis. Obstet Gynecol 2004; 103(3): 551-63.

[81] Myers ER, McCrory DC, Mills AA, *et al.* Effectiveness of assisted reproductive technology (ART). Evid Rep Technol Assess (Full Rep) 2008; 167: 1-195.

[82] McDonald SD, Han Z, Mulla S, Murphy KE, Beyene J, Ohlsson A. Preterm birth and low birth weight among *in vitro* fertilization singletons: a systematic review and meta-analyses. Eur J Obstet Gynecol Reprod Biol 2009; 146(2): 138-48.

[83] Isaksson R, Gissler M, Tiitinen A. Obstetric outcome among women with unexplained infertility after IVF: a matched case-control study. Hum Reprod 2002; 17(7): 1755-61.

[84] Hvidtjorn D, Grove J, Schendel DE, *et al.* Cerebral palsy among children born after *in vitro* fertilization: the role of preterm delivery--a population-based, cohort study. Pediatrics 2006; 118(2): 475-82.

[85] Schieve LA, Meikle SF, Ferre C, Peterson HB, Jeng G, Wilcox LS. Low and very low birth weight in infants conceived with use of assisted reproductive technology. N Engl J Med 2002; 346(10): 731-7.

[86] Katalinic A, Rosch C, Ludwig M. Pregnancy course and outcome after intracytoplasmic sperm injection: a controlled, prospective cohort study. Fertil Steril 2004; 81(6): 1604-16.

[87] Shevell T, Malone FD, Vidaver J, *et al.* Assisted reproductive technology and pregnancy outcome. Obstet Gynecol 2005; 106(5 Pt 1): 1039-45.

[88] Romundstad LB, Romundstad PR, Sunde A, von During V, Skjaerven R, Vatten LJ. Increased risk of placenta previa in pregnancies following IVF/ICSI; a comparison of ART and non-ART pregnancies in the same mother. Human Reprod 2006; 21(9): 2353-8.

[89] Gissler M, Malin Silverio M, Hemminki E. *In-vitro* fertilization pregnancies and perinatal health in Finland 1991-1993. Hum Reprod 1995; 10(7): 1856-61.

[90] Westergaard HB, Johansen AM, Erb K, Andersen AN. Danish National *In-Vitro* Fertilization Registry 1994 and 1995: a controlled study of births, malformations and cytogenetic findings. Hum Reprod 1999; 14(7): 1896-902.

[91] Verlaenen H, Cammu H, Derde MP, Amy JJ. Singleton pregnancy after *in vitro* fertilization: expectations and outcome. Obstet Gynecol 1995; 86(6): 906-10.

[92] Reubinoff BE, Samueloff A, Ben-Haim M, Friedler S, Schenker JG, Lewin A. Is the obstetric outcome of *in vitro* fertilized singleton gestations different from natural ones? A controlled study. Fertil Steril 1997; 67(6): 1077-83.

[93] Howe RS, Sayegh RA, Durinzi KL, Tureck RW. Perinatal outcome of singleton pregnancies conceived by *in vitro* fertilization: a controlled study. J Perinatol 1990; 10(3): 261-6.

[94] Schieve LA, Cohen B, Nannini A, *et al.* A population-based study of maternal and perinatal outcomes associated with assisted reproductive technology in Massachusetts. Matern Child Health J 2007; 11(6): 517-25.

[95] Allen VM, Wilson RD, Cheung A. Pregnancy outcomes after assisted reproductive technology. J Obstet Gynaecol Can 2006; 28(3): 220-50.

[96] Apantaku O, Chandrasekaran I, Bentick B. Obstetric outcome of singleton pregnancies achieved with *in vitro* fertilisation and intracytoplasmic sperm injection: experience from a district general hospital. J Obstet Gynaecol 2008; 28(4): 398-402.

[97] Buckett WM, Chian RC, Holzer H, Dean N, Usher R, Tan SL. Obstetric outcomes and congenital abnormalities after *in vitro* maturation, *in vitro* fertilization, and intracytoplasmic sperm injection. Obstet Gynecol 2007; 110(4): 885-91.

[98] Sheiner E, Shoham-Vardi I, Hershkovitz R, Katz M, Mazor M. Infertility treatment is an independent risk factor for cesarean section among nulliparous women aged 40 and above. Am J Obstet Gynecol 2001; 185(4): 888-92.

[99] Sutcliffe AG, Ludwig M. Outcome of assisted reproduction. Lancet 2007; 370(9584): 351-9.

[100] Basatemur E, Sutcliffe A. Follow-up of children born after ART. Placenta 2008; 29(Suppl B): 135-40.

[101] Schieve LA, Rasmussen SA, Buck GM, Schendel DE, Reynolds MA, Wright VC. Are children born after assisted reproductive technology at increased risk for adverse health outcomes? Obstet Gynecol 2004; 103(6): 1154-63.

[102] Morison IM, Reeve AE. A catalogue of imprinted genes and parent-of-origin effects in humans and animals. Hum Mol Genet 1998; 7(10): 1599-609.

[103] Laprise SL. Implications of epigenetics and genomic imprinting in assisted reproductive technologies. Mol Reprod Dev 2009; 76(11): 1006-18.

[104]   Allen C, Reardon W. Assisted reproduction technology and defects of genomic imprinting. BJOG 2005; 112(12): 1589-94.

[105]   Gosden R, Trasler J, Lucifero D, Faddy M. Rare congenital disorders, imprinted genes, and assisted reproductive technology. Lancet 2003; 361(9373): 1975-7.

[106]   Zhu JL, Basso O, Obel C, Bille C, Olsen J. Infertility, infertility treatment, and congenital malformations: Danish national birth cohort. BMJ 2006; 333(7570): 679.

[107]   Basso O, Baird DD. Infertility and preterm delivery, birthweight, and Caesarean section: a study within the Danish National Birth Cohort. Hum Reprod 2003; 18(11): 2478-84.

[108]   Basso O, Weinberg CR, Baird DD, Wilcox AJ, Olsen J. Subfecundity as a correlate of preeclampsia: a study within the Danish National Birth Cohort. Am J Epidemiol 2003; 157(3): 195-202.

[109]   Zhu JL, Obel C, Hammer Bech B, Olsen J, Basso O. Infertility, infertility treatment, and fetal growth restriction. Obstet Gynecol 2007; 110(6): 1326-34.

[110]   Basso O, Olsen J. Subfecundity and neonatal mortality: longitudinal study within the Danish national birth cohort. BMJ 2005; 330(7488): 393-4.

[111]   Thomson F, Shanbhag S, Templeton A, Bhattacharya S. Obstetric outcome in women with subfertility. BJOG 2005; 112(5): 632-7.

[112]   Williams MA, Goldman MB, Mittendorf R, Monson RR. Subfertility and the risk of low birth weight. Fertil Steril 1991; 56(4): 668-71.

[113]   Henriksen TB, Baird DD, Olsen J, Hedegaard M, Secher NJ, Wilcox AJ. Time to pregnancy and preterm delivery. Obstet Gynecol 1997; 89(4): 594-9.

[114]   Romundstad LB, Romundstad PR, Sunde A, *et al.* Effects of technology or maternal factors on perinatal outcome after assisted fertilisation: a population-based cohort study. Lancet 2008; 372(9640): 737-43.

[115]   Ludwig M, Katalinic A, Gross S, Sutcliffe A, Varon R, Horsthemke B. Increased prevalence of imprinting defects in patients with Angelman syndrome born to subfertile couples. J Med Genet 2005; 42(4): 289-91.

[116]   Preece MA, Moore GE. Genomic imprinting, uniparental disomy and foetal growth. Trends Endocrinol Metab 2000; 11(7): 270-5.

CHAPTER 3

Human Placentation and Maternal Adaptation to Pregnancy: The Role of Trophoblast

Thierry Fournier[1,*], Vassilis Tsatsaris[2], André Malassiné[1] and Danièle Evain-Brion[1]

Unité Mixte de Recherches-Santé UMR-S 767, INSERM and Paris Descartes University, PremUP Foundation, Faculty of Pharmaceutical and Biological Sciences, Paris F-75006, France and [2] Assistance Publique-Hôpitaux de Paris, Centre Hospitalier Universitaire Cochin, and Maternité Port-Royal, Paris F-75014, France

Abstract: Human placentation is characterized by the development of a hemochorial placenta and concomitantly by considerable changes in the vasculature of the uterus. The trophoblast is an essential tissue of the placenta. After blastocyst implantation, it differentiates into villous trophoblast, which ensures exchanges between mother and fetus as well as the endocrine functions of the placenta, and into invasive extravillous trophoblasts, which anchors the placenta in the uterus and participate to the implementation of the utero placental vascularization. We describe here the different stages of the placental morphogenesis and the physiological mechanisms responsible for uterine vascular remodeling. We then consider the main functions of the human placenta and in particular the qualitative and quantitative evolution along pregnancy of trophoblast hormonal functions from a paracrine role during the first trimester of pregnancy involved in the quality of placentation to an endocrine role that allows uterine quiescence and maternal adaptation to pregnancy.

Keywords: Syncytiotrophoblast, invasive extravillous cytotrophoblasts, hormones, preeclampsia, fetal growth.

PLACENTAL DEVELOPMENT

Morphological Development of the Human Placenta

Human placentation is hemomonochorial. Its development can be divided into three stages: prelacunar, lacunar, and villous (Fig. **1**).

Prelacunar Stage

Six days after fertilization, the blastocyst, limited by a cell mass called the trophectoderm, attaches to the epithelium of the uterus. From the trophectoderm differentiates an inner cell mass of cytotrophoblasts, which in contact to the uterus fuse to form a syncytiotrophoblast. This is highly invasive at this stage and its proteolytic activity enables it to penetrate the epithelium of the uterus and invade the endometrium. This results in the implantation of the blastocyst in the mucosa of the uterus.

Lacunar Stage

Around the 8th day after fertilization, vacuoles appear in the syncytiotrophoblast and progressively form lacunae between the finger-like processes of the syncytiotrophoblast. Lacunar networks start to form the future intervillous spaces.

Villous Stage

At 13 days, the cytotrophoblasts, which were still limited to the inner cell mass, invade the finger-like processes of syncytiotrophoblast, thus forming the primary chorionic villi. After 2 weeks, these primary villi are invaded by the embryonic mesenchyme and constitute the secondary villi. Fetal capillaries then appear in the mesenchyme; this vascularization characterizes the formation of the tertiary villi. In parallel,

---

*Address correspondence to Thierry Fournier: INSERM-767, Paris Descartes University, Faculty of Pharmaceutical and Biological Sciences, Paris F-75006, France; Tel: 33-1-53 73 96 03, Fax: 33-1-44 07 39 92, E-mail: thierry.fournier@parisdescartes.fr

the fetal vasculature of the allantois reaches the chorionic plate and joins to the vessels of the villous stems. The chorionic villus reaches its final shape around the third week after fertilization. The villous tree also comprises anchoring villi, which are attached to the endometrium and the floating villi bathing in the intervillous spaces through which the maternal blood circulates after the 12th week of pregnancy.

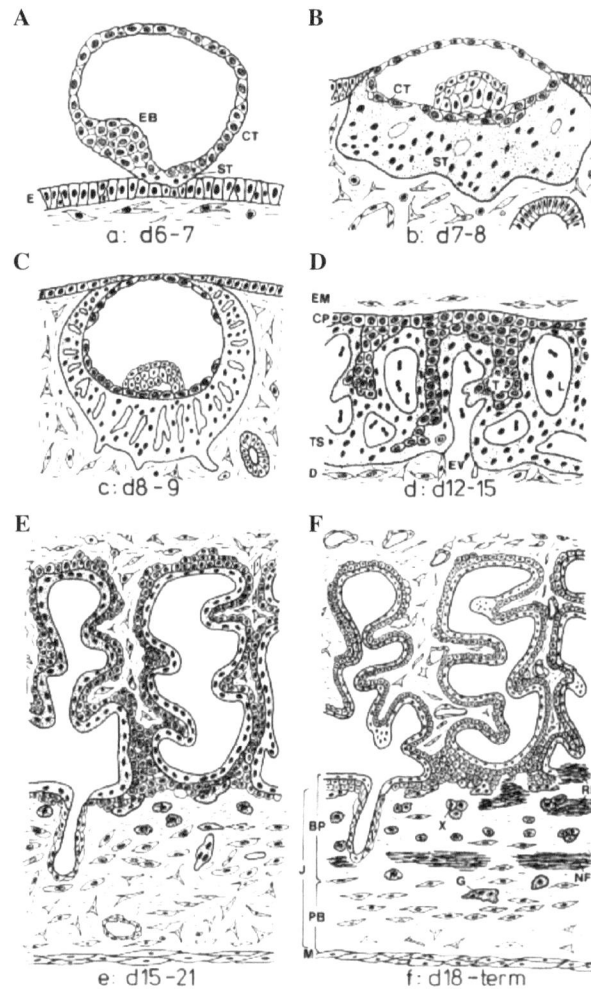

Figure 1: Diagram of the main stages of development of the human placenta (from [1]: Berniscke and Kaufmann, 2000). A: days 6-7, B: days 7-8, C: days 8-9, D: days 12-15, E: days 15-21, F: day 18-term A and B: prelacunar stage; C: lacunar stage; D: villous stage and primary villi; E: villous stage and secondary villi; F: villous stage and tertiary villi. BP: basal plate; CP: chorionic plate; CT: cytotrophoblast; T: trabeculae and primary villi; D: decidua; E: endometrial epithelium; EB: embryonic pole; EM: extraembryonic mesoderm; EV: endometrial vessel; G: giant cells; J: junctional zone; L: maternal blood lacunae; BP: basal plate; PB: placental bed; RF and NF: fibrinoid; ST: syncytiotrophoblast; TS: trophoblastic shell; M: myometrium; X: extravillous trophoblast.

Placental Anatomy

The human placenta is a pancake-shaped transient organ. At term it measures about 25 cm in diameter and 4 cm thick. Fig. **2** shows it at term from the fetal side or chorionic plate (A) and from the maternal side or basal plate (B). The umbilical cord is generally inserted centrally or paracentrally in the chorionic plate. At the insertion, the two arteries and the vein divide into numerous vessels, which run along the chorionic plate before going deeper into the villous tree. The basal plate consists of a fine edge of decidua approximately 2 mm thick, and therefore corresponds to tissue of maternal origin.

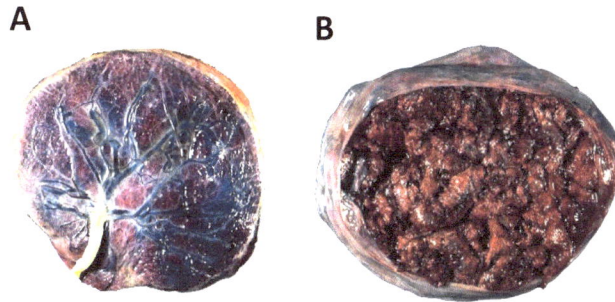

Figure 2: Human placenta at term: side of the chorial plate (A), side of the basal plate (B).

Human Trophoblast Differentiation

The trophoblastic cell is the essential cell of the placenta. It differentiates into villous trophoblast, which ensure exchanges between the fetus and the mother and the endocrine functions of the placenta, and into invasive extravillous trophoblast, which are indispensable for implantation and for remodeling of the uterine arteries. The differentiation of the cytotrophoblast is summarized in Fig. **3**.

The mononucleated villous cytotrophoblasts (VCT) aggregate and fuse to form the syncytiotrophoblast. The extravillous cytotrophoblast (EVCT) proliferates, becomes invasive, and migrates into the decidua and up to the upper third of the myometrium (interstitial EVCT). It colonizes the maternal uterine arteries (endovascular EVCT) or differentiates into giant multinucleated cells within the decidua basalis.

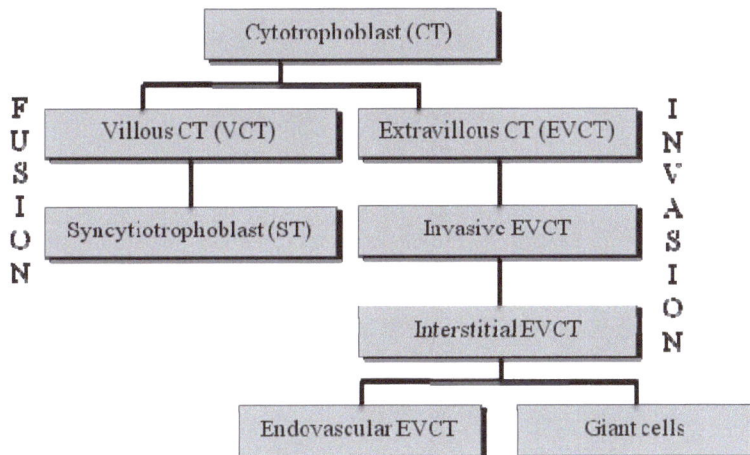

Figure 3: Human cytotrophoblast differentiation pathway.

Villous Trophoblast

The structural and functional unit of the human placenta is the chorionic villus. There are two types of villi: the floating villi, which float freely in the intervillous space, and the anchoring or stem villi, which are anchored in the maternal endometrium. The villi are delimited by a double mass of epithelial cells: the mononucleated villous cytotrophoblast and the multinucleated syncytiotrophoblast, surrounding a mesenchymal core containing fetal blood vessels and immune cells (macrophages: Hofbauer cells) (Cf. Fig. **4**).

The cytotrophoblastic cells remain attached to the villous basement membrane, forming a monolayer of epithelial cells. These cells proliferate and differentiate by fusion to form the syncytiotrophoblast that covers the entire surface of the villus. It has been suggested that once formed, the syncytiotrophoblast evolves towards cell death by apoptosis, leading to the formation of polynuclear syncytial knots and then debris shedding into the intervillous spaces and the maternal circulation [2, 3]. Renewal of the syncytiotrophoblast from the cytotrophoblast occurs throughout pregnancy. The syncytial knots, which are more numerous in various placental diseases (preeclampsia, trisomy 21), are in large part the source of the fetal DNA (deoxyribonucleic acid) and RNA (ribonucleic acid) circulating in the maternal blood. However according to Burton and Jones [4] there is little evidence to support the concept that a turnover of syncytial nuclei takes place in the normal placenta, or that this occurs through an apoptotic-related process. Instead these authors suggested that a proportion of syncytial nuclei are transcriptionally active, that epigenic modifications underlie the changes in chromatin appearance and that syncytial nuclei continue to accumulate until term. However these authors recognized that apoptotic changes can occur in pathologic pregnancies but considered the deportation of trophoblast that has been linked to preeclampsia to be most likely of necrotic origin following ischemic injury. Indeed, necrotic trophoblast debris are able to stimulate the release of the pro298 inflammatory cytokines. Furthermore it was demonstrated that only a minority of the syncytial nuclear aggregates contain apoptotic nuclei, suggesting that they serve different functions rather than just the extrusion of senescent nuclei as has previously been suggested [5].

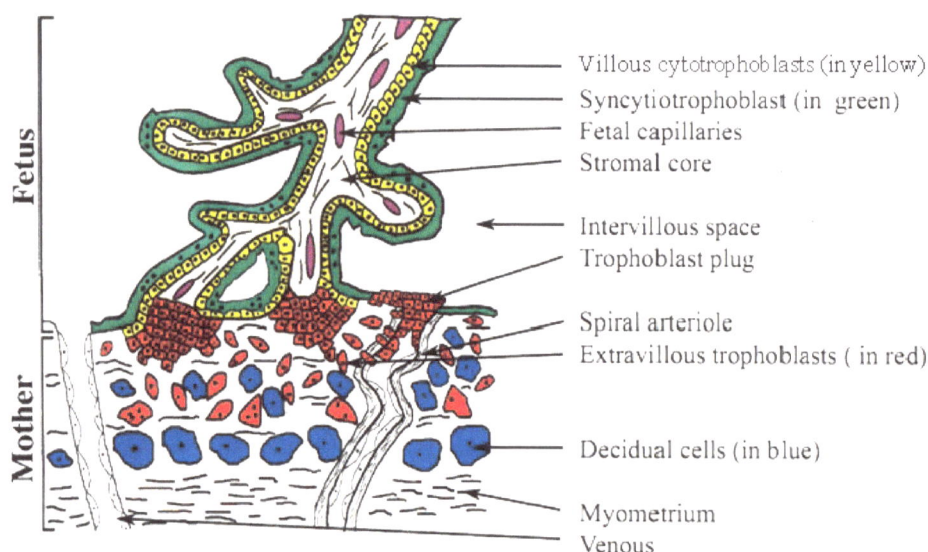

Figure 4: Scheme of human anchoring villous.

The syncytiotrophoblast lines the intervillous space and is in direct contact with the maternal blood from the end of the first trimester of gestation and is the first cellular layer separating the maternal circulation and the fetal circulation. It has metabolic, secretory, endocrine, exchange, and hemostatic functions. The syncytiotrophoblast does not express the classic human leukocyte antigens (HLAs) (A, B, and C) [6, 7].

The mechanisms involved in the differentiation of the villous cytotrophoblast into the syncytiotrophoblast have been much clarified thanks to the possibility of isolating, purifying, and culturing these cells *in vitro* [8-10].

Owing to the specificity of the human placenta (hemomonochorial, strong endocrine function and deep invasion of the trophoblast in the uterine wall), no readily accessible animal models are available for studying human trophoblast differentiation. Therefore, *in vitro* models including explants, cell lines and primary cultures have been established. Fig. **5** illustrates *in vitro* differentiated-cultures of primary villous and extravillous cytotrophoblast isolated from the same first-trimester chorionic villi [11, 12]. The cell line (HIPEC) was obtained by transformation of these primary extravillous cells by Simian Virus 40 large T antigen [13]. These *in vitro* models of human primary-cultured cytotrophoblasts express specific markers of villous (including syncytin 2) and extravillous cytotrophoblasts (including HLA-G) and represent therefore useful tools to study human trophoblast differentiation *in vitro*.

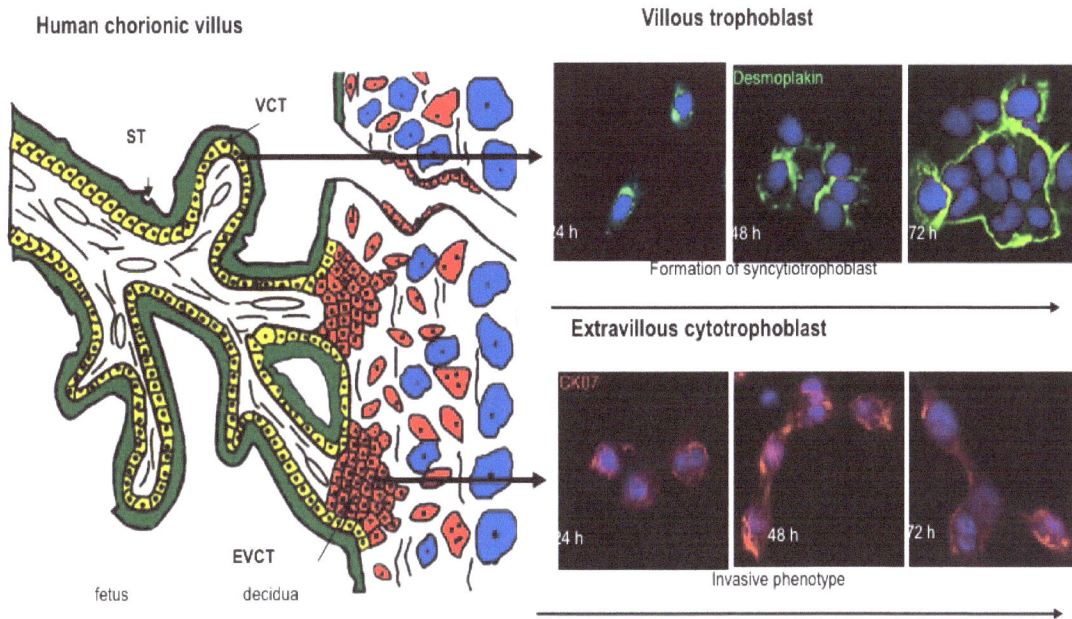

Figure 5: *In vitro* models of human cytotrophoblast differentiation along the endocrine villous or invasive extravillous pathway.

Villous Trophoblast Differentiation

The trophoblastic cell fusion is a multifactorial and dynamic process: cells must leave the proliferative stage and express genes and proteins involved in the fusion process, and then they must recognize and interact with their fusion partner allowing efficient communication and signal exchange. This dynamic process must be tightly regulated and coordinated. Purified cytotrophoblastic cells isolated from human chorionic villi and cultured on plastic dishes aggregate and then fuse, forming the multinucleated syncytiotrophoblast producing pregnancy-specific hormones. However, a realization that the biochemical and morphological features of trophoblast differentiation can be dissociated has surfaced in recent findings [14]. This *in vitro* model coupled with antisense or siRNA strategies, has allowed identifying membrane proteins required for human trophoblast fusion: connexin 43 [15], ZO1 [16] Herv-W (syncytin 1) [17], HERV-FRD (syncytin 2) [18]. Using other *in vitro* models (BeWo cell line, explant cultures), phosphatidylserine flip [19], cadherin 11 [20], CD98 [21], ADAM 12 [22], FGRL1 (fibroblast growth factor receptor-like 1) [23], and caspase 8 expression [24], were also implicated. However, contrary to previously suggested it was recently demonstrated that caspase activation was not required for villous cytotrophoblast fusion into syncytiotrophoblast [25]. Furthermore gap junctional inter-trophoblastic communication mediated by Cx43 channels is also required for trophoblastic cells fusion [26] suggesting that the molecular exchanges (cAMP, Ca^{2+}) between trophoblastic cells are essential for villous trophoblast differentiation.

Some Factors are Highly or Specifically Expressed in the Human Placenta

Retroviral envelop-proteins have been recently shown to be specifically expressed in the placenta and directly involved in trophoblast differentiation. In humans, two *env* genes carried by endogenous proviruses belonging to the HERV-W and HERV-FRD families, and designated *syncytin*-1and *syncytin*-2 respectively, have been identified for which convincing evidence of their involvement in placental physiology can be provided [27-29]. Syncytin 1 and syncytin 2 differ by their receptors. That of syncytin-1 was identified as a sodium-dependent neutral amino acid transporter variously designated as ASCT2/ATB°/SLC1A5 [27]. The receptor for syncytin-2 was identified as encoding a multi-pass transmembrane protein, named Major Facilitator Superfamily Domain Containing 2 (MFSD2) that belongs to a large family of putative carbohydrate transporters conserved in evolution [30]. Syncytin 1 and its receptor are localized in all cell type of human trophoblast [31]. Syncytin-2 is detected only in the cytoplasm of some cytotrophoblastic cells of the villous trophoblast [32] and its MFSD2 receptor is expressed at the level of the syncytiotrophoblast [30]. Syncytin 1 and syncytin 2 are highly fusogenic when over expressed by transfection in various cultured cells and their role in villous trophoblast fusion was demonstrated using antisense strategy for syncytin1 [17] and siRNA strategy for syncytin 2 [18]. The ability of syncytins to induce cell fusion may not be their only physiologic role. Recently, based on the fact that the placenta, expressing feto-paternal antigens, can be considered as a semi-allogenic graft that needs to be tolerated by the mother, Mangeney *et al.* [33] analyzed the immunosuppressive activity of the human syncytins and showed that syncytin 2 was immunosuppressive. Recently it was demonstrated that the presence of syncytin-1 in human placental exosomes present a novel mechanism of retroviral mediated immunosuppression that may be relevant in maternal immune tolerance during pregnancy [34]. Transcriptional regulation of the *syncytin-1* gene has been extensively investigated. The placenta-specific transcription factor Glial-Cell Missing 1 (GCM1; also known as GCMa) has been shown to regulate *syncytin-1* expression. Moreover a selective and temporal unmethylation of ERV-W in placenta during the first trimester may allow syncytin-1-mediated cell fusion [35]. Transcriptional regulation of the *syncytin-2* gene has been recently investigated [36] and GCM1 is also a critical factor for trophoblastic cell fusion. In addition GCM1 may also play a role in the epigenetic regulation of *syncytin-2* gene expression. The fusion of cytotrophoblasts is mediated *in vitro* by various soluble factors from the placenta or decidua, such as human chorionic gonadotropin (hCG), growth factors (EGF: epidermal growth factor, CSF: colony stimulating factor) and cytokines (TGF-β: transforming growth factor-β; TGFα; LIF: leukocyte migration inhibition factor) estradiol, dexamethasone, endothelin, oxygen partial pressure, SOD-1, 15ΔPGJ$_2$ (for review see [37]).

The morphological differentiation of villous cytotrophoblasts by fusion is accompanied by functional differentiation. The syncytiotrophoblast becomes the endocrine unit of the placenta and secretes numerous polypeptide and steroid hormones (human chorionic gonadotropin (hCG), human placental lactogen (hPL)), placental growth hormone (GH), leptin, progesterone, estrogens, and a great variety of growth factors, cytokines, and other peptides involved in the physiology of gestation and maternal adaptation to pregnancy [38-40]. The syncytiotrophoblast develops exchange functions and expresses transport proteins, which enable active transport of amino acids, and transporters involved in the facilitated diffusion of glucose. It is in direct contact with the maternal blood and expresses factors involved in the regulation of hemostasis such as thrombomodulin and annexin V [41-45].

Extravillous Trophoblast [46, 47]

During the first trimester, the human placenta is characterized by deep invasion of the endometrium of the uterus by extravillous cytotrophoblasts. These appear at the base of the anchoring villi as columns of aggregated polarized cells resting on a basal lamina (Fig. **4**). At this stage they are proliferative, but subsequently lose this capacity and differentiate into invasive cytotrophoblasts, at the distal part of the column. These extremely invasive cells colonize the endometrium and the superficial layer of the myometrium. This interstitial invasion ends with the formation of giant multinucleated cells. The invasive trophoblasts also colonize the maternal

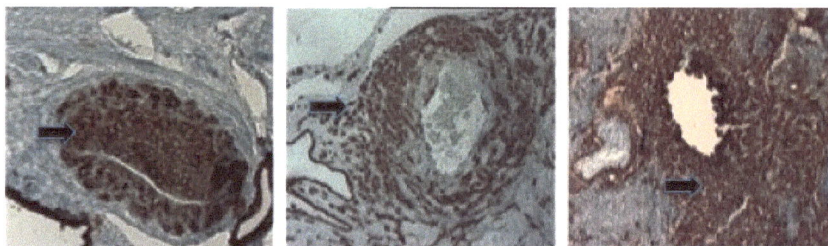

Figure 6: Endovascular invasion by extravillous cytotrophoblasts (plugs, left panel), interstitial trophoblast invasion (center panel) and total remodeling of uterine artery (right panel). Cytokeratin 7, a specific marker of cytotrophoblasts (arrows), is immunostained.

spiral arteries, the lumen of which is blocked by plugs of trophoblastic cells (Fig. **6**). Because of this, the maternal blood cells (notably the erythrocytes) are not found in the intervillous space during the first 8 weeks of gestation [48]. This results in an oxygen-poor placental environment (pO$_2$ or oxygen partial pressure of 20 mm

Hg corresponding to 2-3% O_2 at 8 weeks of gestation). These plugs disappear progressively from 10 weeks of gestation, and so maternal arterial blood gradually enters the intervillous space and pO_2 rise up to 55 mm Hg at 12 weeks corresponding to about 8 % O_2) [49, 50].

This invasion of the arterial wall by extravillous cytotrophoblasts leads to the disappearance of the arterial smooth muscle tunica media and of the maternal endothelial cells, which are replaced by extravillous cytotrophoblasts. The tunica media of the artery no longer responds to vasoactive substances. The endovascular cytotrophoblasts are in contact with the maternal blood, so their secretions act in an endocrine or paracrine manner on the mother's body, and are drawn into the maternal systemic circulation (they circulate in the mother's blood).

Note that these invasive interstitial endovascular and perivascular cytotrophoblasts are in direct contact with maternal immunocompetent cells, particularly of the decidua. It expresses specific HLAs, notably HLA-G, which is not recognized by the mother's immune system [51, 52]. Through the secretion of various cytokines, it also plays a major part in protection of the feto-placental unit against maternal immune rejection [53-56].

Factors that Control Trophoblast Invasion [57]

The human trophoblast invasion is a unique model of a cell invasion process, sharing mechanisms with metastasis. However, in contrast to tumoral invasion, trophoblast invasion is spatially controlled and oriented: it is temporally restricted to early pregnancy and spatially confined to the endometrium, the upper third of the myometrium, and the associated spiral arterioles [58, 59]. Cellular invasion requires different steps such as lost of cell-cell adhesion and communication, modification of receptors to the matrix such as integrins, protease activation promoting matrix degradation, cytoskeleton activation and secretion of soluble factors promoting cell migration. Trophoblast migration and invasive capacity were shown to be modulated by numerous factors (for review see [57]) including oxygen concentration [60], transforming growth factor (TGF-ß), insulin-like growth factor II (IGF-II) and insulin like growth factor binding protein 1 (IGFBP-1) [61, 62], epidermal growth factor [63], hepatocyte growth factor [64], heme oxygenase-1 [65], and activators of the nuclear receptors PPARγ [66] and LXRβ [67]. Peroxisome proliferators-activated receptors (PPARs) are transcription factors belonging to the large ligand-activated nuclear receptor superfamily including the retinoic acid receptors (RAR), the thyroid hormone receptors (TR), the liver X receptors (LXR), the vitamin D3 receptors (VDR), and the steroid receptors (SR) (for review see Fournier *et al.* [68]). Interestingly, at the implantation site, PPARγ is abundantly and specifically expressed in the trophoblast [66, 68] and activation of PPARγ/RXRα heterodimers by either natural (15deoxy-Prostaglandin J_2, oxidized lipids...) or synthetic (rosiglitazone a drug belonging to the thiazolidinedione) PPARγ ligands markedly decreased the cell invasion process in a concentration-dependent manner [13, 66, 67, 69]. Activation of the RXR/LXR heterodimers with specific ligands such as oxysterols also inhibited the trophoblastic cell invasiveness [67]. Analysis of PPARγ-target genes in the human trophoblast led to the discovery of new factors involved in the regulation of human trophoblast invasion [70-72]. Among those, the human placental growth hormone (hPGH), the pregnancy-associated plasma protein A (PAPP-A) [12] and more recently the hCG [73, 74]. Hormones belonging to the GH/prolactin family are expressed at the maternal fetal interface and are involved in cell motility in various models. Invasive extravillous cytotrophoblasts (EVCT) was shown to express both hPGH and human GH receptor (hGHR) and incubation with exogenous hPGH stimulated trophoblast invasiveness through activation of the Janus kinase-2/signal transducer and activator of transcription factor-5 (JAK2/STAT5) signaling pathway [75]. Thus, hPGH participates to the control of trophoblast invasiveness and as a PPARγ target gene, might be involved in the PPARγ-mediated inhibition of trophoblast invasion in an autocrine manner. PAPP-A is a metzincin metalloproteinase that increases in maternal serum during pregnancy. It cleaves the insulin-like growth factor binding protein 4 (IGFBP-4) and consequently modulates the amount of bioactive IGF-II, a factor known to promote trophoblast invasion. The expression of PAPP-A and its regulation by PPARγ were studied *in vitro* using primary cultures of invasive EVCT and endocrine villous cytotrophoblasts (VCT) isolated from the same first trimester chorionic villi. Interestingly, it was shown that invasive EVCT expressed and secreted 10 times more PAPP-A than the endocrine VCT suggesting that PAPP-A might be considered as an early marker of physiological trophoblast invasion. Activation of PPARγ inhibited PAPP-A gene expression and secretion specifically in EVCT, whereas it had no effect in VCT [12]. These results suggest that the PPARγ-induced decrease in PAPP-A secretion might diminish locally the amount of bioactive IGF-II, a factor that promotes trophoblast invasion. It is well established that hCG is secreted by the endocrine VCT (the syncytiotrophoblast) into the maternal compartment. It was recently reported *in situ* and *in vitro* that invasive EVCT also produce and secrete hCG suggesting an autocrine/paracrine role at the implantation site [76]. Indeed, hCG from invasive EVCT stimulated the trophoblastic cell invasion process, whereas hCG from ST had no effect. These results offer evidence that glycoforms of hCG secreted *in vitro* by the invasive EVCT, but not by the ST, promotes trophoblast invasion and may participate as a PPARγ-target gene to the control of the trophoblastic cell invasion process in an autocrine manner [73]. Recently, it was demonstrated that invasive EVCT and endovascular EVCT in particular produced a hyperglycosylated form of hCG (the one produced by the choriocarcinoma JEG-3) that was able to promote cell invasion through a LH/CG receptor independent pathway. Moreover, this hyperglycosylated hCG was found in maternal serum from early pregnancy and was proposed as a serum marker of early human trophoblast invasion [77].

Activation of PPARγ by Human Cytomegalovirus for De Novo Replication Impairs Trophoblast Invasion

The cytomegalovirus (CMV) a virus of the beta herpes family, which generally has no effect on an individual's health, may cause serious disorders in immune deficient individuals and lead to miscarriages and fetus injury in pregnant women. Indeed, an initial infection, or re infection of a mother during pregnancy may be responsible for miscarriage, low birth weight, mental retardation or serious sensory problems in newborn babies. It is known that infection of the fetus is always preceded by infection of the placenta. It was recently shown that when infecting the trophoblasts, CMV activates and uses PPARγ for its own replication, thus upsetting some of the cellular mechanisms such as invasion and migration involved in the physiological process of anchoring the placenta to the uterine wall. This can lead to abnormal development of the placenta resulting, in turn, in insufficient nutrition of the fetus and, as a consequence, the appearance of growth and neurological development disorders, independent of infection of the fetus itself by CMV [78].

UTEROPLACENTAL CIRCULATION

Physiology of the Uteroplacental Circulation [79]

The maternal blood enters the uterus through the uterine arteries and the ovarian arteries. The proportion of the mother's cardiac output that supplies the uterus and the intervillous space increases progressively during pregnancy to as much as 20 to 25% at term. Fetal growth is dependent on the supply of maternal blood to the intervillous space. At the start of pregnancy, the placental blood flow is low, but as the volume of the embryo is one sixth that of the placenta, the embryo can develop and grow. The estimated uterine blood flow at 10 weeks of gestation is 50 mL/min. As pregnancy proceeds, the nutritional needs of the fetus increase. The functional blood flow of the placenta increases as the fetal to placental volume ratio reaches 6 to 1 at the end of pregnancy. The estimated blood flow in the uterine arteries is then 600 mL/min [79]. This considerable increase in uteroplacental blood flow is in part linked to an overall increase in the mother's cardiac output, but above all to remodeling of the uterine vascular network. At the end of pregnancy, the intervillous space contains about 150 mL of maternal blood, which is renewed completely three to four times a minute. When the uterus contracts, the uteroplacental blood flow decreases, but the total placental volume remains unchanged, suggesting that the total volume of maternal blood remains stable (the maternal blood is not expelled from the intervillous space during uterine contractions). Because of this, oxygen transfer from mother to fetus is maintained. The way the blood circulates in the intervillous space is poorly understood. Maternal blood is discharged into the intervillous space as a jet generated by maternal blood pressure, and flows around the placental villi, thus enabling exchanges between mother and fetus. Blood is drained from the systemic maternal circulation by the venous plexuses of the myometrium, which are organized in an anastomotic network. However, regimens of blood flow within the intervillous space and the mechanisms responsible for mixing of maternal blood are unknown. These phenomena nonetheless play a vital role in the exchanges between mother and fetus.

Uterine Artery Remodeling

Vascular remodeling of the uterus is crucial physiologically for appropriate fetal development and growth. Current understanding suggests that changes in vasculature of the gravid uterus can be outlined in three stages:

- Vascular remodeling of the myometrium independent of trophoblastic invasion;

- Vascular remodeling induced by diffusible factors from the interstitial extravillous cytotrophoblast;

- Remodeling induced by a direct interaction between the extravillous cytotrophoblast and components of the arterial wall.

Remodeling Independent of Trophoblastic Invasion

It seems that some of the modifications of the spiral arteries during pregnancy are wholly independent of trophoblastic effects. The initial modifications of the spiral arteries involve their general remodeling, with endothelial vacuolization, disorganization of smooth muscle cells, and luminal dilatation [80]. These structural changes occur very early, from five weeks of gestation onwards, before trophoblastic invasion, and take place in the zone of implantation as well as in that part of the decidua not concerned by placentation [80]. These modifications are also seen in ectopic implantation. The molecules potentially involved in this remodeling of the uteroplacental vasculature are angiogenic factors produced by the villous trophoblast (summarized in Table 1).

Table 1: Angiogenic Factors Produced by the Human Trophoblast

Vascular endothelial growth factors A, B, and C (VEGF-A, B, and C) [82]
Placental growth factor (PIGF) [83]
Fibroblast growth factor (FGF) [89]
Angiopoietin 1 [87]
Angiogenin [88]
Human chorionic gonadotropin (hCG) [84-86]
Platelet-derived growth factor (PDGF) [90]
Epidermal growth factor (EGF) [91]
Insulin-like growth factor 2 (IGF-2) [92]
Leptin [93]

Vascular Remodeling Induced by Diffusible Factors from the Interstitial Extravillous Cytotrophoblast

As mentioned before, arterial dilatation starts before the invasion of the arteries by the trophoblasts [80]. This remodeling combines thinning of the media and fibrinoid deposits within the arterial wall. Some studies suggest that cells neighboring the uterine arteries synthesize and secrete vasodilators such as nitric oxide and carbon monoxide. The extravillous cytotrophoblast secretes angiogenic factors that may be involved in vascular remodeling. The best known is vascular endothelial growth factor A (VEGF-A) [81, 82], which is secreted by villous trophoblasts and by extravillous cytotrophoblasts throughout gestation [83]. It could therefore be responsible for uteroplacental angiogenesis by either a paracrine (VEGF secreted by the extravillous trophoblast) or an endocrine (VEGF secreted by the villous trophoblast) mode of action. The trophoblastic cell also secretes placental growth factor (PIGF) and VEGF-C, which stimulate endothelial survival and vascular remodeling [82]. Furthermore, it has been shown that hCG produced by the villous and extravillous cytotrophoblasts has angiogenic properties similar to those of VEGF, and that the hCG receptor (hCG receptor/luteinizing hormone) is present at the surface of the endothelial cells of the uterine blood vessels [84, 85]. A role for this early embryonic signal (hCG) in vessel maturation by stimulating perivascular cell recruitment, migration, and proliferation in a protein kinase A and phospholipase C/protein kinase C dependent pathway has been recently reported [86]. All these findings suggest that trophoblastic factors are directly involved in uterine angiogenesis and uterine artery remodeling, independently of the invasion of the blood vessel walls by trophoblastic cells.

Remodeling Induced by Direct Interaction Between the Extravillous Trophoblast and Artery Wall Components

Histological studies have shown that vascular remodeling by the (endovascular or interstitial) trophoblast induces a direct interaction between the extravillous cytotrophoblast and artery wall components (smooth muscle cells and endothelial cells) [94, 95]. The smooth muscle wall of these blood vessels is therefore destroyed and replaced by eosinophilic a cellular material [94-99].

PLACENTAL FUNCTIONS

Exchanges Between Mother and Fetus

Transfer Mechanisms

Transplacental transfer is conditioned by physical factors, change in any one of which will modify exchanges:

- Surface of the exchange area: estimated as between 11 and 13 m^2 at term;

- Distance between maternal and fetal circulation, which varies from 2 to 5 μm;

- Maternal blood flow in the intervillous space which is an estimated 600 to 800 mL/min at the end of pregnancy in normal conditions;

- Hydrostatic pressure in the intervillous space: it ranges from 30 to 50 mmHg, like the intra-amniotic pressure;

- Pressure in the fetal capillaries (30 to 35 mmHg);

- Osmotic pressure differences between mother and fetus plasma, osmotic pressure is higher in maternal plasma.

Transplacental transfer increases progressively during gestation and may be perturbed by pregnancy disorders affecting one or other of the physical factors (for example, uterine contraction reduces blood flow in the intervillous space; fibrinoid degeneration of the placenta decreases the exchange area, *etc.*).

Transplacental transfer occurs by classic mechanisms: passive diffusion, facilitated diffusion, active transport, and mechanisms more specific to the placenta, such as trans-endocytosis for immunoglobulins and receptor transferrin mediated endocytosis for iron maternofetal transmission. Most of our understanding of transfer stems from studies on term placentas. However, transfer at the beginning of pregnancy appears to differ from transfer at term. Maternal blood flow, for instance, only supplies the intervillous space from weeks 10-11 onwards. Before this, nutrition is histiotrophic: trophoblastic cells phagocytose glandular secretions of the endometrium [100]. After 10-12 weeks, the maternal blood is in contact with the placental villi and the transfer of gases, nutrients, and waste products can then occur through the cell layers of the villi.

Passive Diffusion

Passive diffusion is governed by Fick's law. The net rate of diffusional transfer (flux) for a particular solute, depends on the surface area available for diffusion per gram of placenta, the diffusion coefficient of the solute in water at 37° C, the path length over which diffusion take place (or membrane thickness) and the maternal fetal concentration difference of that substance. This mechanism is subject to some conditions:

- It only applies to low-molecular-weight molecules that do not bind to blood proteins; it depends on the lipid solubility of the substance, it involves ionic dissociation more than simple weight concentration;

- The molecule transferred must be enzymatically inert and not interfere with fetal or maternal homeostasis.

Respiratory gases are passively transferred and the net transfer will depend on the maternal fetal concentration difference of the gas, which itself depends on the flow rates of the uterine and umbilical circulation.

Facilitated Diffusion

In this mechanism diffusion is facilitated by transporters such as members of glucose gene transporter family (GLUT). Facilitated diffusion by transporters is saturable and specific. It is distinguished from active transport by the fact that it follows an electrochemical gradient and does not involve energy consumption.

In human, GLUT1 is highly expressed in the microvillous and in the basal membrane of the syncytiotrophoblast throughout pregnancy. As a consequence, net transport of glucose across the placenta will be strongly influenced by maternal blood glucose concentration as the fetal plasma glucose concentration is lower than in maternal circulation.

Active Transport

Molecules are also transported against a concentration gradient or an electrical gradient or both. Together the electrical and concentration gradients constitute an electrochemical gradient. This transport mechanism may use energy from the hydrolysis of ATP (adenosine triphosphate). In primary active transport, ATP hydrolysis directly produces the energy used by the ion pumps, such as the Na^+/K^+-ATPase allowing transport of Na^+ and K^+, and Ca^{2+}-ATPase allowing transport of Ca^{2+}. Active transport of solute can be coupled to a passive ion transport mechanism (amino acid/Na^+). If the substance concerned is moving in the same direction as the ion, it is called a symport mechanism; if the ion moves in the opposite direction to the substance, it is called an antiport mechanism. These active transport mechanisms are saturable, more or less specific, and are perturbed if the energy supply is wanting.

Trans-Endocytosis or Receptor-Mediated Transcytosis

In trans-endocytosis, some macromolecules bind to receptors localized on the microvillous membrane and after internalization in clathrin-coated vesicles these molecules are found in multivesicular bodies and then in vesicles close to the basal membrane and finally are found intact into the fetal circulation [101].

Transfer of Natural Substances

Transfer of Respiratory Gases

The placenta is highly permeable to respiratory gases. Given the partial pressure differences, oxygen diffuses passively from the maternal blood to the fetal blood, and carbon dioxide in the opposite direction. In addition, fetal hemoglobin has a greater affinity for oxygen and a lower affinity for carbon dioxide than maternal hemoglobin.

Carbohydrate Transport and Metabolism

The fetus has a much reduced capacity for neoglucogenesis, and so the mother supplies glucose, which is the main sugar transported from mother to fetus. Glucose transport occurs by facilitated diffusion using glucose transporters located in the microvillous and in the basal membrane of the syncytiotrophoblast and in the endothelial membrane of the fetal capillaries. Maternal glucose uptake occurs through the microvillus membrane of the syncytiotrophoblast and the glucose can be transported to the basal membrane of the syncytiotrophoblast for release to the endothelium of the fetal capillaries. In the syncytiotrophoblast, glucose can also be converted into glucose 6-phosphate or into placental glycogen. At term, the glucose transporter GLUT1 is found in the microvillous an in the basal membrane of the syncytiotrophoblast and in endothelial cell membranes of the fetal capillaries. GLUT1 is believed to account for most glucose transfer. GLUT3 is found in the endothelial cells of the fetal capillaries and is important in the regulation of glucose transfer to the fetal blood. Other glucose transporters (GLUT4, GLUT8, and GLUT12) are found in different parts of the placenta. The cellular locations of these transporters change between the first trimester and term, suggesting functional variations between the beginning and end of pregnancy.

As a consequence of the facilitated process for glucose transfer, net transport of glucose across the placenta will be strongly influenced by maternal blood concentration and in diabetes, increased maternal levels expose the fetus to hyper glycemia and consequently to hyper-insulinemia and macrosomia. Interestingly, in isolated human trophoblast, GLUT1 is down regulated by conditions of maternal hyperglycemia, suggesting a mechanism to "protect" the placenta and fetus from excessive glucose exposure [102].

Amino Acid Transport and Metabolism

Amino acids are vital for fetal development as they are components of proteins but also as energy metabolites and as essential precursors for the synthesis of non-protein substance such as nucleotides, heme, nitric oxide, neurotransmitters. Furthermore, the essential amino acids transfer may be very important for fetal development because they cannot be synthesized within the fetus. In healthy fetuses, umbilical blood concentrations of most amino acids are significantly higher than maternal concentration at midgestation and term with the exception of aspartate and glutamate. Therefore amino acid transport occurs against a concentration gradient, and uptake is mediated by transporters localized on the microvillous membrane, while efflux to the fetus is mediated by transporters localized on the basal membrane. Energy is therefore required to transport amino acid into the syncytiotrophoblast against their concentration gradients. Several type of transporters are present in the human placenta: those that co-transport Na^+ with the amino acid (Na^+ dependent) and those that do not (Na^+ independent). Na^+ dependent transporters do not directly utilize ATP: the $Na^+/K^+/ATPase$ creates a Na^+ gradient and the energy of this gradient is used to the transport of the amino acid by its transporter. The driving force for the transport of amino acid by Na^+ independent transporter is not well determined [103].

Transport system L carries some neutral amino acids, system y^+L exchanges cationic amino acids for Na^+, and system $B0^+$ transports neutral or cationic amino acids independently of Na^+. Other transport systems in the human placenta are y^+ (cationic amino acids, Na^+-independent), XAG (for aspartate and glutamate), ASC (alanine, serine, and cysteine, Na^+-dependent) and A (neutral amino acids, Na^+-dependent). These transporters are found in the microvillus membrane and in the basal membrane of the syncytiotrophoblast.

Lipid Transport and Metabolism

Free fatty acids, triacylglycerol, phospholipids, glycolipids, sphingolipids, cholesterol, cholesterol esters, and lipid-soluble vitamins are the principal lipids transported. In the plasma, numerous lipids are bound to proteins: free fatty acids are bound to serum albumin, and phospholipids, triacylglycerol, and cholesterol are constituents of various lipoproteins. Essential fatty acids (EFA) and their long-chain polyunsaturated fatty acids (LCPUFA) are of critical importance in fetal growth and development. These fatty acids are the precursors of eicosanoids and intracellular mediators, and are essential constituents of the membrane lipids that maintain cellular integrity [104].

Free fatty acids and glycerol enter the syncytiotrophoblast either by simple diffusion or by means of fatty acid-binding proteins presents in the microvillus membrane: FAPpm (Fatty Acids Binding Protein plasma membrane), FAT/CD36 (Fatty Acids Translocase), FATP (Fatty Acids Transporter Proteins). The FAT/CD36 and the FATP are also localized on the basal membrane. The internalized fatty acids bind to the FABTP (Fatty Acid Binding Transporter Protein) and then can be oxidized or esterified or exported to the fetal circulation [104]. Maternal plasma lipoproteins can be taken up by syncytiotrophoblast *via* endocytosis mediated by LDL (low density lipoproteins) receptors, VLDL (very low density lipoproteins) receptors localized in the microvillous membrane. Internalization of Very Low Density Lipoprotein (VLDL) by the syncytiotrophoblast is a significant supply of fatty acids for the trophoblast. After internalization, lipoprotein triglycerides are hydrolyzed by lipoprotein lipases and the free fatty acids are released. Alternatively triglycerides present in lipoproteins are hydrolyzed by lipoprotein lipases localized in the microvillous membrane. Furthermore the selective cholesterol uptake pathway using the scavenger receptor B1 (SR-B1) localized on the microvillous membrane allows the trophoblastic uptake of cholesterol esters from various lipoproteins: HDL, LDL, VLDL, modified lipoproteins. In this case, the cholesterol esters are captured by the syncytiotrophoblast without the internalization and degradation of apoproteins [105].

Transfer of Water and Ions

The placenta plays a determinant role in fetal water balance. When placental function is normal, a change in concentration or a dilution of the maternal plasma results in identical changes in the fetal plasma. So, if the mother is dehydrated, the osmolarity of the fetal plasma increases in parallel to that of the maternal plasma [106]. Transplacental exchange between mother and fetus seem to play an important role in the regulation of amniotic fluid volume, which will increase if maternal hydration increases [107]. Transplacental transfer of water occurs passively as a function of hydrostatic and osmotic pressure differences on either side of the chorionic villi. When the maternal blood is injected by the spiral arteries into the intervillous space, its hydrostatic pressure is high and water is transferred from mother to fetus. When the maternal blood arrives at the chorionic plate, it is dispersed laterally and its pressure drops, so water is transferred from the fetal capillaries to the maternal blood. Transfer of water is facilitated by aquaporins (AQPs), transmembrane protein channels, which enable the passage of water through the cell membrane. AQP1 is a water channel protein expressed in the fetal vasculature. AQP3 transports water, urea, and glycerol, and AQP8 mediates the passage of water and glycerol. Both are expressed in the syncytiotrophoblast [108].

Sodium and chloride concentrations are similar in maternal blood and fetal blood; potassium and phosphate concentrations though are higher in the blood of the fetus. Potassium, magnesium, calcium, and phosphates are actively transported. Various active ion transport systems have been found in the placenta, such as Na^+/K^+-ATPase, Ca^{2+}-ATPase, and the Na^+/H^+ exchanger. Ions can also be transported by proteins such as the sodium-dependent amino acid transporters.

Transfer of Drugs and Toxins

Most drugs and exogenous substances or metabolites toxic for the fetus cross the placenta. This transplacental transfer depends on the serum concentration of the substance, its molecular weight, its capacity to bind transporters in the maternal blood, and its lipophilicity.

Endocrine Functions

The Placental Polypeptide Hormones

The syncytiotrophoblast secretes many polypeptide hormones. They are primarily: hCG (see for review [109]), hPL or hCS (human somatomammotropic hormone) [110] and placental GH [111]. The glycoprotein hormone hCG, is the key hormone of human pregnancy. It behaves like a super agonist of LH allowing the transformation of cyclic ovary corpus luteum, in gravidic corpus luteum, ensuring the maintenance of ovarian progesterone secretion during the first 6 weeks of pregnancy [109, 112, 113]. After 6 weeks of pregnancy, the steroidogenic activity of the feto-placental unit compensates for the maternal ovarian functions. Thus, an ovariectomy after 6 weeks of pregnancy has no effect on pregnancy outcome. hCG is made up of two subunits, an alpha sub-unit and a beta sub-unit. The alpha subunit is the same in the other glycoprotein hormones (FSH, LH, TSH). The alpha subunit is made up of 92 acids amino with two N-glycosylation sites. It is encoded by only one gene on the chromosome 6q21.1-23. The beta subunit is made up of 145 amino acids with two sites of N-glycosylation and 4 sites of O-glycosylation. It is encoded by a whole set of genes among a cluster of genes: 4 genes beta (type II encoded by 3,5 and 8 and type I by beta 7 different by 3 aa), 2 pseudogenes CG beta (1 and 2) and a gene LH beta on the chromosome 19q13.3. These genes CG beta evolved by duplication from the gene beta LH and are controlled differently on the level of their promoter. Compared with LH, the 31 additional amino acids in position C-terminal of hCG, and hCG very high glycosylation level allow its intracellular trafficking towards the apical membrane of the syncytiotrophoblast, its secretion directly in maternal circulation and its prolonged half-life [114].

The human trophoblast expresses two types of hCG receptor: a truncated 50 kDa isoform and an 80 kDa full-length isoform [115]. The truncated isoform is expressed during the first trimester of pregnancy and the full-length isoform is expressed in the highly differentiated term trophoblast. HCG receptor is a seven-transmembrane domain receptor coupled with the cAMP signaling pathway and the phospholipase C. Other hCG receptors have been identified in non-gonadal tissue and shown to be involved in the normal course of pregnancy [115, 116]. The secretion of hCG by the trophoblast appears very early, it begins as soon as the 7th day after fecundation, at the time of implantation. The concentrations of maternal hCG increase gradually, pass by a maximum peak about the tenth week, and then decrease very clearly during the 3rd month to remain practically stationary until the childbirth. The reasons of this maternal plasmatic peak of hCG during the first trimester of pregnancy remain discussed. The following hypothesis have been suggested: 1/the presence at this stage of pregnancy of the truncated form of the receptor would block the autocrine regulation of hCG synthesis; 2/the synthesis of hCG by the trophoblast varies during the pregnancy and is higher during the first trimester; 3/the hCG would be controlled by an autocrine/paracrine mechanism by GnRH produced by the cytotrophoblasts present in greater number during the first trimester (see for review: [117]). By an autocrine and paracrine mechanism, hCG plays an essential role in trophoblast differentiation and stimulates *in vitro* the differentiation of the cytotrophoblasts in syncytiotrophoblast [118-120]. Several recent studies have demonstrated the importance of the glycosylation state of hCG, which varies with the stage of pregnancy [121]. Choriocarcinoma cells [122] and trophoblast cells displaying chromosome 21 trisomy [123] produce abnormal glycosylated forms of hCG with low biological activity. It should be noted that no CG beta genes have been found in mice [113].

hCG is the major pregnancy glycoprotein hormone whose maternal concentration and glycan structure change all along pregnancy. hCG is mainly secreted by the syncytiotrophoblast covering the chorionic villi but little is known about the source of hyperglycosylated hCG (H-hCG) production. It was recently shown *in situ* and *in vitro* that H-hCG was specifically expressed and secreted by the invasive extravillous cytotrophoblast and by the endovascular EVCT in particular, while it was weak in mononucleated villous cytotrophoblasts but negative in the syncytiotrophoblast. These observations strongly suggest that H-hCG found in maternal sera from early pregnancy is from endovascular EVCT origin rather than the ST. Therefore, H-hCG represents a serum marker of early human trophoblast invasion [77]. This study together with others point to a differential production in total hCG, α– and β–subunit, and its glycoforms depending on the cytotrophoblast phenotypes and their differentiation pathways *in vitro* and *in vivo* [73, 76, 124, 125]. These different glycoforms exhibit different bioactivity and may act in an autocrine, a paracrine, or an endocrine way during the gestation [73, 123]. *In vitro* data pointed that hCG from invasive EVCT contains high levels of H-hCG whose biological activity seems to trigger trophoblast invasion [73]. This is in agreement with the observation that in the weeks that follow the time of implantation a hyperglycosylated variant of hCG is primarily produced [126] including H-hCG, indicating the interest of H-hCG measurement to predict implantation and the outcome of pregnancy [127]. It is however likely that, in addition to H-hCG, other particular hCG glycoforms are produced by trophoblastic cells depending on the term and cell differentiation. It was also confirmed in this study that maternal H-hCG as well as total hCG are increased in T21 affected pregnancies [123, 128]. All together these data strongly suggest that H-hCG circulating in maternal serum reflects the trophoblastic cell invasion process that occurs during the first trimester of pregnancy. Hence, these results suggest that H-hCG represents a good marker of physiological early placentation process [129].

It is known for many years that the syncytiotrophoblast secretes in the maternal compartment very large amount of hPL. This hormone is also found in fetal blood but in much smaller amount than in maternal blood. The presence of receptors on fetal tissues suggests a role of hPL in fetal growth and metabolism not yet elucidated [130]. The increase in the secretion of hPL during pregnancy follows the evolution of the placental mass, and more particularly the syncytiotrophoblast mass, site of its synthesis. Its real physiological role remains to be elucidated. Indeed normal pregnancies have been described in the absence of hPL secretion.

During the last years several studies underline the important role of a growth hormone, specifically produced by the placenta, the placental growth hormone [111, 129]. This hormone, product of GH-V gene, expressed specifically in the syncytiotrophoblast, differs from the pituitary growth hormone by 13 amino acids. It gradually replaces in the maternal circulation, the pituitary growth hormone, which becomes undetectable during the second trimester of pregnancy. Secreted continuously by the placenta, it seems to control the synthesis of maternal IGF-1. Indeed, maternal IGF1 levels are correlated with placental GH levels. Moreover in pathology, during pregnancies of acromegalic women, maternal IGF-1 increases gradually, thus following the profile of placental GH, in spite of very high stable levels of pituitary GH. The secretion of placental GH but not of hPL or hCG, is inhibited *in vitro* by glucose in explants and in trophoblastic cells. *In vivo*, the levels of placental GH decrease in maternal blood during an oral glucose tolerance test in the event of gestational diabetes. This suggests a metabolic role of placental growth hormone, secreted specifically in the maternal compartment and not detected in fetal circulation. In the event of a fall of maternal glycemia, placental GH secreted then abundantly by the placenta will maintain an energetic flux to the fetus. Recently we demonstrated that this hormone is also involved in the complex mechanisms, which regulate trophoblast invasion into the maternal uterine wall. Indeed placental GH secreted by the invasive trophoblast increases trophoblast invasion by an autocrine/paracrine mechanism [75].

During the last years, the concept of "developmental programming" was introduced and supported by experimental and epidemiological data. This concept supports the idea that the nutritional and hormonal status during pregnancy could irreversibly interfere in metabolism control. The mechanisms responsible for this developmental programming remain poorly documented. However, recent research indicates that adipocytokines may play a critical role in this process. Adipocytokines are small peptides (10-20 kDa) produced by the adipocytes. They regulate the action of insulin and intermediate metabolism. During pregnancy they are produced by the placenta, their secretion increases with the trophoblastic mass and maternal circulating level decrease after the expulsion of the placenta

Leptin is produced by the syncytiotrophoblast, which possesses also leptin receptors. Its circulating levels are high in maternal circulation [132]. Leptin stimulates insulin secretion, glucose uptake and fatty acid metabolism. High levels of maternal circulating leptin are observed in the event of maternal diabetes or of preeclampsia (see for review [133]). The syncytiotrophoblast produces also resistin and possesses receptors. The metabolic action of resistin is the opposite of leptin.

The syncytiotrophoblast also secretes other peptide hormones whose maternal levels increase gradually throughout pregnancy thus reflecting the progressive increase of the syncytiotrophoblastic mass. It is the case of inhibin A and activin A [134]. These two hormones, members of the TGFβ superfamily, are dimeric hormones whose exact role during pregnancy remains not elucidated. Only *in vitro* studies in cultures of trophoblastic cells underline their modulating role on trophoblastic hormonal secretion.

Other Factors

During last years, the production of neuropeptides was highlighted in the placenta, an organ deprived of innervation. These neuropeptides are similar to those found in the hypothalamo-pituitary system or in the digestive tract (TRH, GnRH, CRH, somatostatin, grhelin.). *In vitro* in trophoblastic cultured cells, they modulate by autocrine or paracrine mechanisms the placental hormonal secretion [135]. It must be pointed out that, during pregnancy, the placenta and the fetal membranes produce large amount of CRH (Corticotropin Releasing Hormone). The placental CRH progressively increases during pregnancy due to an increase in its gene expression. It was thus proposed that CRH in interaction with estrogens, fetal adrenal steroids and prostaglandins establishes a stimulating autocrine loop, which would initiate parturition [136]. Lastly, the placenta is the site of expression of many growth factors, such as IGFs and cytokines implicated in its development [137]. Some placental factors implied in angiogenesis, could be early markers of preeclampsia. Thus an increase in the levels of the soluble VEGF receptor (vascular endothelial growth Factor) and a reduction in the levels of PLGF (placental growth Factor) are observed in maternal circulation during the first trimester of pregnancy before the clinical signs of preeclampsia [138, 139].

Hormonal Pathologies of the Pregnancy [140]

The peak of hCG in maternal circulation is associated with a decrease of maternal TSH levels. Indeed, hCG binds to TSH receptors and stimulates thyroid cells. This thyreo-stimulating effect of hCG can lead to the appearance of a maternal goiter, observed more frequently in twin pregnancies where hCG levels are higher. Recently several studies stress the importance of hCG glycosylation state, which varies with the stage of pregnancy. Glycosylation of hCG is modified in the choriocarcinoma and in feto-placental trisomy 21. The increased levels of hCG observed in maternal circulation in case of feto-placental trisomy 21 are used in clinical practice as a maternal serum marker in antenatal screening. It was recently demonstrated that this hCG increase is related to an abnormal glycosylation of this hormone, modifying its biological activity and its clearance in the maternal placental compartment [123]. It is now well established that the levels of placental GH and IGF-1 are lowered in case of intra-uterine growth retardation [141]. The placental sterol sulfatase deficit leads to a very important reduction in estrogens secretion. This enzymatic deficit is linked to X chromosome, affecting the male fetus and associated with ichthyosis [142]. Another genetic abnormality associated with very low levels of maternal estrogens is the deficit in CYP19 (P450 aromatase). In this case, maternal and fetal virilisation are observed due to the weak androgens aromatization [143]. Finally the family deficit of B apolipoproteins is one of the rare conditions of abnormal placental steroidogenesis, related to an insufficient uptake of cholesterol in the syncytiotrophoblast. It is associated apparently with normal pregnancies. The specificity of the human placental steroidogenesis was recently illustrated by the fact that the protein implied in the translocation of cholesterol to the internal mitochondrial membrane (STAR) is not expressed in the trophoblast but in the fetal adrenals [144]. Thus a null mutation of this gene, which is associated with a potentially lethal fetal adrenal lipoid hyperplasia, does not modify the normal course of pregnancy. However the absence of testosterone production by Leydig cells is associated with a female phenotype at birth [145].

In addition maternal or fetal cortisol can be inactivated in cortisone by the placenta. This regulates the quantity of active glucocorticoids available to the fetus. The syncytiotrophoblast expresses the 11β-hydroxysteroid deshydrogenase (type 2) throughout pregnancy. Any defect of syncytiotrophoblast development or function decreases this enzyme inducing therefore a fetal hypercortisolism [146, 147]. Furthermore, intrauterine growth retardation is associated with a null mutation or a reduction in the expression of the 11β-hydroxysteroid deshydrogenase [148]. This trophoblastic enzymatic activity has therapeutic implications. In the antenatal treatment of 21a hydroxylase deficiency in female fetus, the maternal treatment must the unmetabolized dexamethasone instead of hydrocortisone, which is transformed in cortisone by the trophoblast.

Steroid Hormones

The human placenta is the site of an important production of steroid hormones, which are mainly progesterone and estrogens: estriol, estradiol and estrone. At term, the daily placental production is about 300 mg of progesterone and 40 mg of estrogens.

During the first six weeks of pregnancy, the production of progesterone is primarily carried out by the gravidic ovary corpus luteum. It is thus associated with a secretion of 17α hydroxy progesterone, produced exclusively by the ovary at this stage of pregnancy. The placental progesterone production gradually takes over with the appearance within the syncytiotrophoblast of the various enzymatic systems necessary for its synthesis. Therefore as soon as 10 weeks of pregnancy when the trophoblastic plugs start to delete, the synthesis of progesterone is high enough to maintain pregnancy in case of ovariectomy. The precursor of progesterone is cholesterol. The *de novo* synthesis of cholesterol from acetyl CoA is not significant in the placenta and the trophoblast captures cholesterol carried by maternal plasmatic lipoproteins. Second and third trimesters of pregnancy are characterized by high levels of maternal circulating total cholesterol, triglycerides, low-density lipoproteins (LDL), very low-density lipoproteins (VLDL), high-density lipoproteins (HDL). The syncytiotrophoblast apical microvillous membrane, in direct contact with maternal blood presents receptors for these lipoproteins: LDL receptor, scavenger receptor B1. The trophoblast captures and metabolizes LDL by receptor-mediated endocytosis. After internalization, LDL are degraded in the lysosomes to release cholesterol, which will be used for steroidogenesis, and cellular membranes synthesis. The direct involvement of LDL receptors in progesterone synthesis is confirmed by the observation that *in vitro* estrogens stimulate LDL receptor expression, inducing an increase in progesterone synthesis [149]. The scavenger receptor B1 (SR-B1) is involved in the selective cholesterol pathway. The SR-B1 binds HDL, LDL, VLDL as well as modified lipoproteins. In this case, the cholesterol esters are captured by the syncytiotrophoblast without the internalization and degradation of apoproteins.

Free cholesterol is then transported by the Sterol Carrier Protein-2 (SCP2) to the external membrane of the mitochondria and then to the internal membrane by the MLN64 (metastatic lymph node 64). MLN64 presents a final domain similar to the STAR (steroidogenic acute regulatory protein), a protein expressed in the other steroidogenic tissues (corpus luteum, adrenals) [145]. In the internal membrane of the mitochondria, P-450 cytochrome scc (cholesterol side chain cleavage), allows the conversion of cholesterol into pregnenolone. This reaction requires electrons provided by the mitochondrial adrenodoxin (ADX) and adrenodoxin reductase (AdRed) activities. Only one gene (P-450 XIA) coding for P-450scc and localized on chromosome 15 is present in the placenta, as soon as the 10th week of pregnancy. Pregnenolone is then converted into progesterone by the 3β hydroxysteroid-deshydrogenase/isomerase (3β HSD) localized also in mitochondria.

For estrogen synthesis, in contrast to other steroidogenic organs, the placenta does not express the cytochrome P450 17α-hydroxylase-17:20 lyase, and therefore cannot convert pregnenolone and progesterone into androgens. Thus the production of placental estrogens is tributary of a precursor androgen, the sulphate of dehydroepiandrosterone (S-DHA) produced by the maternal and fetal adrenal glands. During pregnancy the estrogen synthesis from fetal adrenal glands origin increases progressively. The S-DHA diffuses from fetal blood to the syncytiotrophoblast and is hydrolyzed by a sterol steroid sulfatase; DHA is then metabolized in androstendione by a 3β HSD. Androstendione is transformed into testosterone by a 17β hydroxysteroid dehydrogenase (17β HSD) encoded by the HSD17B1 gene localized on chromosome 17 (17q11-q21). C19 androsterone and testosterone are then aromatized in C18 estrogens (estrone and estradiol respectively) by the P450 cytochrome aromatase, encoded by CYP19 gene, only present in the syncytiotrophoblast. Fetal adrenal S-DHA may also undergo16α-hydroxylation in the fetal liver leading to the formation of 16α-hydroxy S-DHA, the estriol androgen precursor. Thus 90% of placental estriol arises from fetal adrenal glands and liver activities. This cooperation between the placenta and the fetus has led to the concept of feto-placental unit.

If numerous factors such as hCG, cAMP, prostaglandins, have been described to modulate *in vitro* placental estrogen synthesis, the quality of fetal adrenal glands development remains the essential factor. If progesterone is absolutely required for the well-being of pregnancy, the role of estrogens remains still uncertain. Indeed genetic deficiencies in placental sulfatase or aromatase, leading to very low levels of maternal circulating estrogens are associated with normal pregnancy.

CONCLUSION

The human placenta is an autonomous and transient organ which enables development of the embryo and then of the fetus during intrauterine life. During the first trimester of pregnancy, which occurs in a low oxygen environment, the invasive trophoblast secretes a large amount of hormones directly involved in establishing the placentation. After 10-12 weeks of pregnancy, the endocrine syncytiotrophoblast bathing in maternal blood secretes numerous hormones, which play an essential role in maintaining pregnancy, maternal adaptation to pregnancy, fetal growth and development, and the mechanism of parturition.

REFERENCES

[1]   Berniscke K, Kaufmann P. Early development of the human placenta. In: Berniscke K, Kaufmann P, Eds. Pathology of the human placenta, New-York, Springer-Verlag 2000; p 43.

[2]   Huppertz B, Kingdom JC. Apoptosis in the trophoblast--role of apoptosis in placental morphogenesis [Review]. J Soc Gynecol Investig 2004; 11: 353-62.

[3]   Mayhew TM, Leach L, McGee R, Ismail WW, Myklebust R, Lammiman MJ. Proliferation, differentiation and apoptosis in villous trophoblast at 13-41 weeks of gestation (including observations on annulate lamellae and nuclear pore complexes). Placenta 1999; 20: 407-22.

[4]   Burton GJ, Jones CJ. Syncytial knots, sprouts, apoptosis, and trophoblast deportation from the human placenta [Review]. Taiwan J Obstet Gynecol 2009; 48: 28-37.

[5]   Coleman SJ, Gerza L,Jones CJP, Sibley CP, Aplin JD, Heazell H. Syncytial nuclear aggregates are not universally apoptotic in nature and are closely associated with cytokeratin, ß-actin and ß-tubulin. Placenta 2010; 31: A13.

[6]   LokeYW, Hiby S, King A. Human leucocyte antigen-G and reproduction. J Reprod Immunol 1999; 43: 235-42.

[7]   LokeYW, King A. Immunology of implantation. Baillieres Best Pract Res Clin Obstet Gynaecol 2000; 14: 827-37.

[8]   Kliman HJ, Nestler JE, Sermasi E, Sanger JM, Strauss 3rd JF. Purification, characterization, and *in vitro* differentiation of cytotrophoblasts from human term placentae. Endocrinology 1986; 118: 1567-82.

[9]   Dodeur M, Malassine A, Bellet D, Mensier A, Evain-Brion D. Characterization and differentiation of human first trimester placenta trophoblastic cells in culture. Reprod Nutr Dev 1990; 30: 183-92.

[10]   Evain-Brion D, Alsat E, Mirlesse V, *et al.* Regulation of growth hormone secretion in human trophoblastic cells in culture. Horm Res 1990; 33: 256-9.

[11]   Tarrade A, Lai Kuen R, Malassiné A, Tricottet V, Blain P, Vidaud M, Evain-Brion D. Characterization of human villous and extravillous trophoblasts isolated from first trimester placenta. Lab Invest 2001; 81: 1199-211.

[12]   Handschuh K, Guibourdenche J, Guesnon M, Laurendeau I, Evain-Brion D, Fournier T. Modulation of PAPP-A expression by PPARgamma in human first trimester trophoblast. Placenta 2006; 27 (Suppl A): S127-34.

[13]   Pavan L, Tarrade A, Hermouet A, Delouis C, Titeux M, Vidaud M, Thérond P, Evain-Brion D, Fournier T. Human invasive trophoblasts transformed with simian virus 40 provide a new tool to study the role of PPARgamma in cell invasion process. Carcinogenesis 2003; 24: 1325-36.

[14]   McDonald EA, Wolfe MW. Adiponectin attenuation of endocrine function within human term trophoblast cells. Endocrinology 2009; 150: 4358-65.

[15]   Frendo JL, Cronier L, Bertin G, *et al.* Involvement of connexin 43 in human trophoblast cell fusion and differentiation. J Cell Sci 2003; 116: 3413-21.

[16]   Pidoux G, Gerbaud P, Gnidehou S, *et al.* ZO-1 is involved in trophoblastic cell differentiation in human placenta. Am J Physiol Cell Physiol 2010; 298: C1517-26.

[17]   Frendo JL, Olivier D, CheynetV, *et al.* Direct involvement of herv-w env glycoprotein in human trophoblast cell fusion and differentiation. Mol Cell Biol 2003; 23:3566-74.

[18]   Vargas A, Moreau J, Landry S, LeBellego F, Toufaily C, Rassart E, Lafond J, Barbeau B. Syncytin-2 plays an important role in the fusion of human trophoblast cells. J Mol Biol 2009; 392: 301-18.

[19]   Adler RR, Ng AK, Rote NS. Monoclonal antiphosphatidylserine antibody inhibits intercellular fusion of the choriocarcinoma line, JAR. Biol Reprod 1995; 53: 905-10.

[20]   Getsios S, MacCalman CD. Cadherin-11 modulates the terminal differentiation and fusion of human trophoblastic cells *in vitro.* Dev Biol 2003; 257: 41-54.

[21]   Dalton P, Christian HC, Redman CW, Sargent IL, Boyd CA. Differential effect of cross-linking the CD98 heavy chain on fusion and amino acid transport in the human placental trophoblast (BeWo) cell line. Biochim Biophys Acta 2007; 1768: 401-10.

[22]   Huppertz B, Bartz C, Kokozidou M. Trophoblast fusion: fusogenic proteins, syncytins and ADAMs, and other prerequisites for syncytial fusion [Review]. Micron 2006; 37:509-17.

[23]   Steinberg F, Zhuang L, Beyeler M, Kälin RE, Mullis PE, Brändli AW, Trueb B. The FGFRL1 receptor is shed from cell membranes, binds fibroblast growth factors (FGFs), and antagonizes FGF signaling in Xenopus embryos. J Biol Chem 2010; 285: 2193-202.

[24]   Rote NS, Wei BR, Xu C, Luo L. Caspase 8 and human villous cytotrophoblast differentiation [Review]. Placenta 2010; 31: 89-96.

[25]   Guilbert LJ, Riddell M, Winkler-Lowen B. Caspase activation is not required for villous cytotrophoblast fusion into syncytiotrophoblasts. Placenta 2010; 31: 982-8.

[26]   Cronier L, Bastide B, Defamie N, *et al.* Involvement of gap junctional communication and connexin expression in trophoblast differentiation of the human placenta. Histol Histopathol 2001; 16: 285-95.

[27]   Blond JL, Lavillette D, Cheynet V, Bouton O, Oriol G, Chapel-Fernandes S, Mandrand B, Mallet F, Cosset FL. An envelope glycoprotein of the human endogenous retrovirus HERV-W is expressed in the human placenta and fuses cells expressing the type D mammalian retrovirus receptor. J Virol 2000; 74: 3321-9.

[28]   Mi S, Lee X, Li X, Veldman GM, Finnerty H, Racie L, LaVallie E, Tang XY, Edouard P, Howes S, Keith JC Jr, McCoy JM. Syncytin is a captive retroviral envelope protein involved in human placental morphogenesis. Nature 2000; 403: 785-9.

[29]   Blaise S, de Parseval N, Bénit L, Heidmann T. Genomewide screening for fusogenic human endogenous retrovirus envelopes identifies syncytin 2, a gene conserved on primate evolution. Proc Natl Acad Sci U S A 2003; 100: 13013-8.

[30]   Esnault C, Priet S, Ribet D, Vernochet C, Bruls T, Lavialle C, Weissenbach J, Heidmann T. A placenta-specific receptor for the fusogenic, endogenous retrovirus-derived, human syncytin-2. Proc Natl Acad Sci U S A 2008; 105: 17532-7

[31]   Malassiné A, Handschuh K, Tsatsaris V, Gerbaud P, Cheynet V, Oriol G, Mallet F, Evain-Brion D. Expression of HERV-W Env glycoprotein (syncytin) in the extravillous trophoblast of first trimester human placenta. Placenta 2005; 26: 556-62.

[32]   Malassiné A, Frendo JL, Blaise S, Handschuh K, Gerbaud P, Tsatsaris V, Heidmann T, Evain-Brion D. Human endogenous retrovirus-FRD envelope protein (syncytin 2) expression in normal and trisomy 21-affected placenta. Retrovirology 2008; 5: 6.

[33]   Mangeney M, Renard M, Schlecht-Louf G, Bouallaga I, Heidmann O, Letzelter C, Richaud A, Ducos B, Heidmann T. Placental syncytins: Genetic disjunction between the fusogenic and immunosuppressive activity of retroviral envelope proteins. Proc Natl Acad Sci U S A 2007; 104: 20534-9.

[34]   Tolosa JM, Schjenken JE, Clifton VL, Smith R. The retroviral envelope protein syncytin-1 is immunosuppressive and has hijacked the exosomal pathway in the human placenta. Placenta 2010; 31: A84.

[35]   Gimenez J, Montgiraud C, Oriol G, Pichon JP, Ruel K, Tsatsaris V, Gerbaud P, Frendo JL, Evain-Brion D, Mallet F. Comparative methylation of ERVWE1/syncytin-1 and other human endogenous retrovirus LTRs in placenta tissues. DNA Res 2009; 16: 195-211.

[36]   Liang CY, Wang LJ, Chen CP, Chen LF, Chen YH, Chen H. GCM1 regulation of the expression of syncytin 2 and its cognate receptor MFSD2A in human placenta. Biol Reprod 2010; 83: 387-95.

[37]   Malassiné A, Frendo JL, Evain-Brion D. Trisomy 21-affected placentas highlight prerequisite factors for human trophoblast fusion and differentiation [Review]. Int J Dev Biol 2010; 54:475-82.

[38]   Ashworth CJ, Hoggard N, Thomas L, Mercer JG, Wallace JM, Lea RG. Placental leptin. Rev Reprod 2000; 5: 18-24.

[39]   Evain-Brion D. Maternal endocrine adaptations to placental hormones in humans. Acta Paediatr 1999; 88 (suppl): 12-6.

[40]   Symonds ME, Mostyn A, Stephenson T. Cytokines and cytokine receptors in fetal growth and development. Biochem Soc Trans 2001; 29: 33-7.

[41]   Fazel A, Vincenot A, Malassine A, *et al.* Increase in expression and activity of thrombomodulin in term human syncytiotrophoblast microvilli. Placenta 1998; 19: 261-8.

[42]   Lanir N, Aharon A, Brenner B. Haemostatic mechanisms in human placenta. Best Pract Res Clin Haematol 2003; 16: 183-95.

[43]   Isermann B, Sood R, Pawlinski R, *et al.* The thrombomodulin-protein c system is essential for the maintenance of pregnancy. Nat Med 2003; 9: 331-7.

[44]   Rand JH, Wu XX, Andree HA, *et al.* Pregnancy loss in the antiphospholipid-antibody syndrome--a possible thrombogenic mechanism. N Engl J Med 1997; 337: 154-60.

[45]   Rand JH. Antiphospholipid antibody-mediated disruption of the annexin-v antithrombotic shield: a thrombogenic mechanism for the antiphospholipid syndrome. J Autoimmun 2000; 15: 107-11.

[46]   Aplin JD, Haigh T, Lacey H, Chen CP, Jones CJ. Tissue interactions in the control of trophoblast invasion. J Reprod Fertil 2000; 55(suppl): 57-64.

[47]   Kaufmann P, Castellucci M. Extravillous trophoblast in the human placenta. In: Foidart JM, Aplin JD, Kaufmann P, Schaaps JP, Eds. Trophoblast research. Vol 10. University of Rochester 1997.

[48]   Jaffe R, Jauniaux E, Hustin J. Maternal circulation in the first-trimester human placenta--myth or reality? Am J Obstet Gynecol 1997; 176: 695-705.

[49]   Rodesch F, Simon P, Donner C, Jauniaux E. Oxygen measurements in endometrial and trophoblastic tissues during early pregnancy. Obstet Gynecol 1992; 80: 283-5.

[50]   Jauniaux E, Watson A, Burton G. Evaluation of respiratory gases and acid-base gradients in human fetal fluids and uteroplacental tissue between 7 and 16 weeks' gestation. Am J Obstet Gynecol 2001; 184: 998-1003.

[51]   Blaschitz A, Hutter H, Dohr G. Hla class I protein expression in the human placenta. Early Pregnancy 2001; 5: 67-9.

[52]   Le Bouteiller P. Hla-g in the human placenta: expression and potential functions. Biochem Soc Trans 2000; 28: 208-12.

[53]   Chaouat G. Regulation of t-cell activities at the feto-placental interface--by placenta? Am J Reprod Immunol 1999; 42: 199-204.

[54]   Chaouat G, Assal Meliani A, Martal J, *et al.* Il-10 prevents naturally occurring fetal loss in the cba x dba/2 mating combination, and local defect in il-10 production in this abortion-prone combination is corrected by *in vivo* injection of ifn-tau. J Immunol 1995; 154: 4261-8.

[55]   Chaouat G, Zourbas S, Ostojic S, *et al.* A brief review of recent data on some cytokine expressions at the materno-fetal interface, which might challenge the classical th1/th2 dichotomy. J Reprod Immunol 2002; 53: 241-56.

[56]   Mowbray J, Jalali R, Chaouat G, *et al.* Maternal response to paternal trophoblast antigens. Am J Reprod Immunol 1997; 37: 421-6.

[57]   Knöfler M. Critical growth factors and signalling pathways controlling human trophoblast invasion [Review]. Int J Dev Biol 2010; 54: 269-80.

[58]   Redman CW. Cytotrophoblasts: masters of disguise. Nat Med 1997; 3: 610-11.

[59]   Fisher SJ, Damsky CH. Human cytotrophoblast invasion. Sem Cell Biol 1993; 4: 183-8.

[60]   Zhou Y, Genbacev O, Damsky, CH, Fisher, SJ. Oxygen régulates human cytotrophoblast differentiation and invasion: implications for endovascular invasion in normal pregnancy and in preeclampsia. J Reprod Immunol 1998; 39 : 197-213.

[61]   Irving J, Lala P. Functional role of cell surface integrins on human trophoblast cell migration: regulation by TGF-beta, IGF-II, and IGFBP-1. Exp Cell Res 1995; 21: 419-27.

[62]   Hamilton G, Lysiak J, Han V, Lala P. Autocrine-paracrine regulation of human trophoblast invasiveness by insulin-like growth factor (IGF)-II and IGF-binding protein (IGFBP)-1. Exp Cell Res 1998; 244: 147-56.

[63]   Bass E, Morrish D, Roth I, Bhardwaj D, Taylor R, Zhou Y, Fisher S. Human cytotrophoblast invasion is up-regulated by epidermal growth factor: Evidence that paracrine factors modify this process. Dev Biol 1994; 164: 550-61.

[64] Cartwright J, Holden D, Whitley G. Hepatocyte growth factor regulates human trophoblast motility and invasion: a role for nitric oxide. Br J Pharmacol 1999; 128: 181-89.

[65]   Bilban M, Haslinger P, Prast J, Klinglmüller F, Woelfel T, Haider S, Sachs A, Otterbein LE, Desoye G, Hiden U, Wagner O, Knöfler M. Identification of novel trophoblast invasion-related genes: heme oxygenase-1 controls motility *via* peroxisome proliferator-activated receptor gamma. Endocrinology 2009; 150: 1000-13.

[66]   Tarrade A, Schoonjans K, Pavan L, Auwerx J, Rochette-Egly C, Evain-Brion D, Fournier T. PPARgamma/RXRalpha heterodimers control human trophoblast invasion. J Clin Endocrinol Metab 2001; 86: 5017-24.

[67]   Pavan L, Hermouet A, Tsatsaris V, Therond P, Sawamura T, Evain-Brion D, Fournier T. Lipids from oxidized low-densitylipoprotein modulate human trophoblast invasion: involvement of nuclear liver X receptors. Endocrinology 2004; 145: 4583-91.

[68]   Fournier T, Tsatsaris V, Handschuh K, Evain-Brion D. PPARs and the placenta. Placenta 2007; 28: 65-76.

[69]   Pavan L, Tsatsaris V, Hermouet A, Therond P, Evain-Brion D, Fournier T. Oxidized low-density lipoproteins inhibit trophoblastic cell invasion. J Clin Endocrinol Metab 2004; 89: 1969-72.

[70]   Fournier T, Handschuh K, Tsatsaris V. Guibourdenche J, Evain-Brion D. Role of nuclear receptors and their ligands in human trophoblast invasion. J Reprod Immunol 2008; 77: 161-70.

[71]   Fournier T, Handschuh K, Tsatsaris V, Evain-Brion D. Involvement of PPARgamma in human trophoblast invasion. Placenta 2007; 28(Suppl A): S76-81.

[72]   Fournier T, Thérond P, Handschuh K, Tsatsaris V, Evain-Brion D [Review]. Curr Med Chem 2008; 15: 3011-24.

[73]   Handschuh K, Guibourdenche J, Tsatsaris V, Guesnon M, Laurendeau I, Evain-Brion D, Fournier T. Human chorionic gonadotropin produced by the invasive trophoblast but not the villous trophoblast promotes cell invasion and is down-regulated by peroxisome proliferator-activated receptor-gamma. Endocrinology 2007; 148: 5011-9.

[74]   Handschuh K, Guibourdenche J, Cocquebert M, Tsatsaris V, Vidaud M, Evain-Brion D, Fournier T. Expression and regulation by PPARgamma of hCG alpha-and beta-subunits: comparison between villous and invasive extravillous trophoblastic cells. Placenta 2009; 30: 1016-22.

[75]   Lacroix MC, Guibourdenche J, Fournier T, Laurendeau I, Igout A, Goffin V, Pantel J, Tsatsaris V, Evain-Brion D. Stimulation of human trophoblast invasion by placental growth hormone. Endocrinology 2005; 146: 2434-44.

[76]   Handschuh K, Guibourdenche J, Tsatsaris V, Guesnon M, Laurendeau I, Evain-Brion D, Fournier T. Human chorionic gonadotropin expression in human trophoblasts from early placenta: comparative study between villous and extravillous trophoblastic cells. Placenta 2007; 28: 175-84.

[77] Guibourdenche J, Handschuh K, Tsatsaris V, Gerbaud P, Leguy MC, Muller F, Brion DE, Fournier T. Hyperglycosylated hCG is a marker of early human trophoblast invasion. J Clin Endocrinol Metab 2010; 95: E240-4.

[78] Rauwel B, Mariamé B, Martin H, Nielsen R, Allart S, Pipy B, Mandrup S, Devignes MD, Evain-Brion D, Fournier T, Davrinche C. Activation of peroxisome proliferator-activated receptor gamma by human cytomegalovirus for *de novo* replication impairs migration and invasiveness of cytotrophoblasts from early placentas. J Virol 2010; 84: 2946-54.

[79] Blackburn St. Prenatal period and placental physiology. In: Blackburn St, Eds. Maternal, fetal, neonatal physiology. A clinical perspective. St-Louis: Saunders, 2003.

[80] Craven CM, Morgan T, Ward K. Decidual spiral artery remodeling begins before cellular interaction with cytotrophoblasts. Placenta 1998; 19: 241-52.

[81] Carmeliet P. Mechanisms of angiogenesis and arteriogenesis. Nat Med 2000; 6: 389-95.

[82] Clark DE, Smith SK, Licence D, Evans AL, Charnock-Jones DS. Comparison of expression patterns for placenta growth factor, vascular endothelial growth factor (VEGF), VEGF-B and VEGF-C in the human placenta throughout gestation. J Endocrinol 1998; 159:4 59-67.

[83] Zhou Y, Bellingard V, Feng KT, McMaster M, Fisher SJ. Human cytotrophoblasts promote endothelial survival and vascular remodeling through secretion of Ang2, PlGF, and VEGF-C. Dev Biol 2003; 263: 114-25.

[84] Zygmunt M, Herr F, Keller-Schoenwetter S, *et al.* Characterization of human chorionic gonadotropin as a novel angiogenic factor. J Clin Endocrinol Metab 2002; 87:5290-6.

[85] Berndt S, Perrier d'Hauterive S, Blacher S, Péqueux C, Lorquet S, Munaut C, Applanat M, Hervé MA, Lamandé N, Corvol P, van den Brûle F, Frankenne F, Poutanen M, Huhtaniemi I, Geenen V, Noël A, Foidart JM. Angiogenic activity of human chorionic gonadotropin through LH receptor activation on endothelial and epithelial cells of the endometrium. FASEB J 2006; 20: 2630-2.

[86] Berndt S, Blacher S, Perrier d'Hauterive S, Thiry M, Tsampalas M, Cruz A, Péqueux C, Lorquet S, Munaut C, Noël A, Foidart JM. Chorionic gonadotropin stimulation of angiogenesis and pericyte recruitment. J Clin Endocrinol Metab 2009; 94: 4567-74.

[87] Zhang EG, Smith SK, Baker PN, Charnock-Jones DS. The regulation and localization of angiopoietin-1,-2, and their receptor tie2 in normal and pathologic human placentae. Mol Med 2001; 7: 624-35.

[88] Pavlov N, Hatzi E, Bassaglia Y, Frendo J, Brion DE, Badet J. Angiogenin distribution in human term placenta, and expression by cultured trophoblastic cells. Angiogenesis 2003; 6: 317-30.

[89] Ferriani RA, Ahmed A, Sharkey A, Smith SK. Colocalization of acidic and basic fibroblast growth factor (FGF) in human placenta and the cellular effects of bFGF in trophoblast cell line JEG-3. Growth Factors 1994; 10: 259-68.

[90] Gurski MR, Gonzalez E, Brown EG. Immunochemical localization of platelet-derived growth factor in placenta and its possible role in preeclampsia. J Investig Med 1999; 47: 128-33.

[91] Amemiya K, Kurachi H, Adachi H, *et al.* Involvement of epidermal growth factor (EGF)/EGF receptor autocrine and paracrine mechanism in human trophoblast cells: functional differentiation *in vitro*. J Endocrinol 1994; 143: 291-301.

[92] Hill DJ, Clemmons DR, Riley SC, Bassett N, Challis JR. Immunohistochemical localization of the insulin-like growth factors (IGFs) and IGF binding proteins-1,-2 and-3 in the human placenta and fetal membranes. Placenta 1993; 14: 1-2.

[93] Linnemann K, Malek A, Schneider H, Fusch C. Physiological and pathological regulation of feto/placento/maternal leptin expression. Biochem Soc Trans 2001; 29: 86-90.

[94] Pijnenborg R, Vercruysse L, Verbist L, Van Assche FA. Interaction of interstitial trophoblast with placental bed capillaries and venules of normotensive and preeclamptic pregnancies. Placenta 1998; 19: 569-75.

[95] Pijnenborg R, Bland JM, Robertson WB, Brosens I. Uteroplacental arterial changes related to interstitial trophoblast migration in early human pregnancy. Placenta 1983; 4: 397-413.

[96] Harris LK. Review: Trophoblast-vascular cell interactions in early pregnancy: how to remodel a vessel. Placenta. 2010; 31: S93-8.

[97] Harris LK, Smith SD, Keogh RJ, Jones RL, Baker PN, Knöfler M, Cartwright JE, Whitley GS, Aplin JD. Trophoblast-and vascular smooth muscle cell-derived MMP-12 mediates elastolysis during uterine spiral artery remodeling. Am J Pathol. 2010; 177: 2103-15.

[98] Smith SD, Dunk CE, Aplin JD, Harris LK, Jones RL. Evidence for immune cell involvement in decidual spiral arteriole remodeling in early human pregnancy. Am J Pathol. 2009; 174: 1959-71.

[99] Harris LK, Keogh RJ, Wareing M, Baker PN, Cartwright JE, Aplin JD, Whitley GS. Invasive trophoblasts stimulate vascular smooth muscle cell apoptosis by a fas ligand-dependent mechanism. Am J Pathol. 2006; 169: 1863-74.

[100] Burton GJ,Watson AL, Hempstock J, Skepper JN, Jauniaux E. Uterine glands provide histiotrophic nutrition for the human fetus during the first trimester of pregnancy. J Clin Endocrinol Metab 2002; 87: 2954-9.

[101] Schneider H, Miller RK. Receptor-mediated uptake and transport of macromolecules in the human placenta. Int J Dev Biol 2010; 54: 367-75.

[102] Hahn T, Hahn D, Blaschitz A, Korgun ET, Desoye G, Dohr G. Hyperglycaemia-induced subcellular redistribution of GLUT1 glucose transporters in cultured human term placental trophoblast cells. Diabetologia 2000; 43: 173-80.

[103] Desforges M, Sibley CP. Placental nutrient supply and fetal growth [Review]. Int J Dev Biol 2010; 54: 377-90.

[104] Duttaroy AK. Transport of fatty acids across the human placenta: a review [Review]. Prog Lipid Res 2009; 48: 52-61.

[105] Wadsack C, Hammer A, Levak-Frank S, Desoye G, Kozarsky KF, Hirschmugl B, Sattler W, Malle E. Selective cholesteryl ester uptake from high density lipoprotein by human first trimester and term villous trophoblast cells. Placenta 2003; 24: 131-43.

[106] Wintour E.Water and electrolyte metabolism in the fetal-placental unit. In: Principles of perinatal and neonatal metabolism. New York: Springer-Verlag 1998.

[107] Magann EF, Doherty DA, Chauhan SP, Barrilleaux SP, Verity LA, Martin Jr. JN. Effect of maternal hydration on amniotic fluid volume. Obstet Gynecol 2003; 101: 1261-5.

[108] Damiano A, Zotta E, Goldstein J, Reisin I, Ibarra C. Water channel proteins AQP3 and AQP9 are present in syncytiotrophoblast of human term placenta. Placenta 2001; 22: 776-81.

[109] Jameson JL, Hollenberg AN. Regulation of chorionic gonadotropin gene expression. Endocr Rev 1993; 14: 203-21.

[110] Walker WH, Fitzpatrick S, Barrera-Saldana H, Resendez-Perez D, Saunders G. The human placental lactogen genes: structure, function, evolution and transcriptional regulation. Endocr Rev 1991; 12: 316-28.

[111] Lacroix MC, Guibourdenche J, Frendo JL, Muller F, Evain-Brion D. Human placental growth hormone--a review. Placenta 2002; 23(Suppl A): s87-s94.

[112] Srisuparp S, Strakova Z, Fazleabas AT. The role of chorionic gonadotropin (CG) in blastocyst implantation [Review]. Arch Med Res 2001; 32: 627-34.

[113] Maston GA, Ruvolo M. Chorionic gonadotropin has a recent origin within primates and an evolutionary history of selection. Mol Biol Evol 2002; 19: 320-35.

[114] Jablonka-Shariff A, Garcia-Campayo V, Boime I. Evolution of lutropin to chorionic gonadotropin generates a specific routing signal for apical release *in vivo*. J Biol Chem 2002; 277: 879-82.

[115] Licht P, Russu V,Wildt L. On the role of human chorionic gonadotropin (hCG) in the embryo-endometrial microenvironment: implications for differentiation and implantation. Semin Reprod Med 2001; 19: 37-47.

[116] Rao CV. Tropic effects of LH and hCG on early pregnancy events in women's reproductive tract. Early Pregnancy 2001; 5: 18-9.

[117] Malassiné A, Frendo JL, Evain-Brion D. A comparison of placental development and endocrine functions between the human and mouse model [Review]. Hum Reprod Update 2003; 9: 531-9.

[118] Shi Q, Lei Z, Rao C and Lin J. Novel role of human chorionic gonadotropin in differentiation of human cytotrophoblasts. Endocrinology 1993; 132: 1387-1395.

[119] Yang M, Lei ZM, Rao ChV. The central role of human chorionic gonadotropin in the formation of human placental syncytium. Endocrinology 2003; 144: 1108-20.

[120] Malassiné A, Frendo JL, Evain-Brion D. Trisomy 21-affected placentas highlight prerequisite factors for human trophoblast fusion and differentiation [Review]. Int J Dev Biol 2010; 54: 475-82.

[121] Diaz-Cueto L, Barrios-de-Tomasi J, Timossi C, Mendez JP, Ulloa-Aguirre A. More *in-vitro* bioactive, shorter-lived human chorionic gonadotropin charge isoforms increase at the end of the first and during the third trimesters of gestation. Mol Hum Reprod 1996; 2: 643-650.

[122] Elliott MM, Kardana A, Lustbader JW, Cole LA. Carbohydrate and peptide structure of the alpha-and beta-subunits of human chorionic gonadotropin from normal and aberrant pregnancy and choriocarcinoma. Endocrine 1997; 7: 15-32.

[123] Frendo JL, Guibourdenche J, Pidoux G, Vidaud M, Luton D, Giovangrandi Y, Porquet D, Muller F, Evain-Brion D. Trophoblast production of a weakly bioactive human chorionic gonadotropin in trisomy 21-affected pregnancy. J Clin Endocrinol Metab 2004; 89: 727-32.

[124] Frendo JL, Vidaud M, Guibourdenche J, Luton D, Muller F, Bellet D, Giovagrandi Y, Tarrade A, Porquet D, Blot P, Evain-Brion D. Defect of villous cytotrophoblast differentiation into syncytiotrophoblast in Down syndrome. J Clin Endocrinol Metab 2000; 85: 3700-3707.

[125] Kovalevskaya G, Genbacev O, Fisher SJ, Caceres E, O'Connor JF. Trophoblast origin of hCG isoforms: cytotrophoblasts are the primary source of choriocarcinoma-like hCG. Mol Cell Endocrinol 2002; 194: 147-155.

[126] Lopata A, Oliva K, Stanton PG, Robertson DM. Analysis of chorionic gonadotrophin secreted by cultured human blastocysts. Mol Human Reprod 1997; 3: 517-521.

[127] Bersinger NA, Wunder DM, Nicolas M, Birkhäuser MH, Porquet D, Guibourdenche J. Serum hyperglycosylated human chorionic gonadotropin to predict the gestational outcome in *in vitro* fertilization/intracytoplasmic sperm injection pregnancies. Fetal Diagn Ther 2008; 24: 74-78.

[128] Cole LA, Shahabi S, Oz UA, Bahado-Singh RO, Mahoney MJ. Hyperglycosylated human chorionic gonadotropin (ITA) immunoassay: a new basis for gestational Down syndrome screening. Clin Chem 1999; 45: 2109-2119.

[129] Cole LA. Hyperglycosylated hCG. Placenta 2007; 28: 977-986.

[130] Freemark M. Regulation of maternal metabolism by pituitary and placental hormones: roles in fetal development and metabolic programming [Review]. Horm Res 2006; 65(Suppl 3): 41-9.

[131] Alsat E, Guibourdenche J, Luton D, Frankenne F, Evain-Brion D. Human placental growth hormone [Review]. Am J Obstet Gynecol. 1997; 177: 1526-34.

[132] Hauguel-de Mouzon S, Lepercq J, Catalano P. The known and unknown of leptin in pregnancy [Review]. Am J Obstet Gynecol 2006; 194: 1537-45.

[133] Sagawa N, Yura S, Itoh H, Mise H, Kakui K, Korita D, Takemura M, Nuamah MA, Ogawa Y, Masuzaki H, Nakao K and Fujii S. Role of leptin in pregnancy-a review. Placenta 2002; (Suppl A): S80-86.

[134] Debieve, F., Pampfer, S. and Thomas, K. Inhibin and activin production and subunit expression in human placental cells cultured *in vitro*. Mol Hum Reprod 2000; 6: 743-749.

[135] Petraglia F, Florio P, Nappi C, Genazzani AR. Peptide signaling in human placenta and membranes: autocrine, paracrine, and endocrine mechanisms. Endocr Rev 1996; 17: 156-86.

[136] McLean M, Smith R. Corticotrophin-releasing hormone and human parturition [Review]. Reproduction 2001; 121(4): 493-501.

[137] Fowden AL. The insulin-like growth factors and feto-placental growth. Placenta 2003; 24: 803-12.

[138] Levine RJ, Maynard SE, Qian C, Lim KH, England LJ, Yu KF, Schisterman EF, Thadhani R, Sachs BP, Epstein FH, Sibai BM, Sukhatme VP, Karumanchi SA. Circulating angiogenic factors and the risk of preeclampsia. N Engl J Med 2004; 350: 672-83

[139] Thadhani R, Mutter WP, Wolf M, Levine RJ, Taylor RN, Sukhatme VP, Ecker J, Karumanchi SA. First trimester placental growth factor and soluble fms-like tyrosine kinase 1 and risk for preeclampsia. J Clin Endocrinol Metab 2004; 89: 770-5.

[140] Murphy VE, Smith R, Giles WB, Clifton VL. Endocrine regulation of human fetal growth: the role of the mother, placenta, and fetus [Review]. Endocr Rev 2006; 27: 141-69.

[141] Mirlesse V, Frankenne F, Alsat E, Poncelet M, Hennen G, Evain-Brion D. Placental growth hormone levels in normal pregnancy and in pregnancies with intrauterine growth retardation. Pediatr Res 1993; 34: 439-42.

[142] Bedin M, Pointis G. Steroid sulfatase and placental deficiency. Current data as instigators of new research. Ann Endocrinol 1987; 48: 323-33.

[143] Shozu M, Akasofu K, Harada T, Kubota Y. A new cause of female pseudohermaphroditism: placental aromatase deficiency. J Clin Endocrinol Metab 1991; 72: 560-6.

[144] Tuckey RC, Bose HS, Czerwionka I, Miller WL. Molten globule structure and steroidogenic activity of n-218 mln64 in human placental mitochondria. Endocrinology 2004; 145: 1700-7.

[145] Hasegawa T, Zhao L, Caron KM, *et al.* Developmental roles of the steroidogenic acute regulatory protein (STAR) as revealed by star knockout mice. Mol Endocrinol 2000; 14: 1462-71.

[146] Seckl JR, Cleasby M, Nyirenda MJ. Glucocorticoids, 11beta-hydroxysteroid dehydrogenase, and fetal programming [Review]. Kidney Int 2000; 57: 1412-7.

[147] Murphy VE, Smith R, Giles WB, Clifton VL. Endocrine regulation of human fetal growth: the role of the mother, placenta, and fetus. Endocr Rev 2006; 27: 141-69.

[148] Dave-Sharma S, Wilson RC, Harbison MD, Newfield R, Azar MR, Krozowski ZS, Funder JW, Shackleton CH, Bradlow HL, Wei JQ, Hertecant J, Moran A, Neiberger RE, Balfe JW, Fattah A, Daneman D, Akkurt HI, De Santis C, New MI. Examination of genotype and phenotype relationships in 14 patients with apparent mineralocorticoid excess. J Clin Endocrinol Metab 1998; 83: 2244-54.

[149] Albrecht ED, Pepe GJ. Placental steroid hormone biosynthesis in primate pregnancy. Endocr Rev 1990; 11: 124-50.

CHAPTER 4

Biochemical Markers of Hypertensive Disorders of Pregnancy

Yves Giguère[1,2,*], Marc Charland[1], Dominique Guérette[1], Joël Girouard[1], François Rousseau[1,2] and Jean-Claude Forest[1,2]

[1]*Reproduction, Perinatal Health and Child Health Research Axis, CHUQ Research Center, 10, rue de l'Espinay, Québec City, QC, Canada, G1L 3L5;* [2]*Department of Molecular Biology, Medical Biochemistry and Pathology, Faculty of Medicine, Université Laval, Québec City, QC, Canada, G1K 7P4*

Abstract: Hypertensive disorders of pregnancy, and particularly preeclampsia, remain a leading cause of adverse pregnancy outcomes in both developing and developed countries. Identification of at-risk women, before the emergence of clinical signs, in order to implement preventive measures and early targeted interventions for improving short-and long-term outcomes for the mother and her child, remains a public health priority. The development of validated screening procedures using biological markers is hampered by the limited knowledge of the aetiology and pathophysiology of preeclampsia, despite continuous research efforts. However, recently discovered biochemical markers and ultrasonographic parameters, taken individually or in combination, have shown encouraging potential to better characterize and predict preeclampsia and its adverse outcomes. We provide in this chapter examples of potential markers in relation to their links to pathophysiological processes. We believe there is a need to investigate in large-scale population studies combinations of carefully-selected biochemical, biophysical and maternal determinants to identify early in pregnancy women at risk of developing preeclampsia and its adverse outcomes.

Keywords: Markers, maternal hypertension, pregnancy, blood pressure, proteinuria, foetal.

HYPERTENSIVE DISORDERS OF PREGNANCY

Hypertensive disorders of pregnancy (HDP), and particularly preeclampsia (PE), remain a leading cause of adverse pregnancy outcomes in both developed and developing countries. Using current classifications, their prevalence in nulliparous women varies between 7 and 12% in developed countries [1, 2]. HDP stay a major cause of maternal mortality (15-46%) [3, 4] and is responsible for a five-fold increase of perinatal mortality (up to 65% of fetal deaths) [5, 6]. Adverse outcomes, such as fetal growth restriction (FGR) and preterm birth (PTB), are still responsible for significant newborn morbidity and mortality and can have lifelong consequences for the child [7]. Costs of providing treatment for PE and its adverse outcomes, including the care for child disabilities are enormous [8, 9]. WHO has recognized the importance of PE by launching the "Global Programme to Conquer Preeclampsia-Eclampsia" dedicated to study and to treat this syndrome [10]. A US National Institute of Child Health and Human Development Workshop described PE as "a pressing problem" [11].

Classification and Complications

Over the years, most classifications of HDP proposed by national and international groups [12-14] have considered hypertension (either *de novo* or chronic) and proteinuria as the major clinical issues permitting distinction between them. In Canada, the Society of Obstetricians and Gynaecologists (SOGC) published an updated classification of HDP, reflecting their systemic inflammatory nature [15] HDP encompasses: a) Pre-existing or chronic hypertension (CH) which antedates pregnancy or is diagnosed before 20 weeks of gestation; b) gestational hypertension (GH), which is characterized by hypertension ($\geq$ 90 mmHg diastolic), occurs at or after the 20th week of pregnancy. Both CH and GH can be both sub-divided: i) with co-morbid conditions, such as type I or II diabetes mellitus, renal disease, or an indication for antihypertensive therapy

*Address correspondence to Yves Giguère: Reproduction, Perinatal Health and Child Health Research Axis, CHUQ, 10, rue de l'Espinay, Québec, QC, Canada, G1L 3L5; Tel: 418-525-4444 ext 47261, E-mail: Yves.Giguere@crsfa.ulaval.ca

Julie Lafond and Cathy Vaillancourt (Eds)

outside pregnancy and ii) with preeclampsia (PE) which includes hypertension and abnormal proteinuria (> 0.3 g/d) or other adverse conditions (Table **1**). Specific criteria exist to discriminate between mild and severe forms of PE, mostly related to differences in blood pressure, levels of proteinuria and extent of other clinical signs. PE can also be classified as early-or late-onset, the cut-off being the 34th week of gestation; a classification justified by the fact that early-onset PE is generally associated with more severe adverse outcomes for both the fetus and the mother [16-18].

Table 1: Diagnostic Criteria for Hypertensive Disorders of Pregnancy Following Guidelines from SOGC [15]

	Gestational Hypertension			**Chronic Hypertension**		
Blood pressure before pregnancy	Normal			Diastolic ≥ 90 mmHg		
Blood pressure after pregnancy	Normal			Diastolic ≥ 90 mmHg		
		+ Preeclampsia	**+ Severe Preeclampsia**		**+ Preeclampsia**	**+ Severe Preeclampsia**
Blood pressure during pregnancy	Diastolic ≥ 90 mmHg	Diastolic ≥ 90 mmHg	Systolic ≥ 160 mmHg or Diastolic ≥ 110 mmHg	Diastolic ≥ 90 mmHg	Diastolic ≥ 90 mmHg or resistant/increased hypertension	Systolic ≥160 mmHg or Diastolic ≥ 110 mmHg
Proteinuria	None	≥ 2+ on dipstick or ≥ 0.3 g/24 h or ≥ 30 mg/mmol urinary creatinine	3-5 g/24 h	None	≥ 2+ on dipstick or ≥ 0.3 g/24 h or ≥ 30 mg/mmol urinary creatinine	3-5 g/24 h
Onset	After 20 weeks	After 20 weeks	After 20 weeks (early: before 34 wks)	Before pregnancy	After 20 weeks	After 20 weeks (early: before 34 wks)
Other adverse conditions (the extent of these conditions influences the categorization to severe preeclampsia)		**Maternal symptoms** -persistent or new/unusual headache -visual disturbances; -persistent abdominal or right upper quadrant pain/chest pain/dyspnea; -severe nausea or vomiting. **Maternal signs of end-organ dysfunction** -eclampsia, severe hypertension; -pulmonary oedema; -suspected placental abruption. **Abnormal maternal laboratory testing** -elevated serum creatinine, AST, ALT or LDH [according to local lab. criteria]; -platelet count <100 x10^9/L; -serum albumin < 20 g/L. **Fetal morbidity** -oligohydramnios; -IUGR, Intrauterine fetal death; -absent or reversed end-diastolic flow in UtA by Doppler velocimetry.			**Maternal symptoms** -persistent or new/unusual headache; -visual disturbances; -persistent abdominal or right upper quadrant pain/chest pain/dyspnea; -severe nausea or vomiting. **Maternal signs of end-organ dysfunction** -eclampsia, severe hypertension; -pulmonary oedema; -suspected placental abruption **Abnormal maternal laboratory testing** -elevated serum creatinine, AST, ALT or LDH [according to local lab. criteria]; -platelet count <100 x10^9/L; -serum albumin < 20 g/L. **Fetal morbidity** -oligohydramnios; -IUGR, Intrauterine fetal death; -absent or reversed end-diastolic flow in UtA by Doppler velocimetry.	

PE appears to affect predominantly the kidney, the liver and the neurovascular systems. Hyperuricemia and hypercalciuria are indicative of abnormal reabsorption associated with renal ischemia. The liver may also be affected in PE as detected by elevation of transaminases and by HELLP syndrome which involves hemolysis, elevated liver enzymes and low platelet counts observed in 20% of women with severe PE or eclampsia [19]. However, 15-20% of women affected with HELLP syndrome do not show PE symptoms, meaning that the presentation and manifestations of PE is heterogeneous. The central nervous system can also be affected in PE as manifested by headache or blurred vision. In most severe cases of PE, seizures may arise, leading to eclampsia.

Risk Factors for HDP and PE

PE is generally regarded as a first-pregnancy syndrome for which many risk factors have been identified [18, 20]. Limited sperm exposure with the partner before conception increases the risk, as well as multiple gestation and extremes of maternal age [1, 21]. Since healthy pregnancy itself appears as a state of systemic inflammation, especially during 3rd trimester, any process exacerbating this state increases the risk (*e.g.*: infections) [22]. Maternal characteristics such as obesity (pre-pregnancy BMI [23, 24] or weight gain [25]), gestational diabetes, insulin resistance and existing hypertension [26] also increase PE risk.

Environmental factors influencing pregnancy outcomes have been reviewed [27-29] and sociodemographic characteristics (occupation, marital status, education and economic status) and life habits such as alcohol consumption have been associated with PE [30]. Longitudinal studies have shown effects of maternal psychological conditions such as job stress [31] and anxiety/depression [32-34]. Physical activity [35-37], some nutritional habits [38. 39] as well as smoking [40, 41] decrease HDP and PE risks.

Outcomes and Treatment

The only definitive treatment of PE is delivery. It is therefore a major cause of iatrogenic prematurity, responsible for at least 15% of preterm birth in developed countries [42]. Depending upon severity, PE is commonly associated with intrauterine growth restriction (IUGR-up to 25 % of the cases) [1]. Other complications include *placenta abruptio*, disseminated intravascular coagulation, renal or liver failure, hemorrhages, eclampsia and stroke in the mother, as well as long-term neonate morbidity [1, 43, 44].

Various preventive measures have been investigated such as the use of antioxidants (vitamins C and E), [44-46] and low-dose aspirin which reduces vasospasm and coagulation abnormalities [47]. The former approach appeared controversial [1, 48, 49]. SOGC recommends as preventive measures calcium supplementation for all women with low-calcium intake [15], and low-dose aspirin (75-100 mg/d) prescribed early in pregnancy, for women at high-risk of PE, which agrees with our own recent systematic review [50, 51]. Since excessive hemostasis has been evoked as contributing to the pathological process in PE, especially in severe PE, low molecular weight heparins, which have been associated with reduction of severe PE in selected high-risk women [52], is under investigation [53].

Long-Term Effects

Epidemiological studies have shown an increased long-term cardiovascular risk for both the foetus and the mother who suffered from HDP. We [54, 55] and others have demonstrated that hypertensive pregnancy may be considered as an early manifestation of susceptibility to cardiovascular disease (CVD) for women later in life [56-62]. Moreover, studies have shown that PE is associated with an increased risk of hospitalization due to a number of diseases (endocrine, nutritional and metabolic (incidence rate ratio of 1.6), and of blood and blood-forming organs (incidence rate ratio of 1.5), particularly in children born at term [63]. PE and GH have been shown to be associated with increased risk of stroke in a Finnish adult offspring cohort [64]. The reconnaissance that HDP may represent a signal of future CVD risk is an on-going public health challenge.

Pathophysiology of PE

Abnormal placental implantation seems to be central in the pathophysiology of PE (see relevant chapters in this eBook from Lanoix, Fournier and Asselin as well as recent reviews [18, 65-67] for more details). Indeed, the crucial role of placenta in this syndrome is exemplified by 1) the fact that PE only arises during pregnancy, 2) its appearance in the presence of hydatidiform mole and 3) its resolution after placenta expulsion at delivery.

During normal early pregnancy, extravillous cytotrophoblast cells invade the decidual and myometrial segments of uterus, resulting in artery dilatation and increased uterine blood flow. This transformation is mostly completed around 16 to 20 weeks of gestation. In the setting of PE, trophoblastic invasion is decreased in the decidual region and mostly absent in the myometrial region, leading to diminished placental perfusion [68-70]. As a major consequence, the uterine blood flow is unable to meet the growing placental and fetal demands leading to placental hypoxia, ischemia and oxidative stress [68]. Reduced uterine blood flow impacts both placental and fetal growth, ultimately leading to placental dysfunction and injuries and to IUGR (Fig. **1**). In severe cases, this may lead to intrauterine fetal death.

During normal pregnancy, the placenta releases in maternal circulation a series of metabolites which in turn allows the maternal system to cope with the physiological stress related to pregnancy. The expression of many biochemical factors by trophoblastic cells was found to be modified during PE (Fig. **1**), resulting in deficient cell adhesion, uteroplacental angiogenesis, exaggerated immune response and apoptosis but their relationship as a cause or a consequence of this syndrome is difficult to establish as the diagnosis of PE is clinically established only after the faulty invasion process has occurred. Moreover, the dysfunctional placenta liberates abnormal concentrations of metabolites which specifically affect maternal endothelial function by altering vascular reactivity, coagulation cascade and capillary permeability (Fig. **1**), leading to the clinical manifestations.

Fig. **1** presents a summary of the pathogenesis of preeclampsia, with an emphasis on the involved physiological processes and the related molecules that can ultimately represent potential predictive biomarkers.

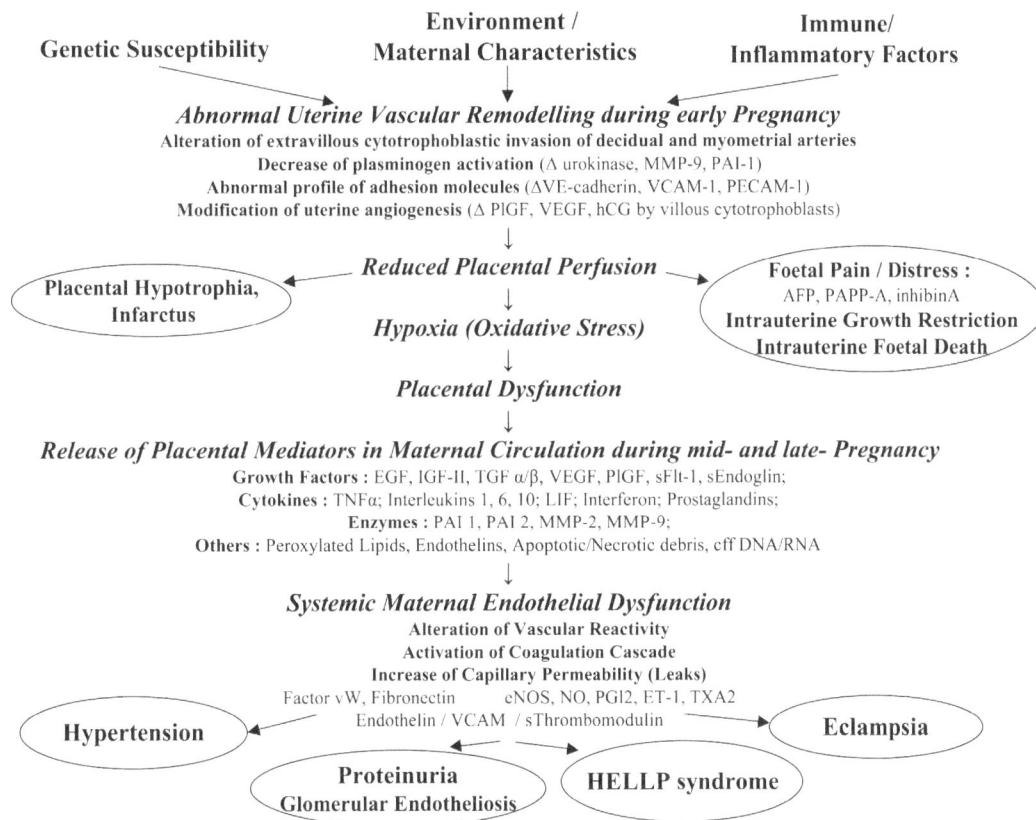

Figure 1: Summary of the pathogenesis of HDP: Major physiological processes and resulting clinical effects. Involved molecules represent potential biomarkers.

AFP: alphafetoprotein; **cff DNA/RNA:** Cell-free fetal DNA or RNA; **EGF:** Epidermal growth factor; **eNOS:** Endothelial NO-synthase; **ET-1:** Endothelin-1; **Factor vW:** vonWillebrand factor; **hCG:** human chorionic gonadotrophin; **IGF-II:** Insulin-like growth factor-II; **LIF:** Leukemia inhibitory factor; **MMP-2:** Matrix metallopeptidase-2; **MMP-9:** Matrix metallopeptidase-9; **NO:** Nitric oxide; **PAI-1:** Plasminogen activator inhibitor-1; **PAI-2:** Plasminogen activator inhibitor-2; **PAPP-A:** Pregnancy associated plasma protein-A; **PECAM-1:** P-endothelial cell adhesion molecule-1; **PGL2:** Prostagnlandin-2; **PlGF:** Placental growth factor; **sFlt-1:** soluble fms-like tyrosine kinase-1; **TGF α/β:** Transforming growth factor α or β; **TNFα:** Tumor necrosis factor α; **TXA2:** Thromboxane-2; **VCAM:** Vascular cell adhesion molecule; **VE-cadherin:** Vascular-E cadherin; **VEGF:** Vascular endothelial growth factor;

POTENTIAL PREDICTIVE PE MARKERS

Until now, antenatal care essentially consisted of serial visits at defined intervals, the primary objective being to detect early clinical signs of PE. Following international guidelines [13, 43], testing for high blood pressure and proteinuria remains the gold standard measurements for the diagnosis of PE, although these clinical manifestations appear only after the onset of the pathophysiological process. Action is then taken when clinically evident signs and symptoms are found or when women present in preterm labour. As a consequence, many affected pregnancies go undetected for a long period, resulting in delayed recognition and worsening complications [71, 72]. Early detection through an efficient procedure is required to enable prevention and intervention. This is emphasized by the benefit of new interventions such as aspirin prophylaxis for high-risk women.

Table 2: Potential biomarkers of preeclampsia: A summary of utilization

Marker	Altered Levels During		Assessed in Combination with			Also Correlated with
	Before onset of PE ($1^{st}/2^{nd}$ trim.)	After onset of PE (3rd trim.)	Other biochemical markers	Ultrasound markers	Maternal characteristics	
VEGF	Decreased	Decreased		UtA PI		GH, GDM, HELLP, T21
PlGF	Decreased	Decreased	sFlt-1; PlGF; PAPP-A	UtA PI	Ethnicity, weight, history CH, smoking, MAP, conception	GH, GDM, HELLP, PTB, IUGR, T21, T18, T13, Triploidy, Turner
sFlt-1	Increased	Increased	PlGF; sEng;	UtA PI		GH, GDM, HELLP, FD, IUGR, stillbirth, T13
sEng	Increased	Increased	PlGF; sFlt-1; PAPP-A	UtA PI	Weight	GH, HELLP, FD, IUGR, SGA,
AFP	Decreased		hCG	UtA PI		GDM, GH, HELLP, PTB, FL, SGA, T21, Neural tube defects
hCG	Decreased		AFP, PAPP-A	UtA PI		GDM, GH, PTB, T21
Inhibin A	Increased	Increased	PAPP-A, activin A	UtA PI	Ethnicity, parity, BMI	GDM, GH, HELLP, PTB, SGA, T21
PAPP-A	Decreased		sEng, PlGF PP-13, inhibinA	UtA PI	Weight, BMI, MAP, ethnicity, history CH, parity conception, maternal age, fetal CRL, smoking	GDM, GH, HELLP, PTB, FD, SGA, T21, T18, Turner
Cell free fetal DNA	Increased	Increased				IUGR
Cell free fetal RNA	Increased	Increased				
P-Selectin	Increased	Increased		UtA PI	Ethnicity, weight, history CH, smoking, MAP, conception	GH, PTB, SGA
VCAM	Increased					GDM, GH, HELLP, SGA
PP-13	Decreased	Decreased	PAPP-A	UtA PI	Weight, smoking	HELLP, PTB, T18, T13, Turner
ADAM-12	Decreased					SGA
Visfatin	Increased	Increased				GDM, PTB, SGA
PTX3	Increased	Increased				GH, PPROM, PTB, IUGR

In a systematic review of screening tests for PE in 2004, WHO reaffirmed that « … there is no clinically useful screening test to predict the development of preeclampsia in either low-risk or high-risk populations. Further prospective, longitudinal studies are needed » [73]. Moreover, systematic reviews supported by the UK NIHR Health Technology Assessment Programme, evaluating the effectiveness of 27 markers related to medical history, biochemistry, physiology of PE and ultrasonography concluded that "…The tests evaluated are not sufficiently accurate, to suggest their routine use in clinical practice"; although some tests appeared to have interesting sensitivity levels, most often at the expenses of compromised specificity [74]. Recent systematic reviews and meta-analyses related to single markers came to similar conclusions [24, 75-78]. However, suggestions from many authors [73, 74, 76, 79] and our own systematic review [80] on effectiveness of combinations of biochemical and biophysical markers to predict PE, including new ultrasonographic measurements and newly-identified candidate biochemical markers, bring us to consider that combinations of markers will be necessary to predict PE and its adverse outcomes early in pregnancy. Such an approach has been successfully applied to screening for trisomy 21.

We present hereafter the principal tests which could be included in a potential screening algorithm based on their actual performance characteristics and their relatedness to PE pathophysiology following recent published data (Table **2**).

Altered Angiogenic Balance During PE: The Case of VEGF, PlGF, sFlt-1 and sEndoglin

Angiogenic factors are thought to be central in the regulation of placental development; any imbalance may contribute to placental dysfunction observed in PE [81, 82]. Extravillous cytotrophoblasts release in their close environment and in maternal circulation some factors that are responsible for angiogenesis, regulating proper invasion of uterine arteries and placental development (Fig. **1**). Mice engineered to have deletions in genes related to the regulation and signaling of angiogenic pathways have defective placental vasculogenesis and early embryonic mortality [66].

Vascular endothelial growth factor (VEGF) and placental growth factor (PlGF) are implicated in signaling pathways that induce angiogenesis and vasculogenesis during embryonic development. Interactions with their receptors (VEGFR-1 or Flt-1, VEGFR-2, Tie-1 and Tie-2) play an essential role in adequate placental angiogenesis. A soluble truncated variant of Flt-1, sFlt-1, secreted by syncytiotrophoblast into the maternal circulation antagonizes both VEGF and PlGF and prevents interaction with their endogenous membrane receptors [66]. Moreover, the decreased expression of transforming growth factor beta (TGF-β) and its receptor, endoglin (Eng), promotes cytotrophoblast invasion and vascular remodeling in early pregnancy. The secretion of a soluble truncated form of this receptor, sEndoglin, by the placenta may interfere with the process. A balance between these factors is the key to normal placental development [83, 84]. In PE, excessive release of antiangiogenic factors, sFlt-1 and sEng, by a dysfunctional placenta and the consequent decrease of angiogenic factors VEGF and PlGF in maternal circulation may be responsible for maternal endothelial dysfunction and clinical manifestations.

Different studies showed that a rise of sFlt-1 and a decrease of VEGF and PlGF are occurring before onset of PE [85-88]. Thus, clinical use of these markers to predict PE becomes very attractive and treatment based on the inhibition of the action of sFlt-1 could be promising. As the balance between angiogenic and antiangiogenic factors is key to placental normal development, ratio of sFlt-1 to VEGF could further increase the predictive potential of PE [88, 89]. sEng was shown to increase earlier and in a significantly greater degree in women who are bound to develop PE [90, 91].

Other molecules related to angiogenesis, such as angiopoietin-1 and -2 and their receptors Tie-1 have recently been evocated and assessed [92-94], but much characterization efforts still have to be made before their clinical use.

To date, angiogenic growth factors correspond to a group of molecules with great potential for clinical use in early prediction of PE. Depending on cut-off concentration used and period of gestation measurement, these factors represent good predictors of PE as shown in different studies [81, 84, 91].

Feto-Placental Unit Dysfunction Markers

Impaired vascular placental development results in fetal stress, which may be followed by the release of a series of biochemical markers in maternal circulation. Although not necessarily related directly to etiopathological pathways, such biomarkers have been found be useful in predicting other clinical manifestations. A good example is given by Down syndrome prenatal screening markers (AFP, hCG,

PAPP-A, inhibin A and activin A); although none of them is causal of the abnormality, they are now widely used in clinical settings. Many of them have also been assessed in screening of PE.

Alpha fetoprotein (AFP), the principal fetal plasma protein, is found in the amniotic fluid and maternal serum secondary to natural fetal exchange. Maternal AFP is used to screen for adverse pregnancy outcomes such as neural tube defect, Down syndrome, anencephaly, IUGR and intrauterine fetal death [95, 96]. Of note, AFP acts as a proangiogenic factor of endothelial cells during fetal development [97]. It has been shown that maternal AFP level in the second trimester has good specificity, but little sensitivity for prediction of PE [98, 99].

Syncytiotrophoblast cells produce human chorionic gonadotropin (hCG) a glycoprotein hormone composed of two subunits (α and β) which is released in maternal circulation: total-hCG, hyperglycosylated hCG and the free beta-subunit of hyperglycosylated hCG. hCG is essential in early pregnancy as it promotes the production of progesterone to maintain the *corpus luteum* and recent research has shown its implication in the differentiation of trophoblast cells during angiogenesis and placental implantation [100]. Unsurprisingly according to this new finding, hCG production is increased during PE but the predictive value of hCG is limited [98, 99, 101].

Inhibin A and activin A are glycoproteins that belong to the transforming growth factor (TGF) alpha protein super-family. Indeed, studies have shown that they are already increased during first trimester, before the onset of clinical signs of PE and GH, although the amplitude of the increase is not of great value when used in univariate analysis [102]. These markers have a greater clinical value when combined with uterine artery Doppler resulting in a good sensitivity and specificity at 14-16 weeks of gestation [103, 104]. Use of activin A and inhibin A could also help to differentiate PE from GH as the levels of these markers are higher in GH.

Pregnancy associated plasma protein A (PAPP-A), a first-trimester marker used in the prenatal screening of Down syndrome, is mainly secreted by the placenta and is implicated in the control of trophoblast invasion during placentation [105]. PAPP-A concentrations are lowered in the first trimester of pregnancy in women bound to develop PE [106]. The use of this marker has low predictive accuracy and combination with other markers increases its potential as a new marker for PE [80, 107]. Placental tissue protein 13 (PP-13) is secreted by syncytiotrophoblast and is implicated in placental implantation and remodeling of maternal uterine arteries [108]. Studies showed that PP-13 is down-regulated in the first trimester in women who will develop PE because of impaired placental functional responsiveness but prospective studies are needed before considering its clinical application [109, 110].

The impaired trophoblastic invasion of spiral arteries leads to placental ischemia and to the release of fragments in maternal circulation containing fetal nucleic acids [111]. Cell-free fetal (cff) DNA increases in maternal blood during pregnancy, especially for women destined to suffer from adverse pregnancy outcomes [112-115]. Studies have shown that cff DNA in plasma from PE women is increased [116-119], even before onset of PE [120, 121]. In order to differentiate between maternal and fetal genes, epigenetic changes have been successfully studied [122]. Hypermethylation patterns of specific genes can be used as a gender-and polymorphism-independent marker of PE [123]. Fetal RNA is also found in circulating maternal plasma [124, 125]; rapid clearance is observed following delivery [125]. Its chemical stability allows handling and study in laboratory settings [126]. Specific placental transcripts have been detected in plasma from third-trimester pregnant women [125, 127, 128], while correlations between severity of PE and amounts of transcripts of CRH, *PLAC1,* selectin-1 [129], VEGF, sFlt1, endoglin [130] and PAI-1, tissue-type plasminogen activator (tPA) [131] have been reported. Recently, a panel of cff mRNA markers was used to detect PE early in pregnancy, yielding a detection rate of 84% at a 5% false-positive rate [119]. Moreover, cff DNA was found to increase in women with pregnancy complicated by IUGR [132, 133] or preterm birth [113].

Maternal System Dysfunction Markers

Although the placenta appears as the starting point of PE, the target organ remains the maternal endothelium. Adrenomedullin, a vasoactive peptide that acts as a vasodilatator, is recognized to increase during normal pregnancy and even more in PE cases [134-136]. Its use as predictive marker however still requests further characterization.

Selectins are part of a super-family of cell surface adhesion molecules (CAM) implicated in the enrolling of leucocytes on activated endothelial cells [137]. P-selectin plays crucial roles in inflammation by supporting the activation of leucocytes and in coagulation [138]. Its soluble form has been shown to be increased in PE women during the first half of pregnancy [139]. Vascular cell adhesion molecules (VCAM) and intracellular adhesion molecules (ICAM) are part of the immunoglobulin gene super-family and are up-regulated in the presence of endothelial dysfunction observed in PE. Their respective predictive values however remain low when used alone [139, 140].

Affection of kidneys during PE may result from glomerular filtration impairment which can be followed through new blood biomarkers such as low molecular weight proteins such as cystatin C [141]. Interestingly, cystatin C originates from placenta where it is involved in the regulation of proteases implicated in placentation [142]. Plasmatic levels of cystatin C have been shown to increase during overt PE [141], but its early predictive performance remains to be assessed.

An increased systemic inflammatory response, mostly due to exaggerated syncytiotrophoblasts shed into the maternal circulation [67] and amplified by periodontal or gastric infections is known to be present in overt PE [143, 144]. C-reactive protein (CRP), a recognized biomarker of inflammation has been shown to be increased in women who suffer from GH or PE [145-147]. Although CRP performs very well as a biomarker of overt PE [148, 149], its use during 1st or 2nd trimesters as a predictive marker (*e.g.* before clinical onset) still requests more investigation [143, 150, 151]. Pentraxin 3 (PTX3), part of the CRP family, another potential pro-inflammatory marker [152], is increased in women with overt PE or IUGR [153] and as early as in the first trimester in women bound to suffer from PE [151, 154].

Many other peptides and proteins implicated in the etiology of PE could also represent candidate predictive markers. For example, homocysteine is implicated in oxidative stress and endothelial dysfunction. However, studies published to date indicate that this marker has poor sensitivity and sensibility and do not appear to be clinically useful in prediction of PE [155]. ADAM-12, a disintegrin and metalloprotease, belongs to a group of molecules related to cell-cell and cell-matrix interactions.

Although promising results were initially observed, further studies are now required since discrepancies between relative amounts of ADAM-12 during pregnancy in women destined or not to develop PE have been reported [156, 157]. Visfatin is an adipokine secreted by adipocytes and an enzyme involved in NAD biosynthesis. Its plasma level has been found to be altered in different pregnancy disorders [158, 159] although it appears unchanged in PE. It would therefore be a good marker allowing predictive distinction between PE and SGA [160]. There is still a need for large-scale studies to confirm initial results obtained with small populations.

Ultrasonographic Markers

As stated above and exemplified in Fig. **1**, abnormal placenta formation results in inadequate uteroplacental blood flow and poor feto-maternal exchanges. Indeed, Doppler ultrasonography can assess the velocity of uterine artery (UtA) blood flow as part of a routine screening process [161]. UtA waveforms are modified during pregnancy as they pass from low end-diastolic velocities and an early diastolic notch in women who are not pregnant or are in their first trimester to the persistence of a diastolic notch (beyond 24 weeks' gestation) or abnormal flow velocity ratios in women with adverse pregnancy outcomes [162, 163]. Cnossen *et al.* in a meta-analysis and systematic review, concluded that pulsatility index and bilateral notching are the most promising Doppler indices and they should be used in daily clinical practice, although the results vary according to patient risk [76]. They also specifically called for research assessing combinations of Doppler ultrasonography with other tests in order to predict early PE.

Combinations of Markers

Due to the heterogeneous nature of PE, combination of two or more independent biomarkers, each of which reflecting a different pathophysiological process, potentially should increase the likelihood to derive suitable predictive algorithms. Our team recently performed a systematic review of the available evidence pertaining to the predictive characteristics of combinations of biochemical and ultrasonographic markers in the first and second trimesters [80].

Among the numerous marker combinations studied during the second trimester, several appeared to have promising predictive characteristics (sensitivity = 60-90%, specificity >90%). Overall, the addition of UtA Doppler data to biochemical marker data improved the predictive performance of biochemical markers alone to a greater extent than did the addition of biochemical markers to UtA Doppler data alone. However, in one study, the addition of PP-13 to first-trimester UtA PI increased sensitivity from 40% to 90% (at a specificity of 90%) [109]. This study was limited to only 10 cases of early-onset PE in a high-risk population. The results are in agreement with those of Romero *et al.* [164] who observed that PP-13 appears to be an interesting marker for risk assessment of preterm PE but a weak marker for severe PE at term, and ineffective for identifying mild PE at term. Also, data from Spencer *et al.* suggested that first-trimester serum PP-13 as a single marker in a low-risk population showed poor predictive performance [165].

First-trimester or early second-trimester PAPP-A, inhibin A and activin A in combination with UtA Doppler measurements may provide good predictive performance for PE in both low-and high-risk populations. Data from recent publications have indicated that these biochemical markers, taken individually, can predict up to 42% of early PE, but up to 89% when combined with maternal characteristics (race, BMI, parity) and UtA PI (at a false-positive rate of 10%) in a low-risk population [166]. PAPP-A and PlGF were recently found significantly decreased during first trimester (0.53 MoM and 0.61 MoM respectively) in women destined to experience early-onset PE, whereas, only mildly diminished in women who developed late PE. When these variables were combined in logistic regression algorithms for early PE, a predictive rate of 94% at a false-positive rate of 5% was observed [167]. Therefore, a growing body of evidence suggests that combination of first-trimester biochemical and ultrasonographic markers may be useful in prediction of early PE.

Furthermore, it has been shown recently that the inclusion of maternal characteristics, namely body mass index, ethnicity, previous maternal medical and obstetrical history, in prediction algorithms further improves predictive accuracy of combinations of biochemical and ultrasonographic markers [110, 167, 168]. These studies used maternal characteristics as *a priori* risk and the results of selected biochemical and biophysical parameters obtained at either first or second trimester as an *a posteriori* risk in logistic multivariate models to derive the patient-specific risk. Such approach was successfully used in the development of prediction algorithms for Down syndrome [169]. Indeed, Akolekar *et al.* [170] used for instance data that were first drawn from maternal characteristics and history, Doppler UtA PI, mean arterial pressure and serum PAPP-A to which they added maternal serum or plasma concentration of PlGF, PP-13, inhibin A, activin A, sEng, pentraxin-3 and P-selectin obtained from case-control studies. The resulting multivariate prediction algorithm reached detection rates of 91.0, 79.4 and 60.9% for early-onset PE, intermediate-onset PE and late-onset PE, respectively. At this stage, since these results are mainly based on a single (still increasing) cohort, there is a clear need to duplicate them in different population and health care environments.

CONCLUSION AND PERSPECTIVES

As of yet, every new potential individual marker has shown relatively poor sensitivity and specificity for the prediction of PE. As in the case of Down syndrome screening, a combination of markers could improve the predictive capacity of some pregnancy outcomes. In the case of PE, many tools are available and a combination of a number of variables could be the key to develop algorithms for the early prediction of women at high risk of PE during pregnancy.

Biomarkers might play critical clinical roles. Since the definition *per se* of PE relies on a series of clinical markers, a diagnosis might be ascertained by adding one or several relevant biomarkers. Moreover, adequate biomarkers will permit the stratification of PE patients in different outcome categories, and thus improve its clinical management. Ultimately, as shown in our recent systematic review on the use of ASA from or before 16 weeks of pregnancy, biomarkers might ensure, particularly in high-risk women, an efficient treatment to decrease PE risk by as much as 80 to 90%.

The advent of OMICS technologies (genomics, proteomics, metabolomics…) undisputedly represents a major source of discovery of new potential biomarkers, since it allows screening molecules from diverse sources. However, their cost, physical and methodological constraints prevent their use in contemporary clinical settings. The rapid development of automated detection and evaluation methods for ELISA and other technologies constitutes a good alternative nowadays.

In the case of hypertensive disorders of pregnancy, and particularly preeclampsia, recent work by many authors should clearly lead researchers to develop risk-algorithms composed of a series of biochemical markers juxtaposed with ultrasonographical parameters and maternal characteristics. The development and assessment of such multivariate algorithms must be made through prospective large-scale studies with rigorous study design criteria to determine the clinical usefulness of combinations of biomarkers in different geographic, population and health care environments.

REFERENCES

[1]   Sibai B, Dekker G, Kupferminc M. Pre-eclampsia. Lancet 2005; 365(9461): 785-99.

[2]   Walker RL, Hemmelgarn B, Quan H. Incidence of gestational hypertension in the Calgary Health Region from 1995 to 2004. Can J Cardiol 2009; 25(8): e284-7.

[3]   RCOG. Why mothers die 2000-2002. The sixth report of the confidential enquires into maternal deaths in the United Kingdom. RCOG Press ed. Northern Ireland: National Institute for Clinical Excellence, S. E. H. D., Department of Health, Social Services and Public Safety 2004.

[4]   Duley L. The global impact of pre-eclampsia and eclampsia. Semin Perinatol 2009; 33(3): 130-7.

[5]   Roberts J. Preeclampsia: is there value in assessing before clinically evident disease? Obstetrics & Gynecology 2001; 98(4): 596-9.

[6]   Moodley J. Maternal deaths due to hypertensive disorders in pregnancy: Saving Mothers report 2002-2004. Cardiovasc J Afr 2007; 18(6): 358-61.

[7]   Goldenberg RL, Culhane JF, Iams JD, Romero R. Epidemiology and causes of preterm birth. Lancet 2008; 371(9606): 75-84.

[8]   Barton JR, Istwan NB, Rhea D, Collins A, Stanziano GJ. Cost-savings analysis of an outpatient management program for women with pregnancy-related hypertensive conditions. Dis Manag 2006; 9(4): 236-41.

[9]   Liu A, Wen SW, Bottomley J, Walker MC, Smith G. Utilization of health care services of pregnant women complicated by preeclampsia in Ontario. Hypertens Pregnancy 2009; 28(1): 76-84.

[10]   WHO. Program of Work 2004-2008 of Department of Reproductive Health and Research. Geneva: WHO2003 July 2003; Contract No.: HRP/PCC(16)/2003/8.1.

[11]   Ilekis JV, Reddy UM, Roberts JM. Preeclampsia--a pressing problem: an executive summary of a National Institute of Child Health and Human Development workshop. Reprod Sci 2007; 14(6): 508-23.

[12]   NHBPEP Working Group. Report of the National High Blood Pressure Education Program Working Group on High Blood Pressure in Pregnancy. Am J Obstet Gynecol 2000; 183(1): S1-S22.

[13]   Brown MA, Lindheimer MD, de Swiet M, Van Assche A, Moutquin JM. The classification and diagnosis of the hypertensive disorders of pregnancy: statement from the International Society for the Study of Hypertension in Pregnancy (ISSHP). Hypertens Pregnancy 2001; 20(1): ix-xiv.

[14]   ACOG. Diagnosis and management of preeclampsia and eclampsia. International Journal of Gynecology & Obstetrics 2002; 77(1): 67-75.

[15]   Magee L, Helewa M, Moutquin J, von Dadelszen P. Diagnosis, evaluation and management of the hypertensive disorders of pregnancy. J Obst Gynaecol Can 2008; 30(3): S1-S50.

[16]   von Dadelszen P, Magee LA, Roberts JM. Subclassification of preeclampsia. Hypertens Pregnancy 2003; 22(2): 143-8.

[17]   Cnossen JS, van der Post JA, Mol BW, Khan KS, Meads CA, Ter Riet G. Prediction of pre-eclampsia: a protocol for systematic reviews of test accuracy. BMC Pregnancy Childbirth 2006; 6: 29.

[18]   Steegers EA, von Dadelszen P, Duvekot JJ, Pijnenborg R. Pre-eclampsia. Lancet 2010; 376(9741): 631-44.

[19]   Joshi D, James A, Quaglia A, Westbrook RH, Heneghan MA. Liver disease in pregnancy. Lancet 2010; 375(9714): 594-605.

[20]   Duckitt K, Harrington D. Risk factors for pre-eclampsia at antenatal booking: systematic review of controlled studies. BMJ 2005; 330(7491): 565.

[21]   Dekker GA. Risk factors for preeclampsia. Clin Obstet Gynecol 1999; 42(3): 422-35.

[22]   Xiong X, Buekens P, Fraser WD, Beck J, Offenbacher S. Periodontal disease and adverse pregnancy outcomes: a systematic review. BJOG 2006; 113(2): 135-43.

[23]   Thadhani R, Stampfer MJ, Hunter DJ, Manson JE, Solomon CG, Curhan GC. High body mass index and hypercholesterolemia: risk of hypertensive disorders of pregnancy. Obstet Gynecol 1999; 94(4): 543-50.

[24]   Cnossen JS, Leeflang MM, de Haan EE, *et al.* Accuracy of body mass index in predicting pre-eclampsia: bivariate meta-analysis. BJOG 2007; 114(12): 1477-85.

[25]   Sibai BM, Ross MG. Hypertension in gestational diabetes mellitus: Pathophysiology and long-term consequences. J Matern Fetal Neonatal Med 2010; 23(3): 229-33.

[26]   Ray J. Dysmetabolic syndrome, placenta-mediated disease and future risk of cardiovascular disease. Fetal Matern Med Rev 2004; 15(3): 231-46.

[27]   Silbergeld EK, Patrick TE. Environmental exposures, toxicologic mechanisms, and adverse pregnancy outcomes. Am J Obstet Gynecol 2005; 192(Suppl 5): S11-21.

[28]   Bale TL. Is mom too sensitive? Impact of maternal stress during gestation. Front Neuroendocrinol 2005; 26(1): 41-9.

[29]   Wadhwa PD. Psychoneuroendocrine processes in human pregnancy influence fetal development and health. Psychoneuroendocrinology 2005; 30(8): 724-43.

[30]   Eskenazi B, Fenster L, Sidney S. A multivariate analysis of risk factors for preeclampsia. JAMA 1991; 266(2): 237-41.

[31]   Klonoff-Cohen HS, Cross JL, Pieper CF. Job stress and preeclampsia. Epidemiology 1996; 7(3): 245-9.

[32]   Kurki T, Hiilesmaa V, Raitasalo R, Mattila H, Ylikorkala O. Depression and anxiety in early pregnancy and risk for preeclampsia. Obstet Gynecol 2000; 95(4): 487-90.

[33]   Sikkema JM, Robles de Medina PG, Schaad RR, *et al.* Salivary cortisol levels and anxiety are not increased in women destined to develop preeclampsia. J Psychosom Res 2001; 50(1): 45-9.

[34]   Qiu C, Sanchez SE, Lam N, Garcia P, Williams MA. Associations of depression and depressive symptoms with preeclampsia: results from a Peruvian case-control study. BMC Womens Health 2007; 7: 15.

[35]   Marcoux S, Brisson J, Fabia J. The effect of leisure time physical activity on the risk of pre-eclampsia and gestational hypertension. J Epidemiol Community Health 1989; 43(2): 147-52.

[36]   Hegaard HK, Pedersen BK, Nielsen BB, Damm P. Leisure time physical activity during pregnancy and impact on gestational diabetes mellitus, pre-eclampsia, preterm delivery and birth weight: a review. Acta Obstet Gynecol Scand 2007; 86(11): 1290-6.

[37]   Gavard JA, Artal R. Effect of exercise on pregnancy outcome. Clin Obstet Gynecol 2008; 51(2): 467-80.

[38]   Qiu C, Coughlin KB, Frederick IO, Sorensen TK, Williams MA. Dietary fiber intake in early pregnancy and risk of subsequent preeclampsia. Am J Hypertens 2008; 21(8): 903-9.

[39]   Xu H, Shatenstein B, Luo ZC, Wei S, Fraser W. Role of nutrition in the risk of preeclampsia. Nutr Rev 2009; 67(11): 639-57.

[40]   Marcoux S, Brisson J, Fabia J. The effect of cigarette smoking on the risk of preeclampsia and gestational hypertension. Am J Epidemiol 1989; 130(5): 950-7.

[41]   Karumanchi SA, Levine RJ. How does smoking reduce the risk of preeclampsia? Hypertension 2010; 55(5): 1100-1.

[42]   Meis PJ, Goldenberg RL, Mercer BM, *et al.* The preterm prediction study: risk factors for indicated preterm births. Maternal-Fetal Medicine Units Network of the National Institute of Child Health and Human Development. Am J Obstet Gynecol 1998; 178(3): 562-7.

[43]   Report of the National High Blood Pressure Education Program Working Group on High Blood Pressure in Pregnancy. Am J Obstet Gynecol 2000; 183(1): S1-S22.

[44]   Dekker G, Sibai B. Primary, secondary, and tertiary prevention of pre-eclampsia. Lancet 2001; 357(9251): 209-15.

[45]   Sibai BM. Prevention of preeclampsia: a big disappointment. Am J Obstet Gynecol 1998; 179(5): 1275-8.

[46]   Chappell LC, Seed PT, Kelly FJ, *et al.* Vitamin C and E supplementation in women at risk of preeclampsia is associated with changes in indices of oxidative stress and placental function. Am J Obstet Gynecol 2002; 187(3): 777-84.

[47]   Knight M, Duley L, Henderson-Smart DJ, King JF. Antiplatelet agents for preventing and treating pre-eclampsia. Cochrane Database Syst Rev 2000; (2): CD000492.

[48]   Poston L, Briley AL, Seed PT, Kelly FJ, Shennan AH. Vitamin C and vitamin E in pregnant women at risk for pre-eclampsia (VIP trial): randomised placebo-controlled trial. Lancet 2006; 367(9517): 1145-54.

[49]   Rumbold AR, Crowther CA, Haslam RR, Dekker GA, Robinson JS, the ASG. Vitamins C and E and the Risks of Preeclampsia and Perinatal Complications. New England Journal of Medicine 2006; pp.1796-806.

[50]   Bujold E, Morency AM, Roberge S, Lacasse Y, Forest JC, Giguere Y. Acetylsalicylic acid for the prevention of preeclampsia and intra-uterine growth restriction in women with abnormal uterine artery Doppler: a systematic review and meta-analysis. J Obstet Gynaecol Can 2009; 31(9): 818-26.

[51]   Bujold E, Roberge S, Lacasse Y, *et al.* Prevention of preeclampsia and intrauterine growth restriction with aspirin started in early pregnancy: a meta-analysis. Obstet Gynecol 2010; 116(2 Pt 1): 402-14.

[52]   Rey E, Garneau P, David M, *et al.* Dalteparin for the prevention of recurrence of placental-mediated complications of pregnancy in women without thrombophilia: a pilot randomized controlled trial. J Thromb Haemost 2009; 7(1): 58-64.

[53]   Rodger MA. Thrombophilia and placenta-mediated pregnancy complications: from the bench to bedside to policy. Thromb Res 2009; 123(Suppl 2): S100-4.

[54]   Forest JC, Girouard J, Masse J, *et al.* Early occurrence of metabolic syndrome after hypertension in pregnancy. Obstet Gynecol 2005; 105(6): 1373-80.

[55]   Girouard J, Giguere Y, Moutquin JM, Forest JC. Previous hypertensive disease of pregnancy is associated with alterations of markers of insulin resistance. Hypertension 2007; 49(5): 1056-62.

[56]   Bellamy L, Casas JP, Hingorani AD, Williams DJ. Pre-eclampsia and risk of cardiovascular disease and cancer in later life: systematic review and meta-analysis. BMJ 2007; 335(7627): 974.

[57]   Garovic VD, Hayman SR. Hypertension in pregnancy: an emerging risk factor for cardiovascular disease. Nat Clin Pract Nephrol 2007; 3(11): 613-22.

[58]   Levesque S, Moutquin JM, Lindsay C, Roy MC, Rousseau F. Implication of an AGT haplotype in a multigene association study with pregnancy hypertension. Hypertension 2004; 43(1): 71-8.

[59]   Bernard N, Girouard J, Forest JC, Giguere Y. The combination of ApoCIII, hepatic lipase and hormono sensitive lipase gene polymorphisms suggests an association with susceptibility to gestational hypertension. J Hum Genet 2007; 52(3): 244-54.

[60]   Craici I, Wagner S, Garovic VD. Preeclampsia and future cardiovascular risk: formal risk factor or failed stress test? Ther Adv Cardiovasc Dis. 2008; 2(4): 249-59

[61]   McDonald SD, Malinowski A, Zhou Q, Yusuf S, Devereaux PJ. Cardiovascular sequelae of preeclampsia/eclampsia: a systematic review and meta-analyses. Am Heart J 2008; 156(5): 918-30.

[62]   Smith GN, Walker MC, Liu A, *et al.* A history of preeclampsia identifies women who have underlying cardiovascular risk factors. Am J Obstet Gynecol 2009; 200(1): 58 e1-8.

[63]   Wu CS, Nohr EA, Bech BH, Vestergaard M, Catov JM, Olsen J. Health of children born to mothers who had preeclampsia: a population-based cohort study. Am J Obstet Gynecol 2009; 201(3): 269 e1-e10.

[64]   Kajantie E, Eriksson JG, Osmond C, Thornburg K, Barker DJ. Pre-eclampsia is associated with increased risk of stroke in the adult offspring: the Helsinki birth cohort study. Stroke 2009; 40(4): 1176-80.

[65]   Hawfield A, Freedman BI. Pre-eclampsia: the pivotal role of the placenta in its pathophysiology and markers for early detection. Ther Adv Cardiovasc Dis 2009; 3(1): 65-73.

[66]   Young BC, Levine RJ, Karumanchi SA. Pathogenesis of preeclampsia. Annu Rev Pathol. 2010;5:173-92.

[67]   Tsatsaris V, Fournier T, Winer N. Pathophysiology of preeclampsia. Ann Fr Anesth Reanim 2010; 29(3): e13-8.

[68]   Osol G, Mandala M. Maternal uterine vascular remodeling during pregnancy. Physiology (Bethesda) 2009; 24: 58-71.

[69]   Burton GJ, Jauniaux E, Charnock-Jones DS. The influence of the intrauterine environment on human placental development. Int J Dev Biol 2010; 54(2-3): 303-12.

[70]   Reynolds LP, Borowicz PP, Caton JS, *et al.* Uteroplacental vascular development and placental function: an update. Int J Dev Biol 2010; 54(2-3): 355-66.

[71]   Lockwood CJ. Inherited thrombophilias in pregnant patients: detection and treatment paradigm. Obstet Gynecol 2002; 99(2): 333-41.

[72]   von Dadelszen P, Magee L. What matters in preeclampsia are the associated adverse outcomes: the view from Canada. Curr Opin Obstet Gynecol 2008; 20(2): 110-5.

[73]   Conde-Agudelo A, Villar J, Lindheimer M. World Health Organization systematic review of screening tests for preeclampsia. Obstet Gynecol 2004; 104(6): 1367-91.

[74]   Meads CA, Cnossen JS, Meher S, *et al.* Methods of prediction and prevention of pre-eclampsia: systematic reviews of accuracy and effectiveness literature with economic modelling. Health Technol Assess 2008; 12(6): 1-270.

[75]   Leeflang MM, Cnossen JS, van der Post JA, Mol BW, Khan KS, ter Riet G. Accuracy of fibronectin tests for the prediction of pre-eclampsia: a systematic review. Eur J Obstet Gynecol Reprod Biol 2007; 133(1): 12-9.

[76]   Cnossen JS, Morris RK, Ter Riet G, *et al.* Use of uterine artery Doppler ultrasonography to predict pre-eclampsia and intrauterine growth restriction: a systematic review and bivariable meta-analysis. CMAJ 2008; 178(6): 701-11.

[77]   Morris RK, Cnossen JS, Langejans M, *et al.* Serum screening with Down's syndrome markers to predict pre-eclampsia and small for gestational age: systematic review and meta-analysis. BMC Pregnancy Childbirth 2008; 8:33.

[78]   Papanna R, Mann LK, Kouides RW, Glantz JC. Protein/creatinine ratio in preeclampsia: a systematic review. Obstet Gynecol 2008; 112(1): 135-44.

[79]   Thangaratinam S, Coomarasamy A, Sharp S, *et al.* Tests for predicting complications of pre-eclampsia: a protocol for systematic reviews. BMC Pregnancy Childbirth 2008; 8(1): 38.

[80]   Giguere Y, Charland M, Bujold E, *et al.* Combining biochemical and ultrasonographic markers in predicting preeclampsia: a systematic review. Clin Chem 2010; 56(3): 361-75.

[81]   Levine R, Maynard S, Qian C, *et al.* Circulating angiogenic factors and the risk of preeclampsia. New Engl J Med 2004; 350(7): 672-83.

[82]   Levine RJ, Lam C, Qian C, *et al.* Soluble endoglin and other circulating antiangiogenic factors in preeclampsia. N Engl J Med 2006; 355(10): 992-1005.

[83]   Kita N, Mitsushita J. A possible placental factor for preeclampsia: sFlt-1. Curr Med Chem 2008; 15(7): 711-5.

[84]   Catarino C, Rebelo I, Belo L, *et al.* Fetal and maternal angiogenic/anti-angiogenic factors in normal and preeclamptic pregnancy. Growth Factors 2009; 27(6): 345-51.

[85]   Hertig A, Berkane N, Lefevre G, *et al.* Maternal serum sFlt1 concentration is an early and reliable predictive marker of preeclampsia. Clin Chem 2004; 50(9): 1702-3.

[86]   Chaiworapongsa T, Romero R, Kim YM, *et al.* Plasma soluble vascular endothelial growth factor receptor-1 concentration is elevated prior to the clinical diagnosis of pre-eclampsia. J Matern Fetal Neonatal Med 2005; 17(1): 3-18.

[87]   Espinoza J, Chaiworapongsa T, Romero R, *et al.* Unexplained fetal death: another anti-angiogenic state. J Matern Fetal Neonatal Med 2007; 20(7): 495-507.

[88]   Stepan H, Unversucht A, Wessel N, Faber R. Predictive value of maternal angiogenic factors in second trimester pregnancies with abnormal uterine perfusion. Hypertension 2007; 49(4): 818-24.

[89]   Kusanovic JP, Romero R, Chaiworapongsa T, *et al.* A prospective cohort study of the value of maternal plasma concentrations of angiogenic and anti-angiogenic factors in early pregnancy and midtrimester in the identification of patients destined to develop preeclampsia. J Matern Fetal Neonatal Med 2009; 22(11): 1021-38.

[90]   Stepan H, Geipel A, Schwarz F, Kramer T, Wessel N, Faber R. Circulatory soluble endoglin and its predictive value for preeclampsia in second-trimester pregnancies with abnormal uterine perfusion. Am J Obstet Gynecol 2008; 198(2): 175 e1-6.

[91]   De Vivo A, Baviera G, Giordano D, Todarello G, Corrado F, D'Anna R. Endoglin, PlGF and sFlt-1 as markers for predicting pre-eclampsia. Acta Obstet Gynecol Scand 2008; 87(8): 837-42.

[92]   Stepan H, Ebert T, Schrey S, *et al.* Serum levels of angiopoietin-related growth factor are increased in preeclampsia. Am J Hypertens 2009; 22(3): 314-8.

[93]   Akolekar R, Casagrandi D, Skyfta E, Ahmed AA, Nicolaides KH. Maternal serum angiopoietin-2 at 11 to 13 weeks of gestation in hypertensive disorders of pregnancy. Prenat Diagn 2009; 29(9): 847-51.

[94]   Leinonen E, Wathen KA, Alfthan H, *et al.* Maternal serum angiopoietin-1 and-2 and tie-2 in early pregnancy ending in preeclampsia or intrauterine growth retardation. J Clin Endocrinol Metab 2010; 95(1): 126-33.

[95]   Wald NJ, Hackshaw AK. Combining ultrasound and biochemistry in first-trimester screening for Down's syndrome. Prenat Diagn 1997; 17(9): 821-9.

[96]   Cuckle H. Biochemical screening for Down syndrome. Eur J Obstet Gynecol Reprod Biol 2000; 92(1): 97-101.

[97]   Chesley LC, Cunningham FG, Lindheimer MD, Roberts JM. Chesley's hypertensive disorders in pregnancy. 3rd ed. Boston: Academic Press 2009.

[98]   Jauniaux E, Gulbis B, Tunkel S, Ramsay B, Campbell S, Meuris S. Maternal serum testing for alpha-fetoprotein and human chorionic gonadotropin in high-risk pregnancies. Prenat Diagn 1996; 16(12): 1129-35.

[99]   Audibert F, Benchimol Y, Benattar C, Champagne C, Frydman R. Prediction of preeclampsia or intrauterine growth restriction by second trimester serum screening and uterine Doppler velocimetry. Fetal Diagn Ther 2005; 20(1): 48-53.

[100] Cole LA. Hyperglycosylated hCG, a review. Placenta 2010; 31(8): 653-64.

[101] Ong C, Liao A, Spencer K, Munim S, Nicolaides K. First trimester maternal serum free B human chorionic gonadotrophin and pregnancy-associated plasma protein A as predictors of pregnancy complications. BJOG 2000; 107(10): 1265-70.

[102] Spencer K, Cowans NJ, Nicolaides KH. Maternal serum inhibin-A and activin-A levels in the first trimester of pregnancies developing pre-eclampsia. Ultrasound Obstet Gynecol 2008; 32(5): 622-6.

[103] Aquilina J, Thompson O, Thilaganathan B, Harrington K. Improved early prediction of pre-eclampsia by combining second-trimester maternal serum inhibin-A and uterine artery Doppler. Ultrasound Obstet Gynecol. Clinical Trial Controlled Clinical Trial 2001; 17(6): 477-84.

[104] Florio P, Reis F, Pezzani I, Severi F, Petraglia F. The addition of activin A and inhibin A measurement to uterine Doppler velocimetry to improve the early prediction of preeclampsia. Ultrasound Obstet Gynecol 2003; 21: 165-9.

[105] Irwin JC, Suen LF, Martina NA, Mark SP, Giudice LC. Role of the IGF system in trophoblast invasion and pre-eclampsia. Hum Reprod 1999; (Suppl 2): 90-6.

[106] Spencer K, Cowans NJ, Nicolaides KH. Low levels of maternal serum PAPP-A in the first trimester and the risk of pre-eclampsia. Prenat Diagn 2008; 28(1): 7-10.

[107] Spencer CA, Allen VM, Flowerdew G, Dooley K, Dodds L. Low levels of maternal serum PAPP-A in early pregnancy and the risk of adverse outcomes. Prenat Diagn 2008; 28(11): 1029-36.

[108] Than NG, Pick E, Bellyei S, *et al.* Functional analyses of placental protein 13/galectin-13. Eur J Biochem 2004; 271(6): 1065-78.

[109] Nicolaides KH, Bindra R, Turan OM, *et al.* A novel approach to first-trimester screening for early pre-eclampsia combining serum PP-13 and Doppler ultrasound. Ultrasound Obstet Gynecol 2006; 27(1): 13-7.

[110] Poon LC, Maiz N, Valencia C, Plasencia W, Nicolaides KH. First-trimester maternal serum pregnancy-associated plasma protein-A and pre-eclampsia. Ultrasound Obstet Gynecol 2009; 33(1): 23-33.

[111] Sifakis S, Zaravinos A, Maiz N, Spandidos DA, Nicolaides KH. First-trimester maternal plasma cell-free fetal DNA and preeclampsia. Am J Obstet Gynecol 2009; 201(5): 472 e1-7.

[112] Lo YM, Corbetta N, Chamberlain PF, *et al.* Presence of fetal DNA in maternal plasma and serum. Lancet 1997; 350(9076): 485-7.

[113] Leung TN, Zhang J, Lau TK, Hjelm NM, Lo YM. Maternal plasma fetal DNA as a marker for preterm labour. Lancet 1998; 352(9144): 1904-5.

[114] Ariga H, Ohto H, Busch MP, *et al.* Kinetics of fetal cellular and cell-free DNA in the maternal circulation during and after pregnancy: implications for noninvasive prenatal diagnosis. Transfusion 2001; 41(12): 1524-30.

[115] Chan LY, Leung TN, Chan KC, *et al.* Serial analysis of fetal DNA concentrations in maternal plasma in late pregnancy. Clin Chem 2003; 49(4): 678-80.

[116] Farina A, Sekizawa A, Sugito Y, *et al.* Fetal DNA in maternal plasma as a screening variable for preeclampsia : A preliminary non-parametric analysis of detection rate in low-risk nonsymptomatic patients. Prenat Diagn 2004; 24: 83-6.

[117] Farina A, Sekizawa A, Rizzo N, *et al.* Cell-free fetal DNA (SRY locus) concentration in maternal plasma is directly correlated to the time elapsed from the onset of preeclampsia to the collection of blood. Prenat Diagn 2004; 24(4): 293-7.

[118] Farina A, Sekizawa A, Iwasaki M, Matsuoka R, Ichizuka K, Okai T. Total cell-free DNA (beta-globin gene) distribution in maternal plasma at the second trimester: a new prospective for preeclampsia screening. Prenat Diagn 2004; 24(9): 722-6.

[119] Purwosunu Y, Sekizawa A, Okazaki S, *et al.* Prediction of preeclampsia by analysis of cell-free messenger RNA in maternal plasma. Am J Obstet Gynecol 2009; 200(4): 386 e1-7.

[120] Diesch CH, Holzgreve W, Hahn S, Zhong XY. Comparison of activin A and cell-free fetal DNA levels in maternal plasma from patients at high risk for preeclampsia. Prenat Diagn 2006; 26(13): 1267-70.

[121] Sekizawa A, Purwosunu Y, Farina A, *et al.* Prediction of pre-eclampsia by an analysis of placenta-derived cellular mRNA in the blood of pregnant women at 15-20 weeks of gestation. BJOG 2010; 117(5): 557-64.

[122] Chim SS, Tong YK, Chiu RW, *et al.* Detection of the placental epigenetic signature of the maspin gene in maternal plasma. Proc Natl Acad Sci U S A 2005; 102(41): 14753-8.

[123] Tsui NB, Dennis Lo YM. Placental RNA in maternal plasma: toward noninvasive fetal gene expression profiling. Ann N Y Acad Sci 2006; 1075: 96-102.

[124] Poon LL, Leung TN, Lau TK, Lo YM. Presence of fetal RNA in maternal plasma. Clin Chem 2000; 46(11): 1832-4.

[125] Ng EK, Tsui NB, Lau TK, *et al.* mRNA of placental origin is readily detectable in maternal plasma. Proc Natl Acad Sci U S A 2003;100(8): 4748-53.

[126] Tsui NB, Ng EK, Lo YM. Molecular analysis of circulating RNA in plasma. Methods Mol Biol 2006; 336: 123-34.

[127] Ng EK, Leung TN, Tsui NB, *et al.* The concentration of circulating corticotropin-releasing hormone mRNA in maternal plasma is increased in preeclampsia. Clin Chem 2003; 49(5): 727-31.

[128] Oudejans CB, Go AT, Visser A, *et al.* Detection of chromosome 21-encoded mRNA of placental origin in maternal plasma. Clin Chem 2003; 49(9): 1445-9.

[129] Purwosunu Y, Sekizawa A, Farina A, *et al.* Cell-free mRNA concentrations of CRH, PLAC1, and selectin-P are increased in the plasma of pregnant women with preeclampsia. Prenat Diagn 2007; 27(8): 772-7.

[130] Purwosunu Y, Sekizawa A, Farina A, *et al.* Evaluation of physiological alterations of the placenta through analysis of cell-free messenger ribonucleic acid concentrations of angiogenic factors. Am J Obstet Gynecol 2008; 198(1): 124 e1-7.

[131] Purwosunu Y, Sekizawa A, Koide K, *et al.* Cell-free mRNA concentrations of plasminogen activator inhibitor-1 and tissue-type plasminogen activator are increased in the plasma of pregnant women with preeclampsia. Clin Chem 2007; 53(3): 399-404.

[132] Alberry MS, Maddocks DG, Hadi MA, *et al.* Quantification of cell free fetal DNA in maternal plasma in normal pregnancies and in pregnancies with placental dysfunction. Am J Obstet Gynecol 2009; 200(1): 98 e1-6.

[133] Al Nakib M, Desbriere R, Bonello N, *et al.* Total and fetal cell-free DNA analysis in maternal blood as markers of placental insufficiency in intrauterine growth restriction. Fetal Diagn Ther 2009; 26(1): 24-8.

[134] Senna AA, Zedan M, el-Salam GE, el-Mashad AI. Study of plasma adrenomedullin level in normal pregnancy and preeclampsia. Medscape J Med 2008; 10(2): 29.

[135] Gratton RJ, Gluszynski M, Mazzuca DM, Nygard K, Han VK. Adrenomedullin messenger ribonucleic acid expression in the placentae of normal and preeclamptic pregnancies. J Clin Endocrinol Metab 2003; 88(12): 6048-55.

[136] Al-Ghafra A, Gude NM, Brennecke SP, King RG. Increased adrenomedullin protein content and mRNA expression in human fetal membranes but not placental tissue in pre-eclampsia. Mol Hum Reprod 2006; 12(3): 181-6.

[137] Chavarria ME, Lara-Gonzalez L, Garcia-Paleta Y, Vital-Reyes VS, Reyes A. Adhesion molecules changes at 20 gestation weeks in pregnancies complicated by preeclampsia. Eur J Obstet Gynecol Reprod Biol 2008; 137(2): 157-64.

[138] Polgar J, Matuskova J, Wagner DD. The P-selectin, tissue factor, coagulation triad. J Thromb Haemost 2005; 3(8): 1590-6.

[139] Poon LC, Akolekar R, Lachmann R, Beta J, Nicolaides KH. Hypertensive disorders in pregnancy: screening by biophysical and biochemical markers at 11-13 weeks. Ultrasound Obstet Gynecol 2010; 35(6): 662-70.

[140] Krauss T, Emons G, Kuhn W, Augustin HG. Predictive value of routine circulating soluble endothelial cell adhesion molecule measurements during pregnancy. Clin Chem 2002; 48(9): 1418-25.

[141] Kristensen K, Wide-Swensson D, Schmidt C, *et al.* Cystatin C, beta-2-microglobulin and beta-trace protein in pre-eclampsia. Acta Obstet Gynecol Scand 2007; 86(8): 921-6.

[142] Kristensen K, Larsson I, Hansson SR. Increased cystatin C expression in the pre-eclamptic placenta. Mol Hum Repro. 2007; 13(3): 189-95.

[143] Ruma M, Boggess K, Moss K, *et al.* Maternal periodontal disease, systemic inflammation, and risk for preeclampsia. Am J Obstet Gynecol 2008; 198(4): 389 e1-5.

[144] UstUn Y, Engin-UstUn Y, Ozkaplan E, Otlu B, Sait TekerekoGlu M. Association of Helicobacter pylori infection with systemic inflammation in preeclampsia. J Matern Fetal Neonatal Med 2010; 23(4): 311-4.

[145] Stefanovic M, Vukomanovic P, Milosavljevic M, Kutlesic R, Popovic J, Tubic-Pavlovic A. Insulin resistance and C-reactive protein in preeclampsia. Bosn J Basic Med Sci 2009; 9(3): 235-8.

[146] Derzsy Z, Prohaszka Z, Rigo J, Jr., Fust G, Molvarec A. Activation of the complement system in normal pregnancy and preeclampsia. Mol Immunol 2010; 47(7-8): 1500-6.

[147] Swellam M, Samy N, Wahab SA, Ibrahim MS. Emerging role of endothelial and inflammatory markers in preeclampsia. Dis Markers 2009; 26(3): 127-33.

[148] Ouyang YQ, Li SJ, Zhang Q, Cai HB, Chen HP. Interactions between inflammatory and oxidative stress in preeclampsia. Hypertens Pregnancy 2009; 28(1): 56-62.

[149] von Versen-Hoeynck FM, Hubel CA, Gallaher MJ, Gammill HS, Powers RW. Plasma levels of inflammatory markers neopterin, sialic acid, and C-reactive protein in pregnancy and preeclampsia. Am J Hypertens 2009; 22(6): 687-92.

[150] Paternoster DM, Fantinato S, Stella A, *et al.* C-reactive protein in hypertensive disorders in pregnancy. Clin Appl Thromb Hemost 2006; 12(3): 330-7.

[151] Cetin I, Cozzi V, Papageorghiou AT, *et al.* First trimester PTX3 levels in women who subsequently develop preeclampsia and fetal growth restriction. Acta Obstet Gynecol Scand 2009; 88(7): 846-9.

[152] Grill S, Rusterholz C, Zanetti-Dallenbach R, *et al.* Potential markers of preeclampsia--a review. Reprod Biol Endocrinol 2009; 7:70.

[153] Cetin I, Cozzi V, Pasqualini F, *et al.* Elevated maternal levels of the long pentraxin 3 (PTX3) in preeclampsia and intrauterine growth restriction. Am J Obstet Gynecol 2006; 194(5): 1347-53.

[154] Akolekar R, Casagrandi D, Livanos P, Tetteh A, Nicolaides KH. Maternal plasma pentraxin 3 at 11 to 13 weeks of gestation in hypertensive disorders of pregnancy. Prenat Diagn 2009; 29(10): 934-8.

[155] Mignini LE, Latthe PM, Villar J, Kilby MD, Carroli G, Khan KS. Mapping the theories of preeclampsia: the role of homocysteine. Obstet Gynecol 2005; 105(2): 411-25.

[156] Poon LC, Chelemen T, Granvillano O, Pandeva I, Nicolaides KH. First-trimester maternal serum a disintegrin and metalloprotease 12 (ADAM12) and adverse pregnancy outcome. Obstet Gynecol 2008; 112(5): 1082-90.

[157] Spencer K, Cowans NJ, Stamatopoulou A. ADAM12s in maternal serum as a potential marker of pre-eclampsia. Prenat Diagn 2008; 28(3): 212-6.

[158] Mazaki-Tovi S, Vaisbuch E, Romero R, *et al.* Maternal plasma concentration of the pro-inflammatory adipokine pre-B-cell-enhancing factor (PBEF)/visfatin is elevated in pregnant patients with acute pyelonephritis. Am J Reprod Immunol 2010; 63(3): 252-62.

[159] Gok DE, Yazici M, Uckaya G, *et al.* The Role of Visfatin in the Pathogenesis of Gestational Diabetes Mellitus. J Endocrinol Invest 2011; 34(1): 3-7.

[160] Mazaki-Tovi S, Romero R, Kim SK, *et al.* Could alterations in maternal plasma visfatin concentration participate in the phenotype definition of preeclampsia and SGA? J Matern Fetal Neonatal Med 2010; 23(8): 857-868.

[161] Steel SA, Pearce JM, Nash G, Christopher B, Dormandy J, Bland JM. Maternal blood viscosity and uteroplacental blood flow velocity waveforms in normal and complicated pregnancies. Br J Obstet Gynaecol 1988; 95(8): 747-52.

[162] Papageorghiou AT, Leslie K. Uterine artery Doppler in the prediction of adverse pregnancy outcome. Curr Opin Obstet Gynecol 2007; 19(2): 103-9.

[163] Sciscione AC, Hayes EJ. Uterine artery Doppler flow studies in obstetric practice. Am J Obstet Gynecol 2009; 201(2): 121-6.

[164] Romero R, Kusanovic JP, Than NG, *et al.* First-trimester maternal serum PP13 in the risk assessment for preeclampsia. Am J Obstet Gynecol 2008; 199(2): 122 e1-e11.

[165] Spencer K, Cowans NJ, Chefetz I, Tal J, Kuhnreich I, Meiri H. Second-trimester uterine artery Doppler pulsatility index and maternal serum PP13 as markers of pre-eclampsia. Prenat Diagn 2007; 27(3): 258-63.

[166] Akolekar R, Minekawa R, Veduta A, Romero XC, Nicolaides KH. Maternal plasma inhibin A at 11-13 weeks of gestation in hypertensive disorders of pregnancy. Prenat Diagn 2009; 29(8): 753-60.

[167] Poon LC, Kametas NA, Maiz N, Akolekar R, Nicolaides KH. First-trimester prediction of hypertensive disorders in pregnancy. Hypertension 2009; 53(5): 812-8.

[168] Savvidou MD, Akolekar R, Zaragoza E, Poon LC, Nicolaides KH. First trimester urinary placental growth factor and development of pre-eclampsia. BJOG 2009; 116(5): 643-7.

[169] Cuckle HS. Screening for pre-eclampsia--lessons from aneuploidy screening. Placenta 2011; (Suppl 32): S42-8.

[170] Akolekar R, Syngelaki A, Sarquis R, Zvanca M, Nicolaides KH. Prediction of early, intermediate and late pre-eclampsia from maternal factors, biophysical and biochemical markers at 11-13 weeks. Prenat Diagn 2011; 31(1): 66-74.

CHAPTER 5

Immune System and Perinatal Outcomes

Shigeru Saito*

Department of Obstetrics and Gynecology, University of Toyama, 2630 Sugitani Toyama-shi, Toyama 930-0194 Japan

Abstract: Pregnancy represents a semiallograft to a maternal host. To prevent semiallograft rejection, the maternal immune system dramatically changes to a unique immune system during pregnancy. Maladaptation of this system could cause implantation failure, recurrent spontaneous abortion, preeclampsia and preterm delivery. The objective of this report is to review the pathophysiology of these events in human pregnancy from the aspects of reproductive immunology.

Keywords: Miscarriage, preeclampsia, pregnancy, preterm labor, reproductive immunology.

INTRODUCTION

Successful embryo implantation requires the synchronization of embryo development and uterine preparation. The major histocompatibility complex (MHC) antigens are already expressed on the surface of the fetal cells or trophoblasts; therefore, maternal (endometrial) immune cells play a role in the maintenance of pregnancy *via* a tolerance system. Thus, the process of implantation should include mechanisms that prevent allograft rejection. For preventing allograft rejection, the maternal immune system dramatically changes after pregnancy, especially at the feto-maternal interface. Decidual lymphocyte subsets are quite different from those of non-pregnant endometrium and those of peripheral blood. Placental tissue produces a variety of cytokines and hormones that are essential for the regulation of the feto-maternal unit. To understand the immune system during pregnancy, it is helpful to know the pathophysiology of abnormal pregnancy such as implantation failure, unknown recurrent spontaneous abortion (URSA), preeclampsia (PE), and preterm delivery (PTD).

IMMUNE SYSTEM DURING PREGNANCY

The immune system is classified into the innate immune system and adaptive (specific) immune system (Fig. **1**). Pathogens are firstly recognized by the pattern recognition receptors such as Toll-like receptors (TLR) on neutrophils and monocytes belonging to the innate immune system. The TLRs are related to immune responses to Gram negative bacteria, Gram positive bacteria, mycoplasma, fungus and virus, and stimulation of TLRs result in the production of inflammatory cytokines. NK cells are classified into $CD16^+CD56^{dim}$ NK cells and $CD16\text{-}CD56^{bright}$ NK cells (Fig. **1**). These NK cells are characterized by cytoplasmic granules that contain cytotoxic molecules such as perforin, granzymes, and granulysin, and they have cytolytic activity against cells lacking surface major histocompatibility complex (MHC) class I antigen, virus infected cells or tumor cells.

Complement is a core component of the immune system, and over 30 proteins act in concert to protect the host against invading organisms. They promote chemotaxis of inflammatory cells, and generate proteolytic fragments that enhance phagocytosis by neutrophils and monocytes (Fig. **1**). Dendritic cells (DCs) are a heterogeneous population of cells that initiate and coordinate the innate and adaptive immune responses (Fig. **1**). DCs firstly phagocytose bacterial pathogens and digest them. DCs present these digested peptides to adaptive immune cells inducing antibody production or cell-mediated immunity.

In the adaptive immune system, T cells and B cells play central roles. T cells are classified into $CD4^+$ helper

---

*Address correspondence to Shigeru Saito: Department of Obstetrics and Gynecology, University of Toyama, 2630 Sugitani Toyama-shi, Toyama 930-0194 Japan; Tel: +81-76-434-7355, Fax: +81-76-434-5036, E-mail: s30saito@med.u-toyama.ac.jp

T cells and CD8$^+$ cytotoxic T cells (Fig. **1**). CD4$^+$ T helper T cells are further classified into Th1 cells involved in cell-mediated immunity or rejection, Th2 cells involved in antibody production, Th3 and Tr1 cells involved in immunosuppression, and Th17 cells involved in inflammation and autoimmune disease, based on their cytokine profile (Fig. **1**). CD4$^+$CD25$^+$ regulatory T (Treg) cells play a central role for induction and maintenance of tolerance (Fig. **1**). Murine studies show that depletion of Treg cells leads to autoimmune diseases and abortion in allogeneic pregnancy [1-3]. B cells differentiate into plasma cells and produce antigen-specific antibodies. In this step, DCs, T cells and B cells interact.

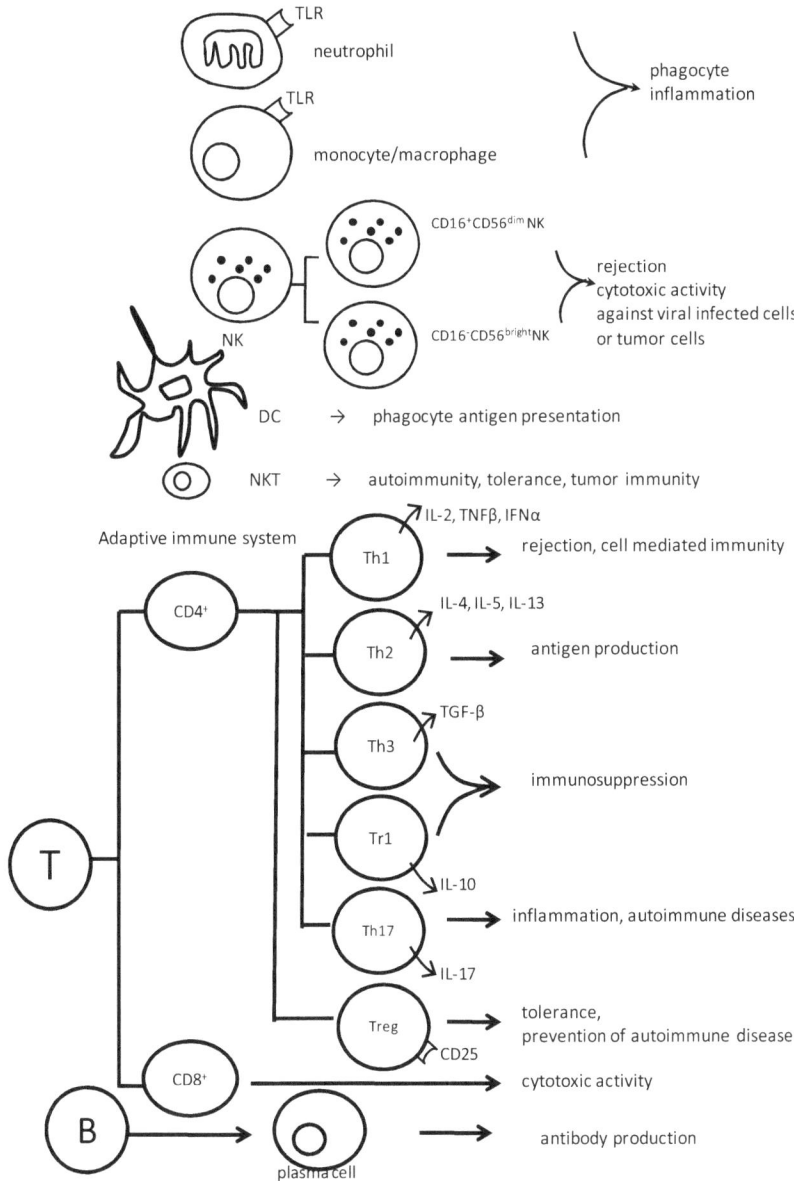

Figure 1: Immune system.

During pregnancy, the numbers of peripheral blood neutrophils and monocytes increase and these functions are also up-regulated [4] because cell-mediated immune systems such as Th1 cells and CD8$^+$T cells are suppressed (Table **1**). This is recognized as a complementary effect in the immune system during pregnancy. NK cell-cytotoxic activity is decreased during the pregnancy period especially in late pregnancy (Table **1**). Augmented NK cell-cytotoxic activity by IL-2 or TNFα induces abortion in mice, and NK cells could induce apoptosis in extravillous trophoblasts in human miscarriage cases [5]. Therefore, NK cell cytotoxic activity during pregnancy is suppressed in order to prevent pregnancy loss. One of the major roles of NK cells is to protect against viral infection, and therefore decreased NK cell-cytotoxic activity induces susceptibility to viral infection. Indeed, we know viral infection such as influenza or measles in pregnant women induces serious illness. We have experienced that pregnant women have an extremely high risk for H1N1 influenza infection [6]. TLR is expressed not only on neutrophils and monocytes but also on trophoblast [7, 8]. Virus-derived double-stranded RNA could stimulate the innate immune system and trophoblasts. The innate immune system is primed during pregnancy [9], and therefore excessive inflammation easily appears during pregnancy, resulting in miscarriage or preterm delivery in viral infection during pregnancy. This is derived from the specific immune environment in pregnancy.

The adaptive immune system also changes during pregnancy. Th1 type immunity is suppressed for preventing fetal rejection, and therefore the symptoms of rheumatoid arthritis (RA), which involves Th1 type cells, are decreased during pregnancy [10] (Table **1**).

These specialized immune conditions play important roles for maintenance of pregnancy, but maladaptation of this system might cause implantation failure, recurrent pregnancy loss, preeclampsia (PE) or preterm delivery (PTD).

CONTRIBUTION OF IMMUNOCOMPETENT CELLS TO EMBRYO IMPLANTATION

Human decidua contains potent HLA-DR$^+$CD83$^+$ immunostimulatory-and CD123-myeloid lineage DCs and these DC cells contact uterine NK cells [11, 12]. This contact is important to induce proliferation of uterine cells and to reduce the production of Th1 type cytokines such as IL-12 and TNF-α. Human myeloid DCs produce proangio-genic factors, such as vascular endothelial growth factor (VEGF), fibroblast growth factor (FGF)-2 and endothelin-1 (ET-1), and mouse CD11C$^+$ DCs mediate VEGF-dependent vascular growth, which is necessary for successful implantation. DC-SIGN$^+$-DCs are absent in the non-pregnant uterus, but these cells increase in number within 1 week of implantation in Rhesus monkey [13]. Very importantly, DCs are only found adjacent to the implantation. These findings suggest that DC function seems to be of great importance for a successful pregnancy. Recent data show that uterine DCs are crucial for successful implantation [14, 15]. Depletion of DCs using CD11C-diphtheria toxin receptor transgenic mice resulted in severe impairment of the implantation process, impairment of NK cell maturation, and abnormal placental development, leading to embryo resorption. DC is an antigen-presenting cell, and therefore fetal antigen presentation by DCs might be necessary for successful pregnancy in allogeneic pregnancy.

Table 1: Immune System During Pregnancy

Innate immunity		
neutrophils :	number↑ function↑ priming(+)	
monocytes :	number↑ function↑ priming(+)	
NK cells :	CD16$^+$CD56^{dim}NK cells : number↓ cytotoxic activity↓	
	CD16$^-$CD56^{bright}NK cells: •increase in decidua	
	•produce variety of cytokines	
	•induce angiogenesis	
complements:	enhance	
DCs :	accumulate in pregnant uterus,	
	induce tissue remodeling and angiogenesis	
Adaptive immunity		
CD4 cells Th1 cells :	suppressed↓	
Th2 cells :	increased↑	
Th3 cells :	increased↑	
Tr1 cells :	increased↑	
Th17 cells :	unchanged or suppressed in late pregnancy	
Treg cells :	increased↑	
CD8 cells :	the function is slightly suppressed	
B cells :	the function and number is not changed	

However, Placks *et al.* reported that depletion of uterine DCs also caused embryo resorption in syngeneic and T-cell deficient pregnancies [15]. These findings suggest that DCs appear to govern principal uterine receptivity by regulating tissue remodeling and angiogenesis, independent of the immunological tolerance. They showed that uterine DCs directly induce decidual angiogenesis.

$CD4^+CD25^+$ Treg cells play central roles for induction and maintenance of pregnancy [2, 3, 16]. Interestingly, $CD4^+CD25^+$ Treg cells increased in number in uterine draining lymph nodes before the implantation period (2 days after mating) [17]. At the implantation period (4.5 days after mating), accumulation of Treg cells is observed in the uterus. Seminal plasma priming is necessary for this Treg cells expansion in draining lymph nodes and uterus [17]. Treg cell expansion is observed in syngeneic pregnancy [2] suggesting that pregnancy hormone such as estrogen [18] or hCG [19] might accumulate Treg cells at the feto-maternal interface. But an increased number of Treg cells is observed in allogeneic pregnancy compared with syngeneic pregnancy [20] suggesting that increased Treg size might play a role in successful pregnancy. Depletion of Treg cells using anti CD25 monoclonal antibody during the implantation period induced implantation failure in an allogeneic pregnancy model [3, 21] or abortion prone model [22]. This antibody treatment induced an increase in activated $CD4^+$-and $CD8^+$-T cells in the uterine draining lymph node in an allogeneic pregnancy model [4] suggesting that T cells are activated in the Treg cell depletion state. But this antibody treatment does not affect the implantation in a syngeneic pregnancy mice model [3, 21]. These findings clearly show that fetal alloantigens are recognized by maternal T cells, and embryos are easily rejected when Treg cells are absent.

Possible contributions of hormone, cytokine and immunocompetent cells in implantation are shown in Fig. **2**. Progesterone is an essential factor for the decidualization. Leukemia inhibitory factor (LIF) is a cytokine discovered to be essential for implantation in mice. LIF expression in the uterine gland induces endometrial receptivity, and LIF also enhances extravillous trophoblast (EVT) adhesion and invasion (Fig. **2**). In addition, DCs are essential cells for the induction of successful implantation [14, 15]. DCs produce sFlt-1 and TGF-β [15], and NK cells produce VEGF [12]. Therefore DCs and NK cells control angiogenesis resulting in successful implantation (Fig. **2**). Interestingly, Th1-induced IL-12 production by uterine DCs is dramatically abrogated in the presence of uterine NK cells [12]. Therefore, DC and NK cell interaction regulates Th1-cell induced rejection resulting in successful implantation (Fig. **2**). Robertson *et al.* reported that seminal plasma drives expansion of Treg cells in uterine draining lymph nodes before implantation [17]. And human chorionic gonadotropin attracts Treg cells into the fetomaternal interface [19] (Fig. **2**). These Treg cells protect the fetus from maternal T cell-attack. Jasper *et al.* reported that primary unexplained infertility is associated with reduced expression of the Treg-cell transcription factor Foxp3 in endometrium [23] suggesting that reduced Treg cell numbers might be one of the causes of implantation failure in humans.

RECURRENT PREGNANCY LOSS

Recurrent spontaneous abortion (RSA) is defined as the occurrence of three or more spontaneous abortions and occurs in about 2-4% of women. About 50% of these cases are unexplained. Maladaptation of immunological tolerance might be the cause of these cases. And about 10% of RSA cases express antiphospholipid antibodies (aPL), and experimental animal models revealed that antiphospholipid antibodies induce fetal loss and growth restriction (IUGR).

Antiphospholipid Antibody in RSA

The antiphospholipid syndrome (APS) is defined by recurrent pregnancy loss and thrombosis in the presence of aPL antibodies [24]. The most frequently serological markers for APS are anticardiolipin antibodies (aCL), anti-β_2-glycoprotein I antibody and lupus anticoagulant. When aCL or anti-β_2 GP1 antibodies bind to β_2 GP1 molecules expressed on trophoblast, a complement cascade is activated (Fig. **3**). C5a activates endothelial cells and platelets, resulting in formation of thrombosis in blood vessel [25] (Fig. **2**). On the other hand, C5a activates neutrophils and induces cell injury of trophoblast by neutrophil attack resulting in abortion (Fig. **3**). C5a also stimulates monocytes and augments sFlt-1 production by monocytes. Soluble Flt-1 inhibits VEGF, resulting in poor angiogenesis and growth restriction in preeclampsia [26] (Fig. **3**).

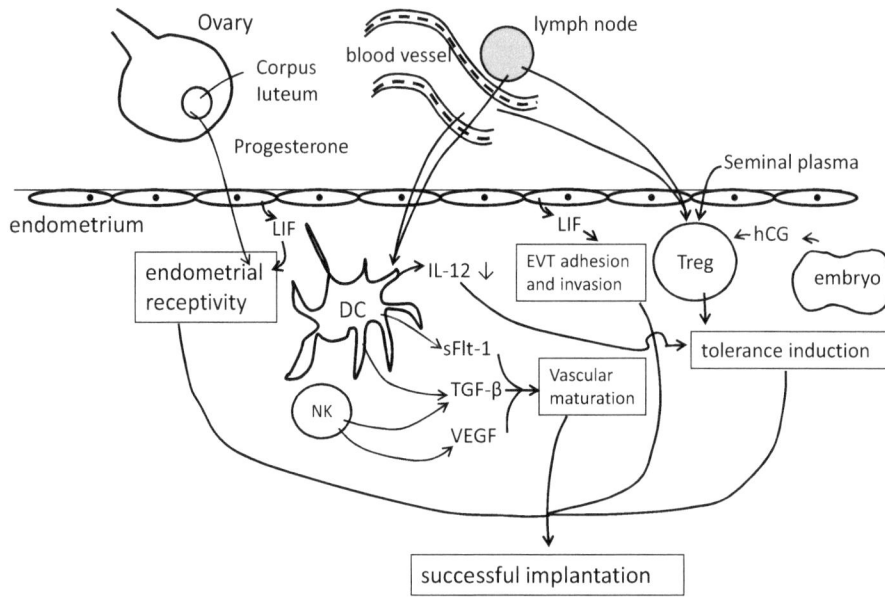

Figrue 2: Possible contribution of hormone, cytokine and immunocompetent cells in implantation.

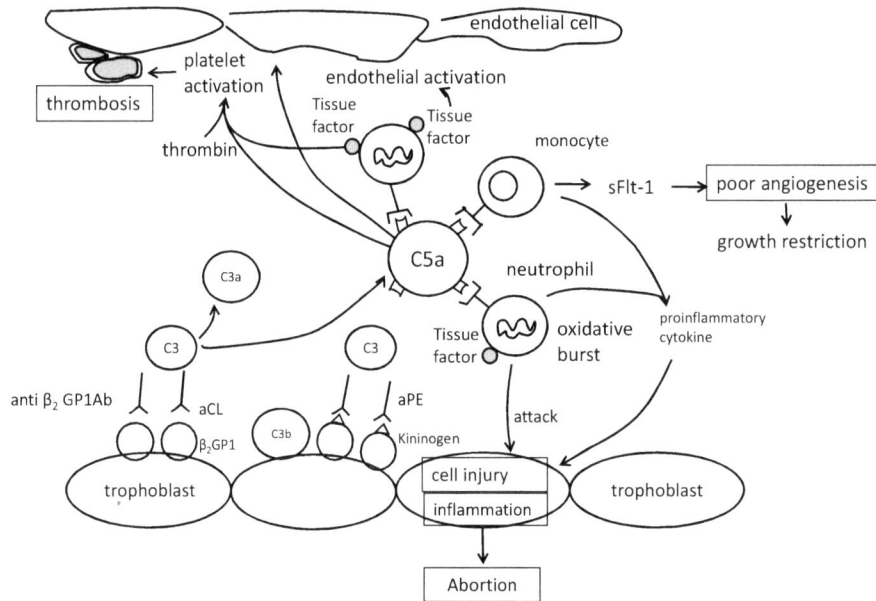

Figure 3: Mechanism of aPL induced abortion or IUGR.

Heparin is widely used for anticoagulant treatment and is used to prevent recurrent pregnancy loss in aPA positive cases. Recently, Girardi *et al.* reported that treatment with heparin prevented complement activation and protected mice from pregnancy complications induced by aPL antibodies [27]. Anticoagulant therapy such as fondaparinux or hirudin treatment did not protect pregnant mice from aPL antibody.

Immunological Changes in Unexplained Recurrent Spontaneous Abortion

Th1/Th2 Balance in Normal Pregnancy and Recurrent Spontaneous Abortion

Th1-dependent effector mechanisms such as cytotoxic T lymphocyte (CTL) activity play a role in acute allograft rejection (Fig. **1**). Wegmann *et al.* hypothesized that physiological fetal-protection from maternal rejection is due to a Th2-type response at the maternal-fetal interface in mice [10]. In humans, peripheral blood Th1/Th2 balance during pregnancy is controversial because the amplitude of this balance is very small [28]. On the other hand, the Th1/Th2 balance in decidua changes to a Th2-predominant state [28]. Thus, the local immune condition shifts to a Th2 predominant state in human pregnancy, but it is very difficult to determine the endometrial immune condition by checking peripheral blood-Th1/Th2 balance. This is a dilemma in clinical medicine. Hill *et al.* first reported that Th1 type cytokine secretion by peripheral blood was observed in RSA patients [29]. Piccinni *et al.* also reported decreased Th2 type immunity in the decidua of RSA cases [30]. After that, several conflicting studies have been published [31]. Therefore it is not known whether predominant Th1 type immunity is the major cause of RSA or not. In my opinion, the etiology of RSA is heterogeneous, and therefore excessive Th1 type immunity may cause abortion in some limiting RSA cases.

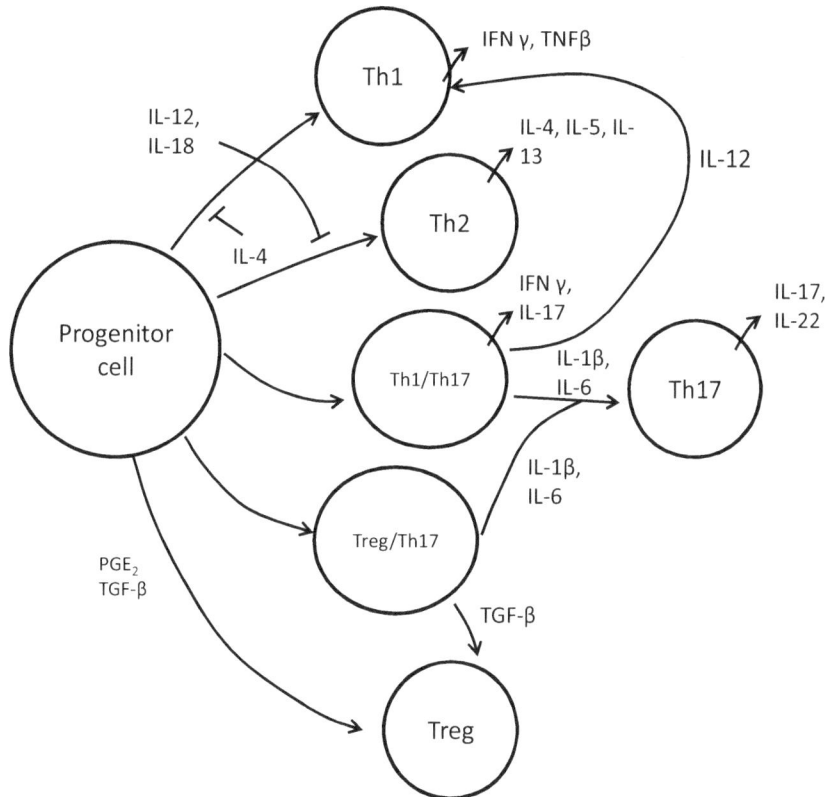

Figure 4: Th1, Th2, Th17 and Treg cell development from CD4+ progenitor cells.

Th1/Th2/Th17 and Treg Balance in Normal Pregnancy and Recurrent Spontaneous Abortion

The Th1/Th2 paradigm has now developed into the Th1/Th2/Th17 and Treg paradigm (Figs. **4** and **5**). Th1 cells are involved in cellular immunity and Th2 cells are involved in humoral immunity. Th17 cells produce the proinflammatory cytokine IL-17 and play important roles for induction of inflammation and autoimmune diseases. IL-17 also plays an important role for the defense system to bacterial and fungal infection. Treg cells are potent suppressors of autoimmunity and allograft rejection. Treg cells are increased in the peripheral blood, decidual tissue and lymph nodes draining into the uterus in murine and human pregnancy [2, 3, 17, 22, 32]. Allogeneic pregnancy leads to a greater increase in Treg cell numbers in mice [20], and HLA-C mismatch leads to increased numbers of decidual Treg number in humans [33], suggesting that Treg cells should play an essential role for maintenance of allogeneic pregnancy (Fig. **5**). Deletion or depletion of Treg cells induces abortion in an allogeneic pregnancy model in mice [2, 3]. Furthermore, abortion-prone CBA/J mice mated with DBA/2J males show a decreased number of Treg cells, and adoptive transfer of Treg cells purified from normal pregnancy mice prevent abortion [22]. Transfer of exogenous Treg cells into abortion-prone mice induces the production of leukemic inhibitory factor (LIF) and TGF-β, but does not affect the production of Th1 type cytokine such as IFNγ and TNFα

[34]. Very interestingly, paternal antigen-specific Treg cells accumulate in uterine draining lymph nodes before the implantation and in the uterus after implantation in mice [17]. In humans, immunosuppressive activity of Treg cells against neonatal lymphocytes is more powerful in decidual Treg cells compared with that in peripheral blood [35], showing paternal antigen-specific Treg cells accumulate in decidua for protecting rejection. Cyclosporin A, a potent immunosuppressant, prevents abortion in abortion-prone mice, and this treatment enhances the expression of CTLA-4 [36]. CTLA-4 is expressed in Treg cells, and therefore this treatment might induce Treg cell expansion. CTLA-4 Ig gene transfer [37] and TGF-β_3 [38] administration also expand Treg cells in abortion-prone mice. Lymphocyte therapy in RSA patients induces the expansion of Treg cells in peripheral blood, and Treg cells are significantly higher in successful pregnancy than in those with pregnancy loss after therapy in humans [38]. These therapeutic trials for preventing abortion show that expansion of Treg cells in RSA cases might be useful therapy for unexplained RSA.

Recent data have revealed important developmental and functional links between induced Treg (iTreg) and Th17 cells. Increased Th17 cells and decreased Treg cells are observed in peripheral blood and decidua of unexplained RSA cases [39] (Fig. **5**). But accumulation of Th17 cells are observed in inevitable abortion cases but not in missed abortion cases [40] suggesting that Th17 cells are involved in the induction of inflammation in the late stage of abortion, but not in the early stage of abortion.

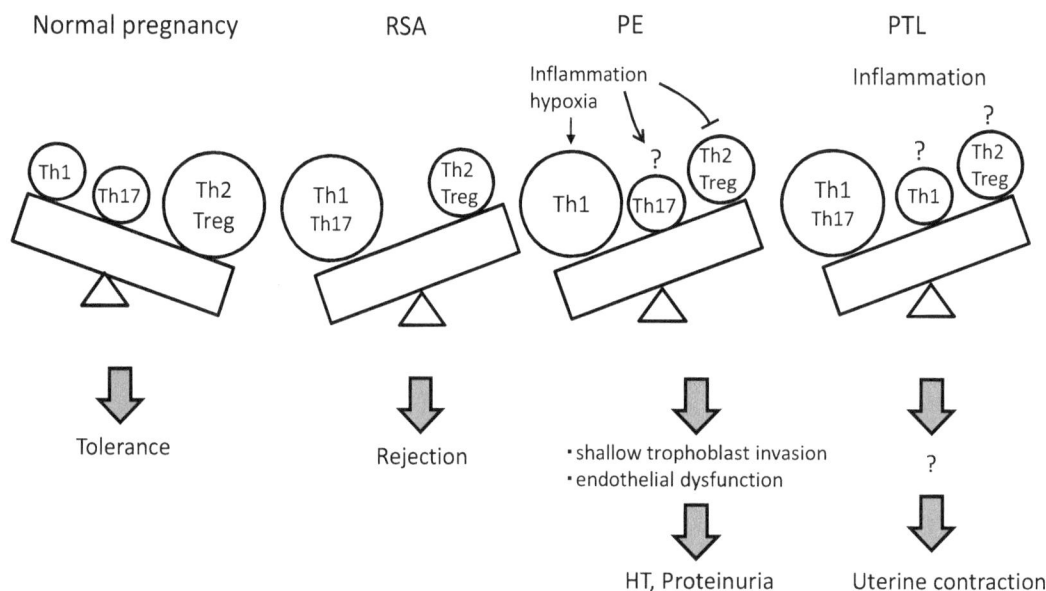

Figure 5: The balance of Th1/Th2/Th17 and Treg cells in normal pregnancy and complicated pregnancy.

NK Cells Profile in RSA

NK cells are found in major components of endometrial lymphocytes in the early pregnancy period. Uterine NK (uNK) cells have less cytotoxic activity and have high capacity to produce immunoregulatory cytokines such as TGF-β and IL-10, and angiogenic growth factors such as VEGF-C, placental growth factor (PlGF), angiopoietin (Ang)-1 and Ang-2 [41]. These NK cells play very important roles for maintenance of pregnancy. But recent data show increased number of uNK cells in RSA. Quenby *et al.* proposed that RSA with increased uNK cell density may appear to be increased angiogenesis and peri-implantation blood flow, which may lead to maternal circulation and hence pregnancy loss due to excessive oxidative stress [42]. Uterine-and peripheral blood-NK cells can be classified into NK1, NK2, NK3 and NKr$_1$ cells by their cytokine profiles [43]. In normal pregnancy, the main populations of decidual NK cells are TGF-β producing NK 3 cells and IL-10 producing NKr$_1$ cells, but IFN-γ or TNF-α producing NK 1 cells increase in miscarriage. Therefore, we should compare not only the number but also the character of uNK cells in RSA.

Our group recently reported that granulysin level in uNK cells was increased, and these NK cells induce apoptosis of extravillous trophoblasts (EVTs) *in vitro* [5]. We also observed nuclear staining of granulysin in EVTs of abortion cases suggesting that activated uNK cells could attack EVTs in human miscarriage [5]. NK cells express activating or inhibitory killer immunoglobulin like receptors on their surface. These profiles are now controversial. The NK cell function is regulated by Treg cells, therefore we should clarify the NK cell and Treg cell profile in detail in the near future.

PATHOPHYSIOLOGY OF PREECLAMPSIA WITH A VIEW POINT OF IMMUNOLOGY

Preeclampsia (PE) occurs in 3-5% of pregnancies and is a major cause of maternal and neonatal morbidity and mortality. Epidemiological evidence strongly support that the immune system is involved in pathophysiology of PE [44] (Table **2**). PE occurs more commonly in first conception, and when the partner is changed, the risk of PE is the same as that in a first pregnancy.

Additionally, an interval from the last delivery is associated with an increasing risk of PE [45]. These findings suggest that memory lymphocytes that induce paternal antigen-specific tolerance are present, and these cells might expand quickly after the next pregnancy, resulting in decreased risk of PE [46]. Only T cells have memory function, and Treg cells play a central role for induction and maintenance of tolerance. Therefore Treg cells might play an important role for reducing PE. Indeed, many papers reported the decreased number of peripheral blood-and decidual-Treg cells in PE [47-49].

The second important epidemiological finding is that short duration of sexual cohabitation or condom use are risk factors for PE. In donated spermatozoa, semen exposure is negative, and the risk of PE is very high [50]. Paternal MHC-class I soluble antigens are present in seminal fluid. It is well known that continuous antigen exposure in mucosal tissue induces tolerance, and therefore sexual cohabitation for a long time might establish paternal antigen-specific tolerance before the pregnancy [46].

A fetus is a semi-allograft to the maternal host. In ovum donation cases, the fetus is a complete allograft, but seminal exposure is positive. The frequency of PE in ovum donation is very high (11.1%) suggesting that complete allograft fetus is a risk for PE [50]. In donated embryos, the fetus is a complete allograft, and semen exposure is negative, and the frequency of PE is elevated to 25% [50]. These findings clearly show that absence of semen exposure and allografted fetus are the greatest risk of PE [44, 46]. These findings suggest that inadequate tolerance induction to paternal alloantigens might induce PE. T cells and NK cells play central roles for induction of tolerance.

Villous trophoblast do not express MHC-class I and MHC-class II antigens on their surface, but extravillous trophoblasts (EVTs) express MHC-class I antigens such as HLA-C, HLA-G, HLA-E. Therefore, EVTs only express polymorphic HLA-C antigens on their surface. These HLA-C molecules are recognized by KIR on NK cells. KIR-A lack activation receptor, and KIR-B possess both activation receptors and inhibitory receptors. These KIR recognize HLA-C1 or HLA-C2. Hiby *et al.* reported that maternal KIR AA genotype is significantly increased in PE when the fetus has an HLA-C2 gene [51]. The prevalence of PE decrease accompanies the increase of the activation receptor of KIR-B. This finding is very interesting in the pathophysiology of PE, but this hypothesis does not explain why the first conception, short cohabitation or donate embryo transfer are risk factors of PE. The frequency of HLA-C2 and KIR-AA are negatively correlated. For example, Japanese people have the highest frequency of KIR-AA genotype and the lowest frequency of HLA-C2 genotype, and Caucasians have moderate frequency of KIR-AA and HLA-C2 genotype. If Hiby's hypothesis is correct, the couples consisting of Japanese women and Caucasian men should have a high risk for PE, because the frequency of maternal KIR AA and fetal HLA-C2 genotype is increased 4 to 5 times higher compared to that in Japanese women and Japanese men couples. Regrettably, the risk of PE in couples consisting of Japanese women and Caucasian men is the same to that of Japanese women and Japanese men couples [52]. The etiology of PE is multifactorial, therefore the combination of KIR AA on maternal NK cells and fetal HLAC2 genotype might explain the pathophysiology in limited PE cases.

Table 2: Epidemiological evidence supporting the relationship between immune maladaptation and PE

1. PE occurs more commonly in first conception. →	Inadequate tolerance induction might induce PE.
2. An increasing interval from the last delivery is associated with an increasing risk of PE. →	Memory T cells that induce paternal antigen specific tolerance decrease in size when the interval from the last delivery is too long.
3. The protective effect of multiparity in PE is lost with the change of partner. →	Paternal antigen-specific Treg cells might decrease the risk of PE.
4. A short duration of sexual cohabitation or condom use increases risk of PE →	Sperm or seminal fluid exposure for a long period might induce paternal Ag-specific tolerance.
5. Frequency of PE in the cases of donated gametes is very high especially in donated embryo. →	Absence of semen exposure and allograft pregnancy induce the greatest risk of PE.
6. Histological changes in the placental bed of women with PE resemble that of acute graft rejection →	Inadequate tolerance induction might induce PE.

In normal pregnancy, all the steps from implantation to the fetal growth period are well organized, but several abnormal findings are observed in the second stage of EVT-invasion period (GW 9-18) and fetal growth period (Fig. **5**). The abnormalities at implantation period and first stage of EVT invasion period in PE are unexplained. Placental bed biopsy at delivery in PE shows shallow EVT invasion and inadequate vascular remodeling in spiral artery causing decreased blood supply to the fetus. Th1 predominant immune condition and decreased Treg cells have been reported in PE cases [44, 47-49] (Fig. **5**). Placental indoleamine-2, 3 dioxygenase (IDO) expression also decreased in PE. As IDO is an enzyme that induces tolerance, this also supports the idea in that PE is associated with inadequate tolerance. Indeed, peripheral blood T cells and NK cells are activated in PE [44]. Activated T cells and NK cells might attack EVT, resulting in shallow trophoblast invasion. But a prospective study to examine these immunological conditions in early pregnancy period has not been performed. If Th1 type immunity or decreased Treg cells are present in the early stage of pregnancy, these markers would be very useful to estimate the risk of PE (Figs. **5** and **6**). Fetal growth speed accelerates after 20 weeks of gestation, and the fetus require a strong nutrient and oxygen supply. In PE cases, vascular remodeling is inadequate, and therefore hypoxic conditions induce aponecrosis of trophoblasts, causing systemic inflammation by the innate immune system [9].

Soluble Flt-1 and sEndoglin 1 are produced by trophoblast in PE. These factors inhibit angiogenesis by regulating VEGF-, PlGF-and TGF-β induced angiogenesis. Interestingly, sEndoglin inhibits TGF-β signal. Recent data have revealed developmental and functional links between induced Treg (iTreg) cells and Th17 cells. TGF-β is a key cytokine that induces Treg cells from Treg/Th17 cells and progenitor T cells (Fig. **7**). Santner-Nannan *et al.* reported an increased number of Th17 cells and decreased number of Treg cells in PE [49]. This finding might be caused by excessive amounts of sEndoglin, which inhibits the differentiation of Treg cells from progenitor cells or Th17/Treg cells (Fig. **6**). Decreased Treg cells in PE induce inadequate tolerance [44] and auto-antibody production [1]. Angiotensin binds to the AT 1 receptor. Recent data show that AT-1 autoantibodies (AT1-AA) have been reported in PE [53]. AT1-AA binds to a 7-amino acid sequence on the second extracellular loop of the AT1 receptor. AT1-AA treatment in pregnant mice induces PE-like symptoms. AngII stimulates sFlt-1 production by human trophoblast through the AT-1 receptor, and therefore AT1-AAs are possible candidates for a stimulus of enhanced synthesis and secretion of sFlt-1 associated with PE (Fig. **7**). Furthermore, we have recently reported a decreased proportion of peripheral blood VEGF-expressing T and NK cells in PE [54]. In standard methods, intracytokine level is evaluated by flow cytometry in activated lymphocytes. In our study, we evaluated intracellular VEGF level without stimulation. Therefore this result directly reflects an *in vivo* cytokine profile. As shown in Fig. **6**, many factors are involved in the pathogenesis of PE.

	Normal pregnancy	PE
Implantation	good	? DC ↓ ? Treg ↓ ?
↓	↓	↓
Placentation 1st stage of EVT invasion (GW ∼9)	good	good
↓	↓	↓ Th1 cells? NK cells
Placentation 2nd stage of EVT invasion (GW 9∼18)	•good •Deep EVT invasion •Adequate blood vessel formation •Normoxia	•disturbed •Shallow EVT invasion •Inadequate blood vessel formation •Hypoxia
↓	↓	ATI-AA ↓ Th1 cells ↑ Treg cells ↓ sFlt-1 ↑, sEndoglin ↑
Fetal growth period (GW 20∼40)	Normotension No protein urea Adequate fetal growth	Hypertension Proteinuria IUGR

Figure 6: Sequential pathophysiology of preeclampsia.

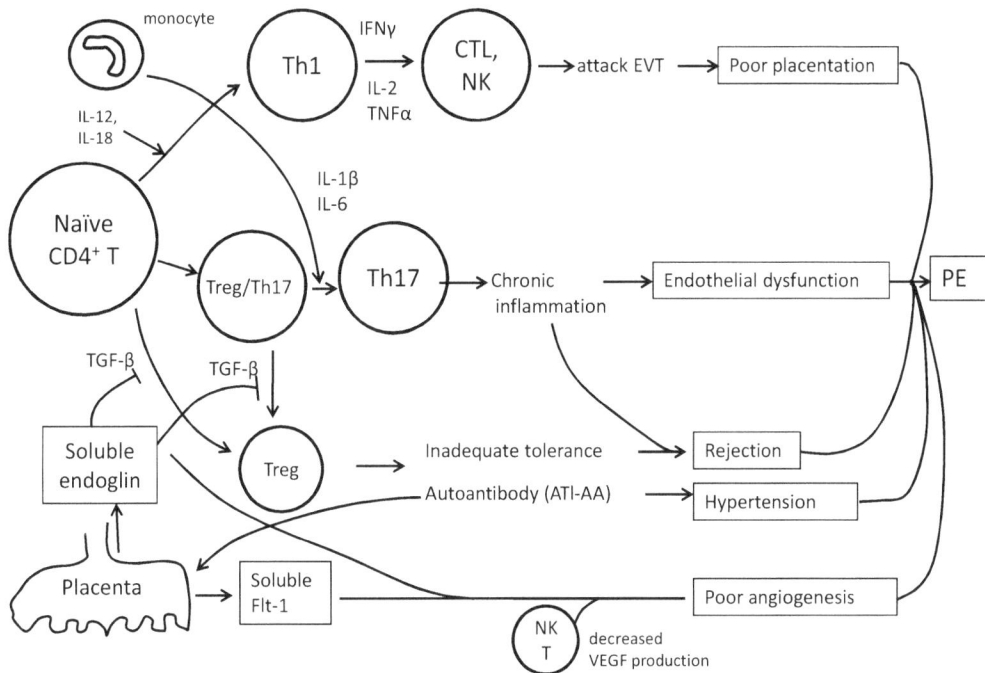

Figure 7: An imbalance in Th1/Th2/Th17 and Treg cells might induce preeclampsia.

PRETERM DELIVERY

Preterm delivery is associated with elevated production of pro-inflammatory cytokines such as IL-1, TNF-α, IL-6 and IL-8 [55]. Progesterone is used for the prevention of preterm birth (PTB) in women with prior PTB and short cervical length [56]. Progesterone reduces the proinflammatory cytokines by macrophage or cervical epithelial cells in response to bacterial products. Progesterone also alters cytokine production of T cell to produce IL-10 [57]. Polymorphisms in the genes that encode the TLRs have been associated with the risk of PTB [58]. And genetic background such as polymorphism in the TNFα gene and environmental factors such as bacterial vaginosis synergistically increased the risk of PTB [59].

Th1/Th2 balance is not dramatically changed in PTB, and the frequency of Treg cells has not been reported. Th17 cells are increased in the chorionic membrane of severe chorioamnionitis complicated cases. IL-17 produced by Th17 cells and TNFα produced by monocytes significantly augment IL-8 secretion by primary cultured amniotic mesenchymal cells [60], suggesting that Th17 cells play an important role for induction of inflammation at the feto-maternal interface.

T and B cell deficient RAG1-/-mice are more susceptible to PTD by LPS treatment than control mice. This increased susceptibility is partially reversed by transfer of purified CD4$^+$ T cells [61]. Transfer of CD4$^+$ T cells to RAG1-/-mice resulted in increased Treg cells in uterine draining lymph nodes, suggesting that Treg cells might regulate inflammation to bacterial pathogens. Depletion of Treg cells does not induce PTD [3], and therefore decreased Treg cells during pregnancy might enhance the susceptibility for PTD by chorioamnionitis. Low dose LPS treatment triggered PTD in IL-10-/-mice [62]. These mice had an increased number and placental infiltration of cytotoxic NK cells and placental cell death. Depletion of NK cells or TNFα neutralization in these mice restored term delivery [62]. These findings suggest NK cells play a role for induction of PTL by producing TNFα, and Treg cells might regulate this reaction.

ACKNOWLEDGEMENTS

Grant support: This work was supported by Grant from the Ministry of Education, Culture, Sports, Science and Technology, Japan [Grant-in-Aid for Scientific Research (B)-23390386] and [Grant-in-Aid for challenging Exploratory Research-22659297], and Grants from the Ministry of Health Labour and Welfare, Japan [Health Labour Sciences Research Grant-H22-jisedai-ippan-008,H22-nanchi-ippan-159, H22-kagaku-ippan-006, H22-rinkensui-ippan-013, H23-shinkou-ippan-016, H23-jisedai-shitei-008].

REFERENCES

[1]   Sakaguchi S, Sakaguchi N, Asano M, Itoh M, Toda M. Immunologic self-tolerance maintained by activated T cells expressing IL-2 receptor alpha-chains (CD25). Breakdown of a single mechanism of self-tolerance causes various autoimmune diseases. J Immunol 1995; 155: 1151-1164.

[2]   Aluvihare VR, Kallikourdis M, Betz AG. Regulatory T cells mediate maternal tolerance to the fetus. Nat Immunol 2004; 5: 266-271.

[3]   Shima T, Sasaki Y, Ito M, Nakashima A, Ishii N, Sugamura K, Saito S. Regulatory T cells are necessary for implantation and maintenance of early pregnancy but not late pregnancy in allogeneic mice. J Reprod Immunol 2010; 85(2): 121-9

[4]   Saito S, Motoyoshi K, Ichijo M, Saito M, Takaku F. High serum human macrophage colony-stimulating factor level during pregnancy. Int J Hematol 1992; 55: 219-225.

[5]   Nakashima A, Shiozaki A, Myojo S, Ito M, Tatematsu M, Sakai M, Takamori Y, Ogawa K, Nagata K, Saito S. Granulysin produced by uterine natural killer cells induces apoptosis of extravillous trophoblasts in spontaneous abortion. Am J Pathol 2008; 173: 653-664.

[6]   Siston AM, Rasmussen SA, Honein MA, Fry AM, Seib K, Callaghan WM, Louie J, Doyle TJ, Crockett M, Lynfield R, Moore Z, Wiedeman C, Anand M, Tabony L, Nielsen CF, Waller K, Page S, Thompson JM, Avery C, Springs CB, Jones T, Williams JL, Newsome K, Finelli L, Jamieson DJ. Pandemic 2009 influenza A(H1N1) virus illness among pregnant women in the United States. JAMA 2010; 303: 1517-1525.

[7]   Koga K, Cardenas I, Aldo P, Abrahams VM, Peng B, Fill S, Romero R, Mor G. Activation of TLR3 in the trophoblast is associated with preterm delivery. Am J Reprod Immunol 2009; 61: 196-212.

[8]   Lin Y, Ren L, Wang W, Di J, Zeng S, Saito S. Effect of TLR3 and TLR7 activation in uterine NK cells from non-obese diabetic (NOD) mice. J Reprod Immunol 2009; 82: 12-23.

[9]   Sacks G, Sargent I, Redman C. An innate view of human pregnancy. Immunol Today 1999; 20: 114-118.

[10]   Wegmann TG, Lin H, Guilbert L, Mosmann TR. Bidirectional cytokine interactions in the maternal-fetal relationship: is successful pregnancy a TH2 phenomenon? Immunol Today 1993; 14: 353-356.

[11]   Kammerer U, Kruse A, Barrientos G, Arck PC, Blois SM. Role of dendritic cells in the regulation of maternal immune responses to the fetus during mammalian gestation. Immunol Invest 2008; 37: 499-533.

[12]   Blois SM, Barrientos G, Garcia MG, Orsal AS, Tometten M, Cordo-Russo RI, Klapp BF, Santoni A, Fernández N, Terness P, Arck PC. Interaction between dendritic cells and natural killer cells during pregnancy in mice. J Mol Med 2008; 86: 837-852.

[13]   Breburda EE, Dambaeva SV, Slukvin II, Golos TG. Selective distribution and pregnancy-specific expression of DC-SIGN at the maternal-fetal interface in the rhesus macaque: DC-SIGN is a putative marker of the recognition of pregnancy. Placenta 2006; 27: 11-21.

[14]   Krey G, Frank P, Shaikly V, Barrientos G, Cordo-Russo R, Ringel F, Moschansky P, Chernukhin IV, Metodiev M, Fernández N, Klapp BF, Arck PC, Blois SM. *In vivo* dendritic cell depletion reduces breeding efficiency, affecting implantation and early placental development in mice. J Mol Med 2008; 86: 999-1011.

[15]   Plaks V, Birnberg T, Berkutzki T, Sela S, BenYashar A, Kalchenko V, Mor G, Keshet E, Dekel N, Neeman M, Jung S. Uterine DCs are crucial for decidua formation during embryo implantation in mice. J Clin Invest 2008; 118: 3954-3965.

[16]   Guerin LR, Prins JR, Robertson SA. Regulatory T-cells and immune tolerance in pregnancy: a new target for infertility treatment? Hum Reprod Update 2009; 15: 517-535.

[17]   Robertson SA, Guerin LR, Bromfield JJ, Branson KM, Ahlström AC, Care AS. Seminal fluid drives expansion of the CD4+CD25+ T regulatory cell pool and induces tolerance to paternal alloantigens in mice. Biol Reprod 2009; 80: 1036-1045.

[18]   Arruvito L, Sanz M, Banham AH, Fainboim L. Expansion of CD4+CD25+and FOXP3+ regulatory T cells during the follicular phase of the menstrual cycle: implications for human reproduction. J Immunol 2007; 178: 2572-2578.

[19]   Schumacher A, Brachwitz N, Sohr S, Engeland K, Langwisch S, Dolaptchieva M, Alexander T, Taran A, Malfertheiner SF, Costa SD, Zimmermann G, Nitschke C, Volk HD, Alexander H, Gunzer M, Zenclussen AC. Human chorionic gonadotropin attracts regulatory T cells into the fetal-maternal interface during early human pregnancy. J Immunol 2009; 182: 5488-5497.

[20]   Zhao JX, Zeng YY, Liu Y. Fetal alloantigen is responsible for the expansion of the CD4(+)CD25(+) regulatory T cell pool during pregnancy. J Reprod Immunol 2007; 75: 71-81.

[21]   Darrasse-Jèze G, Klatzmann D, Charlotte F, Salomon BL, Cohen JL. CD4+CD25+ regulatory/suppressor T cells prevent allogeneic fetus rejection in mice. Immunol Lett 2006; 102 :106-109.

[22]   Zenclussen AC, Gerlof K, Zenclussen ML, Sollwedel A, Bertoja AZ, Ritter T, Kotsch K, Leber J, Volk HD. Abnormal T-cell reactivity against paternal antigens in spontaneous abortion: adoptive transfer of pregnancy-induced CD4+CD25+ T regulatory cells prevents fetal rejection in a murine abortion model. Am J Pathol 2005; 166: 811-822.

[23]   Jasper MJ, Tremellen KP, Robertson SA. Primary unexplained infertility is associated with reduced expression of the T-regulatory cell transcription factor Foxp3 in endometrial tissue. Mol Hum Reprod 2006; 12: 301-308.

[24]   Levine JS, Branch DW, Rauch J. The antiphospholipid syndrome. N Engl J Med 2002; 346: 752-763.

[25]   Girardi G. Complement inhibition keeps mothers calm and avoids fetal rejection. Immunol Invest 2008; 37: 645-659.

[26]   Levine RJ, Lam C, Qian C, Yu KF, Maynard SE, Sachs BP, Sibai BM, Epstein FH, Romero R, Thadhani R, Karumanchi SA. Soluble endoglin and other circulating antiangiogenic factors in preeclampsia. Engl J Med 2006; 355: 992-1005.

[27]   Girardi G, Redecha P, Salmon JE. Heparin prevents antiphospholipid antibody-induced fetal loss by inhibiting complement activation. Nat Med 2004; 10: 1222-1226.

[28]   Saito S, Miyazaki S, Sasaki Y. Th1/Th2 balance of the implantation site in human in Immunology of Pregnancy. Gil Mor Edt. Landes Bioscience, Texas USA. 2006;37-48.

[29]   Hill JA, Polgar K, Anderson DJ. T-helper 1-type immunity to trophoblast in women with recurrent spontaneous abortion. JAMA 1995; 273: 1933-1936.

[30]   Piccinni MP, Beloni L, Livi C, Maggi E, Scarselli G, Romagnani S. Defective production of both leukemia inhibitory factor and type 2 T-helper cytokines by decidual T cells in unexplained recurrent abortions. Nat Med 1998; 4: 1020-1024.

[31]   Bates MD, Quenby S, Takakuwa K, Johnson PM, Vince GS. Aberrant cytokine production by peripheral blood mononuclear cells in recurrent pregnancy loss? Hum Reprod 2002; 17: 2439-2444.

[32]   Sasaki Y, Sakai M, Miyazaki S, Higuma S, Shiozaki A, Saito S. Decidual and peripheral blood CD4+CD25+ regulatory T cells in early pregnancy subjects and spontaneous abortion cases. Mol Hum Reprod 2004; 10: 347-353.

[33]   Tilburgs T, Scherjon SA, van der Mast BJ, Haasnoot GW, Versteeg-V D Voort-Maarschalk M, Roelen DL, van Rood JJ, Claas FH. Fetal-maternal HLA-C mismatch is associated with decidual T cell activation and induction of functional T regulatory cells. J Reprod Immunol 2009; 82: 148-157.

[34]   Zenclussen AC, Gerlof K, Zenclussen ML, Ritschel S, Zambon Bertoja A, Fest S, Hontsu S, Ueha S, Matsushima K, Leber J, Volk HD. Regulatory T cells induce a privileged tolerant microenvironment at the fetal-maternal interface. Eur J Immunol 2006; 36: 82-94.

[35]   Tilburgs T, Roelen DL, van der Mast BJ, de Groot-Swings GM, Kleijburg C, Scherjon SA, Claas FH. Evidence for a selective migration of fetus-specific CD4+CD25bright regulatory T cells from the peripheral blood to the decidua in human pregnancy. J Immunol 2008; 180: 5737-5745.

[36]   Zhou WH, Dong L, Du MR, Zhu XY, Li DJ. Cyclosporin A improves murine pregnancy outcome in abortion-prone matings: involvement of CD80/86 and CD28/CTLA-4. Reproduction 2008; 135: 385-395.

[37]   Li W, Li B, Fan W, Geng L, Li X, Li L, Huang Z, Li S. CTLA4Ig gene transfer alleviates abortion in mice by expanding CD4+CD25+ regulatory T cells and inducing indoleamine 2,3-dioxygenase. J Reprod Immunol 2009; 80 :1-11.

[38]   Yang H, Qiu L, Di W, Zhao A, Chen G, Hu K, Lin Q. Proportional change of CD4+CD25+ regulatory T cells after lymphocyte therapy in unexplained recurrent spontaneous abortion patients. Fertil Steril 2009; 92: 301-305.

[39]   Wang WJ, Hao CF, Yi-Lin, Yin GJ, Bao SH, Qiu LH, Lin QD. Increased prevalence of T helper 17 (Th17) cells in peripheral blood and decidua in unexplained recurrent spontaneous abortion patients. J Reprod Immunol 2010; 84: 164-170.

[40]   Nakashima A, Ito M, Shima T, Bac ND, Hidaka T, Saito S. Accumulation of IL-17-positive cells in decidua of inevitable abortion cases. Am J Reprod Immunol 2010; 64(1): 4-11

[41]   Moffett-King A. Natural killer cells and pregnancy. Nat Rev Immunol 2002; 2: 656-663.

[42]   Quenby S, Nik H, Innes B, Lash G, Turner M, Drury J, Bulmer J. Uterine natural killer cells and angiogenesis in recurrent reproductive failure. Hum Reprod 2009; 24: 45-54.

[43]   Higuma-Myojo S, Sasaki Y, Miyazaki S, Sakai M, Siozaki A, Miwa N, Saito S. Cytokine profile of natural killer cells in early human pregnancy. Am J Reprod Immunol 2005; 54: 21-29.

[44]   Saito S, Shiozaki A, Nakashima A, Sakai M, Sasaki Y. The role of the immune system in preeclampsia. Mol Aspects Med 2007; 28: 192-209.

[45]   Skjaerven R, Wilcox AJ, Lie RT. The interval between pregnancies and the risk of preeclampsia. N Engl J Med 2002; 346: 33-38.

[46]   Saito S, Nakashima A, Myojo-Higuma S, Shiozaki A. The balance between cytotoxic NK cells and regulatory NK cells in human pregnancy. J Reprod Immunol 2008; 77: 14-22.

[47]   Sasaki Y, Darmochwal-Kolarz D, Suzuki D, Sakai M, Ito M, Shima T, Shiozaki A, Rolinski J, Saito S. Proportion of peripheral blood and decidual CD4(+) CD25(bright) regulatory T cells in pre-eclampsia. Clin Exp Immunol 2007; 149: 139-145.

[48]   Steinborn A, Haensch GM, Mahnke K, Schmitt E, Toermer A, Meuer S, Sohn C. Distinct subsets of regulatory T cells during pregnancy: is the imbalance of these subsets involved in the pathogenesis of preeclampsia? Clin Immunol 2008; 129: 401-412.

[49]   Santner-Nanan B, Peek MJ, Khanam R, Richarts L, Zhu E, Fazekas de St Groth B, Nanan R. Systemic increase in the ratio between Foxp3+ and IL-17-producing CD4+ T cells in healthy pregnancy but not in preeclampsia. J Immunol 2009; 183: 7023-7030.

[50]   Salha O, Sharma V, Dada T, Nugent D, Rutherford AJ, Tomlinson AJ, Philips S, Allgar V, Walker JJ. The influence of donated gametes on the incidence of hypertensive disorders of pregnancy. Hum Reprod 1999; 14: 2268-2273.

[51]   Hiby SE, Walker JJ, O'shaughnessy KM, Redman CW, Carrington M, Trowsdale J, Moffett A. Combinations of maternal KIR and fetal HLA-C genes influence the risk of preeclampsia and reproductive success. J Exp Med 2004; 200: 957-965.

[52]   Saito S, Takeda Y, Sakai M, Nakabayahi M, Hayakawa S. The incidence of pre-eclampsia among couples consisting of Japanese women and Caucasian men. J Reprod Immunol 2006; 70: 93-98.

[53]   Verlohren S, Muller DN, Luft FC, Dechend R. Immunology in hypertension, preeclampsia, and target-organ damage. Hypertension 2009; 54: 439-443.

[54]   Molvarec A, Ito M, Shima T, Yoneda S, Toldi G, Stenczer B, Vasarhelyi B, Rigo Jr J, Saito S. Decreased proportion of peripheral blood vascular endothelial growth factor-expressing T and natural killer cells in preeclampsia. Am J Obstet Gynecol. 2010; 203(6): 567.e1-8.

[55]   Romero R, Espinoza J, Gonçalves LF, Kusanovic JP, Friel LA, Nien JK. Inflammation in preterm and term labour and delivery. Semin Fetal Neonatal Med 2006; 11: 317-326.

[56]   Mackenzie R, Walker M, Armson A, Hannah ME. Progesterone for the prevention of preterm birth among women at increased risk: a systematic review and meta-analysis of randomized controlled trials. Am J Obstet Gynecol 2006; 194: 1234-1242.

[57]   Szekeres-Bartho J, Wilczynski JR, Basta P, Kalinka J. Role of progesterone and progestin therapy in threatened abortion and preterm labour. Front Biosci 2008; 13: 1981-1990.

[58]   Orsi NM, Gopichandran N, Simpson NA. Genetics of preterm labour. Best Pract Res Clin Obstet Gynaecol 2007; 21: 757-772.

[59]   Macones GA, Parry S, Elkousy M, Clothier B, Ural SH, Strauss JF 3rd. A polymorphism in the promoter region of TNF and bacterial vaginosis: preliminary evidence of gene-environment interaction in the etiology of spontaneous preterm birth. Am J Obstet Gynecol 2004; 190: 1504-1508.

[60]   Ito M, Nakashima A, Hidaka T, Okabe M, Bac ND, Ina S, Yoneda S, Shiozaki A, Sumi S, Tsuneyama K, Nikaido T, Saito S. A role for IL-17 in induction of an inflammation at the fetomaternal interface in preterm labour. J Reprod Immunol 2010; 84: 75-85.

[61]   Bizargity P, Del Rio R, Phillippe M, Teuscher C, Bonney EA. Resistance to lipopolysaccharide-induced preterm delivery mediated by regulatory T cell function in mice. Biol Reprod 2009; 80: 874-881.

[62]   Murphy SP, Hanna NN, Fast LD, Shaw SK, Berg G, Padbury JF, Romero R, Sharma S. Evidence for participation of uterine natural killer cells in the mechanisms responsible for spontaneous preterm labor and delivery. Am J Obstet Gynecol 2009; 200: 308.e1-9.

CHAPTER 6

Gestational Diabetes Affects Placental-Fetal Development

Evemie Dubé[1,2], Cathy Vaillancourt[2,3], Julie Lafond[1,2,*] and Louiza Belkacemi[4,*]

[1]Department of Sciences Biologiques, Université du Québec à Montréal, Montréal, Québec, Canada, H3C 3P8; [2]BioMed Research Centre, Montréal, Québec, Canada; [3]INRS-Institut Armand-Frappier, Laval, Québec, Canada; [4]Department of Obstetrics and Gynecology, Harbor-UCLA Medical Center, Los Angeles Biomedical Research Institute at Harbor-UCLA, and David Geffen School of Medicine at UCLA, Torrance, California 90502, USA

Abstract: Gestational diabetes mellitus occurs only during pregnancy, and usually disappears shortly after delivery. Although, GDM is a common disorder, its pathophysiology is not well understood. Impaired placental function is probably a contributing factor as the placenta hinders insulin signaling and produce increased levels of cytokines that affect placental transport and metabolism of glucose and lipids. This in turn negatively impacts on fetal growth and development with significantly increased risk of a number of short-and long-term adverse consequences for the fetus, and the most significant of which is a predisposition to the development of metabolic syndrome and Type 2 diabetes. This article will describe placental changes in gestational diabetes related to glucose and lipids following placental insulin and cytokines dysfunction, and subsequent effects on the offspring development.

Keywords: Diabetes, gestation, glucose, receptors, lipids, insulin, cytokines.

INTRODUCTION

Gestational diabetes mellitus (GDM) is a condition in which women without previously diagnosed diabetes exhibit high blood glucose levels during pregnancy [1]. The prevalence of GDM has increased dramatically in developed countries over the last 20 years, particularly in populations emigrating from less-developed areas [2]. Although, most women with GDM return to normal glucose tolerance after delivery, some of the women have an increased risk of developing type 2 diabetes mellitus (T2DM) later in life. GDM is therefore classified as a pre-diabetic state [3]. The incidence of developing T2DM later in life is even greater if obesity is present. The offspring of women with GDM are prone to adverse side-effects such as macrosomia (which is strongly associated with fetal death), prematurity, birth trauma and respiratory distress syndrome, and more importantly, have a higher risk of developing obesity, impaired glucose tolerance, and T2DM later in life [4]. Owing to its position, as a maternal-fetal exchange organ, the human placenta is exposed to metabolic and hormonal diabetes-associated alterations from both mother and fetus. These alterations are more likely at the origin of disturbances in placental function and metabolic performances [5].

In this review, we will focus on placental changes in GDM pregnancies that are related to glucose and lipid metabolism and transfer, as glucose and lipids represent crucial nutrients for fetal growth and development. We will also discuss alterations in levels of insulin, and placental inflammatory cytokines since insulin is essential for glucose metabolism, and cytokines have the ability to interfere with insulin signaling and lipid metabolism. Finally, we will review the consequences of short and long term effects of GDM on fetal growth and development.

GESTATIONAL DIABETES, PLACENTAL NUTRIENT METABOLISM AND TRANSPORT

Changes in glucose and lipid metabolism occur during pregnancy to ensure a continuous supply of nutrients to the growing fetus despite intermittent maternal food intake. These metabolic changes are progressive and may be accentuated in women who develop GDM [6].

*Addresss correspondence to Julie Lafond and Louiza Belkacemi: Département des Sciences Biologiques, Université du Québec à Montréal, Montréal, Québec, Canada, H3C 3P8; Tel: 514-987-3000, Fax: 514-987-6367. E-mail: Lafond.julie@uqam.ca and Los Angeles Biomedical Research Institute at Harbor-UCLA, Torrance, California 90502, USA; E-mail: lbelkacemi@obgyn.humc.edu

Glucose

During normal pregnancy, glucose is the primary energy substrate for the developing fetus. Glucose is supplied to the fetus either by passing from the mother through the placenta or by metabolism in the placenta itself. The transport of glucose across the plasma membrane of the cell is mediated by a family of glucose membrane-spanning glycoproteins transporters (GLUT). In humans, during the first trimester, GLUT1 and GLUT3 are both expressed by the microvillous membrane of the syncytiotrophoblast and the plasma membrane of the cytotrophoblast, while GLUT4 is localized in perinuclear membranes in the syncytiotrophoblast cytosol [7]. The insulin-regulated GLUT4 expression in the cytosol of first trimester syncytiotrophoblast is compatible with a role for GLUT4 in placental glucose transport in early pregnancy [7]. At term human pregnancy, GLUT1 is expressed abundantly, due perhaps to increasing glucose concentrations over the physiological range. On the other hand, the expression of GLUT3 and 4 is markedly reduced at term compared with first trimester [7]. The presence of GLUT4 in placenta at term pregnancy may be important for transporting glucose and conversion to glycogen and response to insulin in the fetal circulation [8].

GDM is a condition associated with alterations in placental glucose uptake, circulation, utilization, and transfer to fetal circulation [9-12]. Placentas of diet controlled GDM pregnancies have not only reduced glucose uptake but also decreased transfer and utilization [10]. Interestingly, glucose handling by the placenta is different depending on whether the woman insulin therapy status. Insulin-treated GDM pregnancies without macrosomia, have decreased placental glucose utilization compared to the control group, whereas in insulin-treated GDM with macrosomia no change was observed [13]. This indicates that placental glucose utilization is different between insulin-treated GDM placentas with and without fetal macrosomia [13]. In streptozocin treated rats, an animal model of diabetes, circulating glucose is elevated, whereas insulin is decreased [14]. Notably, alteration in glucose associated with GDM occurs in conjunction with altered glucose transporters (GLUTs) expression. In humans, GLUT1 protein expression is increased in the basal membrane vesicles in insulin-controlled GDM placentas as compared with normal controls [15] suggesting that GLUT1 is the main GLUT involved in placental glucose transport in the presence of defective insulin signaling. This is supported by *in vitro* culture studies showing a down-regulation of GLUT1 protein expression and its translocation from the membrane to intracellular sites of the trophoblast cell during hyperglycemia [16]. Furthermore, in insulin-controlled GDM, GLUT4 mRNA expression was lower in comparison with normal controls. These results indicate that basal GLUT1 responsible for cellular metabolism and glucose transport may actually be the major glucose transporter into the cell in placental tissue rather than GLUT4, which is likely affected by defective insulin signaling upstream.

Lipids

Fatty acids are critical for fetal development and growth due not only to their importance as a source of energy but also their involvement in several structural and metabolic functions. Fetal fatty acids are mostly derived from the maternal circulation, as free fatty acids or as fatty acids incorporated into lipoproteins, and have to cross the placenta before entering the fetal circulation [17]. Fatty acids uptake by the placenta is facilitated by the presence of several lipoprotein receptors and fatty acid transport proteins expressed by human placental cells. Lipoproteins receptors include the LDL receptor (LDLr), the VLDL receptor (VLDLr), the scavenger receptor class B type I (SR-BI) and the lectin-like oxidized LDL receptor-1 (OLR1) [18-21]. The main fatty acid transport proteins are FAT/CD36 (fatty acid translocase), FABPpm (plasma membrane fatty acid binding protein) and FATPs (fatty acid transfer proteins) [22-25]. FAT/CD36 and FATP1 are located on both the placental microvillous and basal membranes [22] while the human placental FABPpm (p-FABPpm) is only present on the microvillous membranes of the syncytiotrophoblast [26, 27]. Fatty acids dissociate from lipoproteins by the placental lipoprotein lipase (LPL) [28]. Once fatty acids enter the cytoplasm, two cytosolic binding proteins the heart-FABP (H-FABP) and the liver-FABP (L-FABP) transfer the fatty acids, by simple diffusion or through fatty acid transport proteins, to the fetal circulation through the basal membrane [22-25].

GDM pregnancies are associated with alterations in maternal lipid profile, and placental lipid uptake, synthesis and transport to the fetus. Indeed maternal hypertriglyceridemia, hypercholesterolemia, higher serum VLDL concentrations and lower LDL cholesterol concentrations have been detected in GDM pregnancies compared to normal pregnancies [19, 29, 30]. In humans, cholesterol, which is an important nutrient involved in structural functions and in the synthesis of steroid hormones, is mainly derived from LDL-cholesterol and *de novo* synthesis [31]. Several placental genes involved in cholesterol synthesis are increased in GDM pregnancies [32]. GDM also increases the level of the fatty acid synthase (FAS) protein expression, a key enzyme in *de novo* lipid synthesis, in human full-term placenta [33]. In addition, hypercholesterolemia has been shown to reduce the expression of LDLr, which is involved in the binding and internalization of LDL-cholesterol [34]. Several lines of evidence suggest an enhanced flux of fatty acids to the fetus in case of GDM. Indeed the expression of several genes encoding proteins involved in placental fatty acid uptake and transport are up-regulated in GDM pregnancies as well as L-FABP protein expression [32, 35]. Overall these data reflect the increased availability of lipids at the maternal-placental interface that could contribute to fetal fat depot accumulation. Moreover GDM seems to enhance the risk of oxidative stress and lipid peroxidation. This is suggested by the increase in GDM pregnancies of the expression of OLR1 protein, involved in the uptake of oxidized LDL [19], and ApoD protein, implicated in lipid transport and possibly in the response to stress and lipid peroxidation [36, 37]. I would delete this last sentence because it does not fit well with the rest.

Collectively, these data show that maternal and fetal influences can discordantly alter placental function in women with GDM and consequently, hinder transport of nutrients such as glucose and lipids, vital for normal fetal growth. We postulate that defects present in placental tissue which increase inflammatory cytokines, and hinder insulin signaling and subsequent glucose and lipid transport may be contributing factors to short and long-term developmental risks for the offspring.

ROLE OF INSULIN AND CYTOKINES

Insulin

Insulin is the hormone essential for glucose metabolism. The human placenta expresses high amounts of insulin receptors (IR) relative to other tissues in the body. Their location undergoes developmental changes. At the beginning of gestation, they are located on the microvillous membrane of the syncytiotrophoblast, whereas at term, they are predominantly found in the endothelium [38]. This spatio-temporal shift in insulin sensitivity throughout pregnancy suggests a shift in control of insulin-dependent processes from the mother at the beginning of pregnancy to the fetus at the end [39]. Insulin signaling is essential for the regulation of intracellular and blood glucose levels. Insulin increases glucose uptake mainly by inducing the translocation of the GLUT4 proteins to the plasma membrane, rather than by increasing the intrinsic activity of the transporter [40]. Hence, when insulin concentrations are low, GLUT4 is present in cytoplasmic vesicles. The binding of insulin to cell receptors leads rapidly to fusion of those vesicles with the plasma membrane and insertion of GLUT4 thereby giving the cell an ability to efficiently take up glucose. When blood levels of insulin decrease and insulin receptors are no longer occupied, the GLUT4 is recycled back into the cytoplasm. In the placenta, stimulation of GLUT4 by insulin results in more glucose passing to the fetus. Inversely, if the placenta produces more insulin, the supply of glucose to the fetus is decreased.

Insulin resistance usually begins about 20 to 24 weeks into the normal pregnancy. As the placenta grows, more placental hormones are produced, and insulin resistance becomes greater. Normally, the pancreas is able to make additional insulin to overcome insulin resistance, however when the production of insulin is not enough to overcome the effect of placental hormones including estrogen, cortisol, and human placental lactogen, GDM results.

Cytokines

Virtually all known cytokines are expressed by the placenta and associated fetal and maternal membranes during normal gestation [41]. The human placenta expresses virtually all known cytokines including tumor necrosis factor-alpha (TNF-α), resistin and leptin, which are also produced by adipose cells. Some of these adipokines are major players in the regulation of insulin action which may indicate probable novel interactions between the placenta and adipose tissue in understanding pregnancy-induced insulin resistance. The type and the location of the cytokine receptors on the placental cells determine whether signals are generated by the placenta, maternally (presumably adipose-derived), or by the fetus. This highlights the possibility of an external control of placental function that can become deregulated when the cytokine levels are increased, such as in GDM.

Thus, an abnormal maternal metabolic environment including GDM generates stimuli within the adipose tissue and the placenta cells that result in increased production of inflammatory cytokines. This was reflected in studies of transcriptional profiling showing that the adipose tissue and the placenta overexpress common cytokines and inflammation-related genes, in a diabetic environment [42]. The deregulation of inflammatory pathways, in GDM pregnancies, is supported by increased circulating concentration of inflammatory molecules [43, 44]. In these pregnancies the serum concentration of TNF-α is elevated [45]. Conversely, adipose and placental tissue TNF-α release in women with GDM is lower compared to normal pregnant women [45]. Notably, the overexpression of placental TNF-α is associated with increased fetal adiposity [46]. Although, the mechanisms responsible for increased TNF-α gene expression and production are still unknown; the consequences of their overproduction are just beginning to be resolved [32]. A possibility is that in GDM pregnancies the activation of the proximal cytoplasmic proteins of TNF-α signaling such as TNF receptor 1 (TNFR1), tumor necrosis factor receptor type 1-associated death domain (TRADD) protein, TNF receptor 2 (TNFR2)-associated death domain (TRAF2) protein, and Fas-associated death domain (FADD) protein is an indication of the recruitment of TNF-α R1 and R2 receptors in the placenta [46]. This indicates that placental TNF-α down-regulates insulin action through serine phosphorylation of placental insulin receptors, such as in skeletal muscle of women with GDM [47]. Moreover TNF-α activates phospholipase A2 (PLA$_2$), a family of lipolytic enzymes that generate eicosanoid precursors such as docosahexaenoic acid, an essential omega (ω)-3 polyunsaturated fatty acid. Recent evidence demonstrates an accumulation of ω-3 fatty acids in placenta of offspring of GDM mothers with increased adiposity at birth [48]. This may represent a potential mechanism linking local placental inflammatory responses with increased lipid substrate availability for fetal fat deposition, besides increased maternal supply.

EFFECT OF GDM ON THE OFFSPRING

Short Term Effects

Infants of mothers suffering from GDM are vulnerable to major health problems during pregnancy including macrosomia, hypoglycemia, respiratory distress and oxidative stress.

Macrosomia

Macrosomia refers to a baby that is considerably larger than normal. This occurs when there is excessive placental transport of glucose and other nutrients from the mother to the fetus. Macrosomia is divided into a symmetric and asymmetric type. Symmetric fetal overgrowth may be due to genetic factors, whereas asymmetric fetal overgrowth is induced in a diabetic intra-uterine environment with an increased maternal-fetal nutrient transfer [49]. Macrosomia is characterized by an enlarged thoracic and abdominal circumference, which is relatively larger than the head circumference. The disproportionate fetal growth is associated with increased fetal morbidity at the time of delivery, including an increased rate of cesarean deliveries [50]. Other associated delivery complications include shoulder dystocia, where the shoulder becomes pressed against the mother's pubic bone and can result in permanent neurologic injuries, clavicle fractures, brachial plexus injuries, damage to the network of nerves within the neck and shoulder that are supplied by nerves exiting from the spine, as well as asphyxia, and oxygen deprivation [51]. These occur as the result of the large size of the neonate in comparison to the birth canal.

Hypoglycemia and Respiratory Distress Syndrome

Hypoglycemia (low blood glucose levels) in neonates can occur within a few hours after delivery. This short supply of blood glucose in the neonate may be present in up to 35% of infants born to diabetic mothers [52]. This problem arises when the mother's blood sugar levels have been consistently high, causing the fetus to have a high level of insulin in its circulation. The severity of the neonatal hypoglycemia is dependent upon the maternal glucose control in late gestation as well as during parturition [51]. After delivery, the baby continues to have a high insulin level, but it has no longer access to the high sugar level from its mother, resulting in the newborn's blood sugar level becoming very low. Thus it may be necessary to give the baby glucose. Animal models studies show that this results from the maternal hyperglycemic state, which induces fetal hyperinsulinemia [51]. Insulin is stored and released from the β cells of the fetal pancreas. However, with the excessive stimulation that is caused by hyperglycemia in fetuses of diabetic mothers, pancreatic β cells eventually lose their stores of insulin. The hypoglycemia resulting from a large maternal insulin response may cause fetal defects including respiratory distress syndrome in the fetus [53].

Respiratory distress syndrome is caused by increasing difficulty in breathing due to lung air sac collapse. Because of the fatal consequences of respiratory distress syndrome, lung maturity should be checked at delivery. It is recommended that before doing any delivery before 38.5 weeks of gestation for other than the most urgent fetal and maternal indications, an amniocentesis to document pulmonary maturity should be performed.

Oxidative Stress

Oxidative stress is a state in which oxygen free radicals in the body exceed natural antioxidant defenses [54]. Hyperglycemia causes the depletion of antioxidants and the generation of reactive oxygen species [55]. The presence of increased oxidative components in samples taken from the umbilical cord blood of women with GDM suggests that this environment is also shared with the fetus [45, 56-58]. In animal models, oxyradicals play an essential role in the timing and progression of neuronal development, differentiation [59] and synaptic plasticity [60]. Changes in the balance of these signals may lead to alterations in major neurodevelopmental processes. The brain, in particular, is susceptible to oxidative damage due owing to its high oxygen consumption and poor antioxidant defenses [61]. Free radicals cause oxidation of lipids, proteins [62] and DNA, which result in the inactivation of the biological functions of these molecules, and potentially leading to cell death. Oxidative stress may also contribute to increased risk of schizophrenia observed in offspring of diabetic pregnancies. Therefore, we postulate that OS during pregnancy may play a role in fetal 'programming' and the transmission of a diabetogenic tendency to the next generation through permanent alteration of DNA and tissue damage in the developing fetus.

LONG-TERM CONSEQUENCES FOR THE OFFSPRING

Offspring from GDM pregnancies are likely to develop diabetes, obesity and neurological deficits later in life.

Diabetes

Epidemiological studies indicate that long range complications of GDM include an increased risk of impaired glucose tolerance in the offspring. Similarly, several animal model studies imply that GDM results in an increased risk of diabetes in the offspring [63]. The maternal glucose intolerance may impair fetal insulin sensitivity, and consequently "program" the susceptibility to T2DM [64]. Despite the existence of genetic predisposing factors, glucose control during pregnancy will probably reduce frequency of these disorders in the offspring.

Obesity

Obesity is a complication in offspring born to mothers with GDM. Compared to offspring of mothers with type 1 diabetes (T1DM) and of non-diabetic mothers, offspring of mothers with GDM have significantly increased weight [65]. A prospective singleton pregnancy cohort study performed by Boerschmann *et al.* [65] found overweight prevalence at ages 2, 8 and 11 years in the offspring of GDM. They also found that insulin resistance was increased in offspring of GDM mothers compared to offspring of non-GDM mothers, and was associated with the child's BMI. Therefore, fetal hyperinsulinemia was suggested as a good predictor of childhood obesity [51].

Neuropsychological Deficits

Abnormal glucose levels during pregnancy have been implicated as potential teratogenic agents for fetal organ development. The altered glucose environment long-term effects on the offspring include neuropsychological deficits [53] since the brain is an important consumer of glucose. In humans the brain requires about 20% of the body's metabolic consumption for its normal functioning. If deprived of this, even temporarily, brain function is negatively affected. Because glucose is a requirement for brain function and development, the different GLUT isoforms are expressed at different times of brain development. Glucose availability may act within cells to up or down regulate the expression of GLUT proteins, and hence its presence in the brain. These effects may be irreversible [66]. In humans, differentiation and maturation of the brain cortex increase near the end of the second trimester; this is also a time of vulnerability for the brain, and any alteration to its environment may lead to an altered neurology [67]. Hypoglycemia that results from hyperinsulinemia in the offspring of diabetic mothers may cause damage to the neurons of the medial temporal region of the brain [68]. Severe perfusion defects can also affect memory processing in the brain [68]. These neurological effects of altered glucose levels may explain the findings that offspring of diabetic mothers tend to have poorer academic performance as well as other neuropsychological deficits [69]. Experimentally, the importance of glucose in brain development has been shown by Smoak and Sadler [70] in mouse embryos. When glucose levels were reduced by 50% for 2 hours in neurulating mice, dysmorphogenesis resulted. Those mice undergoing gastrulation were also more sensitive to even shorter periods of hypoglycemia [70].

SUMMARY

Maternal environment during pregnancy is an important determinant of optimal fetal development, pregnancy outcome, and adult health. Normal placental function facilitates the maternal-fetal transfer of nutrients that are critical for the development of a healthy fetus [71] Thus, an abnormal maternal metabolic environment such as in GDM generates stimuli that elicit changes in insulin sensitivity and a prominent increase in cytokines in the placenta that alter placental function, particularly with respect to the uptake, transfer, and/or utilization of glucose and lipids. The plasticity of the placenta allows this pivotal tissue to respond to exogenous insults and compensate for varying maternal environmental insults. When this response is insufficient the fetus is at higher risks for suboptimal outcomes that will persist into adulthood.

As studies of the offspring of diabetic mothers have provided unequivocal evidence that alterations in the nutritional environment *in utero* leads to chronic disease in the offspring, optimal diabetic control, good antenatal and perinatal care for women and adequate lactation and nutrition after birth are priorities.

REFERENCES

[1]   Metzger BE, Coustan DR. Summary and recommendations of the Fourth International Workshop-Conference on Gestational Diabetes Mellitus. The Organizing Committee. Diabetes Care 1998; 21(Suppl 2): B161-7.

[2]   Beischer NA, Wein P, Sheedy MT, Steffen B. Identification and treatment of women with hyperglycaemia diagnosed during pregnancy can significantly reduce perinatal mortality rates. Aust N Z J Obstet Gynaecol 1996; 36(3): 239-47.

[3]   Colomiere M, Permezel M, Riley C, Desoye G, Lappas M. Defective insulin signaling in placenta from pregnancies complicated by gestational diabetes mellitus. Eur J Endocrinol 2009; 160(4): 567-78.

[4]   Cox NJ. Maternal component in NIDDM transmission. How large an effect? Diabetes 1994; 43(1): 166-8.

[5]   Desoye G, Shafrir E. Placental metabolism and its regulation in health and diabetes. Mol Aspects Med 1994; 15(6): 505-682.

[6]   Butte NF. Carbohydrate and lipid metabolism in pregnancy: normal compared with gestational diabetes mellitus. Am J Clin Nutr 2000; 71(Suppl 5): 1256S-61S.

[7]   Ericsson A, Hamark B, Powell TL, Jansson T. Glucose transporter isoform 4 is expressed in the syncytiotrophoblast of first trimester human placenta. Hum Reprod 2005; 20(2): 521-30.

[8]   Xing AY, Challier JC, Lepercq J, et al. Unexpected Expression of Glucose Transporter 4 in Villous Stromal Cells of Human Placenta. J Clin Endocrinol Metab 1998; 83(11): 4097-101.

[9]   Osmond DT, King RG, Brennecke SP, Gude NM. Placental glucose transport and utilisation is altered at term in insulin-treated, gestational-diabetic patients. Diabetologia 2001; 44(9): 1133-9.

[10] Osmond DT, Nolan CJ, King RG, Brennecke SP, Gude NM. Effects of gestational diabetes on human placental glucose uptake, transfer, and utilisation. Diabetologia 2000; 43(5): 576-82.

[11] Challier JC, Hauguel S, Desmaizieres V. Effect of insulin on glucose uptake and metabolism in the human placenta. J Clin Endocrinol Metab 1986; 62(5): 803-7.

[12] Hauguel S, Desmaizieres V, Challier JC. Glucose uptake, utilization, and transfer by the human placenta as functions of maternal glucose concentration. Pediatr Res 1986; 20(3): 269-73.

[13] King RG, Osmond DT, Brennecke SP, Gude NM. Effect of fetal macrosomia on human placental glucose transport and utilization in insulin-treated gestational diabetes. J Perinat Med 2003; 31(6): 475-83.

[14] Al-Achi A, Greenwood R. A brief report on some physiological parameters of streptozocin-diabetic rat. Drug Dev Ind Pharm 2001; 27(5): 465-8.

[15] Jansson T, Wennergren M, Powell TL. Placental glucose transport and GLUT 1 expression in insulin-dependent diabetes. Am J Obstet Gynecol 1999; 180(1 Pt 1): 163-8.

[16] Hahn T, Hahn D, Blaschitz A, Korgun ET, Desoye G, Dohr G. Hyperglycaemia-induced subcellular redistribution of GLUT1 glucose transporters in cultured human term placental trophoblast cells. Diabetologia 2000; 43(2): 173-80.

[17] Haggarty P. Fatty acid supply to the human fetus. Annu Rev Nutr. Aug 21;30:237-55.

[18] Cummings SW, Hatley W, Simpson ER, Ohashi M. The binding of high and low density lipoproteins to human placental membrane fractions. J Clin Endocrinol Metab 1982; 54(5): 903-8.

[19] Ethier-Chiasson M, Forest JC, Giguere Y, *et al.* Modulation of placental protein expression of OLR1: implication in pregnancy-related disorders or pathologies. Reproduction 2008; 136(4): 491-502.

[20] Wittmaack FM, Gafvels ME, Bronner M, *et al.* Localization and regulation of the human very low density lipoprotein/apolipoprotein-E receptor: trophoblast expression predicts a role for the receptor in placental lipid transport. Endocrinology 1995; 136(1): 340-8.

[21] Cao G, Garcia CK, Wyne KL, Schultz RA, Parker KL, Hobbs HH. Structure and localization of the human gene encoding SR-BI/CLA-1. Evidence for transcriptional control by steroidogenic factor 1. J Biol Chem 1997; 272(52): 33068-76.

[22] Campbell FM, Bush PG, Veerkamp JH, Dutta-Roy AK. Detection and cellular localization of plasma membrane-associated and cytoplasmic fatty acid-binding proteins in human placenta. Placenta 1998; 19(5-6): 409-15.

[23] Paulussen RJ, van Moerkerk HT, Veerkamp JH. Immunochemical quantitation of fatty acid-binding proteins. Tissue distribution of liver and heart FABP types in human and porcine tissues. Int J Biochem 1990; 22(4): 393-8.

[24] Biron-Shental T, Schaiff WT, Ratajczak CK, Bildirici I, Nelson DM, Sadovsky Y. Hypoxia regulates the expression of fatty acid-binding proteins in primary term human trophoblasts. Am J Obstet Gynecol 2007; 197(5): 516 e1-6.

[25] Daoud G, Simoneau L, Masse A, Rassart E, Lafond J. Expression of cFABP and PPAR in trophoblast cells: effect of PPAR ligands on linoleic acid uptake and differentiation. Biochim Biophys Acta 2005; 1687(1-3): 181-94.

[26] Campbell FM, Dutta-Roy AK. Plasma membrane fatty acid-binding protein (FABPpm) is exclusively located in the maternal facing membranes of the human placenta. FEBS Lett 1995; 375(3): 227-30.

[27] Campbell FM, Taffesse S, Gordon MJ, Dutta-Roy AK. Plasma membrane fatty-acid-binding protein in human placenta: identification and characterization. Biochem Biophys Res Commun 1995; 209(3): 1011-7.

[28] Huter O, Wolf HJ, Schnetzer A, Pfaller K. Lipoprotein lipase, LDL receptors and apo-lipoproteins in human fetal membranes at term. Placenta 1997; 18(8): 707-15.

[29] Koukkou E, Watts GF, Lowy C. Serum lipid, lipoprotein and apolipoprotein changes in gestational diabetes mellitus: a cross-sectional and prospective study. J Clin Pathol 1996; 49(8): 634-7.

[30] Knopp RH, Chapman M, Bergelin R, Wahl PW, Warth MR, Irvine S. Relationships of lipoprotein lipids to mild fasting hyperglycemia and diabetes in pregnancy. Diabetes Care 1980; 3(3): 416-20.

[31] Woollett LA. Maternal cholesterol in fetal development: transport of cholesterol from the maternal to the fetal circulation. Am J Clin Nutr 2005; 82(6): 1155-61.

[32] Radaelli T, Lepercq J, Varastehpour A, Basu S, Catalano PM, Hauguel-De Mouzon S. Differential regulation of genes for fetoplacental lipid pathways in pregnancy with gestational and type 1 diabetes mellitus. Am J Obstet Gynecol 2009; 201(2): 209 e1-e10.

[33] Marseille-Tremblay C, Ethier-Chiasson M, Forest JC, *et al.* Impact of maternal circulating cholesterol and gestational diabetes mellitus on lipid metabolism in human term placenta. Mol Reprod Dev 2008; 75(6): 1054-62.

[34] Ethier-Chiasson M, Duchesne A, Forest JC, *et al.* Influence of maternal lipid profile on placental protein expression of LDLr and SR-BI. Biochem Biophys Res Commun 2007; 359(1): 8-14.

[35] Magnusson AL, Waterman IJ, Wennergren M, Jansson T, Powell TL. Triglyceride hydrolase activities and expression of fatty acid binding proteins in the human placenta in pregnancies complicated by intrauterine growth restriction and diabetes. J Clin Endocrinol Metab 2004; 89(9): 4607-14.

[36]   Navarro A, Alonso A, Garrido P, *et al.* Increase in placental apolipoprotein D as an adaptation to human gestational diabetes. Placenta 2010; 31(1): 25-31.

[37]   Muffat J, Walker DW, Benzer S. Human ApoD, an apolipoprotein up-regulated in neurodegenerative diseases, extends lifespan and increases stress resistance in Drosophila. Proc Natl Acad Sci U S A 2008; 105(19): 7088-93.

[38]   Desoye G, Hartmann M, Jones CJ, *et al.* Location of insulin receptors in the placenta and its progenitor tissues. Microsc Res Tech 1997; 38(1-2): 63-75.

[39]   Hiden U, Maier A, Bilban M, *et al.* Insulin control of placental gene expression shifts from mother to foetus over the course of pregnancy. Diabetologia 2006; 49(1): 123-31.

[40]   Chang L, Chiang SH, Saltiel AR. Insulin signaling and the regulation of glucose transport. Mol Med 2004; 10(7-12): 65-71.

[41]   Bowen JM, Chamley L, Mitchell MD, Keelan JA. Cytokines of the placenta and extra-placental membranes: biosynthesis, secretion and roles in establishment of pregnancy in women. Placenta 2002; 23(4): 239-56.

[42]   Hauguel-de Mouzon S, Guerre-Millo M. The placenta cytokine network and inflammatory signals. Placenta 2006; 27(8): 794-8.

[43]   Retnakaran R, Hanley AJ, Raif N, Connelly PW, Sermer M, Zinman B. C-reactive protein and gestational diabetes: the central role of maternal obesity. J Clin Endocrinol Metab 2003; 88(8): 3507-12.

[44]   Ramsay JE, Ferrell WR, Crawford L, Wallace AM, Greer IA, Sattar N. Maternal obesity is associated with dysregulation of metabolic, vascular, and inflammatory pathways. J Clin Endocrinol Metab 2002; 87(9): 4231-7.

[45]   Lappas M, Permezel M, Rice GE. Release of proinflammatory cytokines and 8-isoprostane from placenta, adipose tissue, and skeletal muscle from normal pregnant women and women with gestational diabetes mellitus. J Clin Endocrinol Metab 2004; 89(11): 5627-33.

[46]   Radaelli T, Varastehpour A, Catalano P, Hauguel-de Mouzon S. Gestational diabetes induces placental genes for chronic stress and inflammatory pathways. Diabetes 2003; 52(12): 2951-8.

[47]   Barbour LA, McCurdy CE, Hernandez TL, Kirwan JP, Catalano PM, Friedman JE. Cellular mechanisms for insulin resistance in normal pregnancy and gestational diabetes. Diabetes Care 2007; 30(Suppl 2): S112-9.

[48]   Varastehpour A, Radaelli T, Minium J, *et al.* Activation of phospholipase A2 is associated with generation of placental lipid signals and fetal obesity. J Clin Endocrinol Metab 2006; 91(1): 248-55.

[49]   Van Assche FA, Holemans K, Aerts L. Long-term consequences for offspring of diabetes during pregnancy. Br Med Bull 2001; 60: 173-82.

[50]   Paramsothy P, Lin YS, Kernic MA, Foster-Schubert KE. Interpregnancy weight gain and cesarean delivery risk in women with a history of gestational diabetes. Obstet Gynecol 2009; 113(4): 817-23.

[51]   Weintrob N, Karp M, Hod M. Short-and long-range complications in offspring of diabetic mothers. J Diabetes Complications 1996; 10(5): 294-301.

[52]   Alam M, Raza SJ, Sherali AR, Akhtar AS. Neonatal complications in infants born to diabetic mothers. J Coll Physicians Surg Pak 2006; 16(3): 212-5.

[53]   ter Braak EW, Evers IM, Willem Erkelens D, Visser GH. Maternal hypoglycemia during pregnancy in type 1 diabetes: maternal and fetal consequences. Diabetes Metab Res Rev 2002; 18(2): 96-105.

[54]   Feng   A,   Steele   D.   Pediatrics,   respiratory   distress   syndrome.   2006;   Available   from: http://www.emedicine.com/emerg/topic398.htm. [Accessed June 15, 2011]

[55]   Mehta JL, Rasouli N, Sinha AK, Molavi B. Oxidative stress in diabetes: a mechanistic overview of its effects on atherogenesis and myocardial dysfunction. Int J Biochem Cell Biol 2006; 38(5-6): 794-803.

[56]   Kinalski M, Sledziewski A, Telejko B, *et al.* Lipid peroxidation, antioxidant defence and acid-base status in cord blood at birth: the influence of diabetes. Hormone and metabolic research Hormon-und Stoffwechselforschung 2001; 33(4): 227-31.

[57]   Bis-Gluchowska M, Marciniak B, Szpringer-Bogun E, Rola R, Leszczynska-Gorzelak B, Oleszczuk J. [Determination of antioxidative-peroxidative balance in the cord blood of newborns delivered to mothers with diabetes type G1] Ginekol Pol 2001; 72(12A): 1255-8.

[58]   Biri A, Onan A, Devrim E, Babacan F, Kavutcu M, Durak I. Oxidant status in maternal and cord plasma and placental tissue in gestational diabetes. Placenta 2006; 27(2-3): 327-32.

[59]   Allen RG, Venkatraj VS. Oxidants and antioxidants in development and differentiation. J Nutr 1992; 122(3 Suppl): 631-5.

[60]   Rafalowska U, Liu GJ, Floyd RA. Peroxidation induced changes in synaptosomal transport of dopamine and gamma-aminobutyric acid. Free Radic Biol Med 1989; 6(5): 485-92.

[61]   Mahadik SP, Mukherjee S. Free radical pathology and antioxidant defense in schizophrenia: a review. Schizophr Res 1996; 19(1): 1-17.

[62]   Stadtman ER. Protein oxidation and aging. Science 1992; 257(5074): 1220-4.

[63]   Boney CM, Verma A, Tucker R, Vohr BR. Metabolic syndrome in childhood: association with birth weight, maternal obesity, and gestational diabetes mellitus. Pediatrics 2005; 115(3): e290-6.

[64]   Luo ZC, Delvin E, Fraser WD, *et al.* Maternal Glucose Tolerance in Pregnancy Affects Fetal Insulin Sensitivity. Diabetes Care 2010; 33(9): 2055-2061.

[65]   Boerschmann H, Pfluger M, Henneberger L, Ziegler AG, Hummel S. Prevalence and predictors of overweight and insulin resistance in offspring of mothers with gestational diabetes mellitus. Diabetes Care 2010; 33(8): 1845-9.

[66]   Lampl M, Jeanty P. Exposure to maternal diabetes is associated with altered fetal growth patterns: A hypothesis regarding metabolic allocation to growth under hyperglycemic-hypoxemic conditions. Am J Hum Biol 2004; 16(3): 237-63.

[67]   Carrapato M. The offspring of gestational diabetes. Journal of Perinatal Medicine 2003; 31: 5-11.

[68]   Akyol A, Kiylioglu N, Bolukbasi O, Guney E, Yurekli Y. Repeated hypoglycemia and cognitive decline. A case report. Neuro Endocrinol Lett 2003; 24(1-2): 54-6.

[69]   Rizzo TA, Metzger BE, Dooley SL, Cho NH. Early malnutrition and child neurobehavioral development: insights from the study of children of diabetic mothers. Child Dev 1997; 68(1): 26-38.

[70]   Smoak IW, Sadler TW. Embryopathic effects of short-term exposure to hypoglycemia in mouse embryos *in vitro*. Am J Obstet Gynecol 1990; 163(2): 619-24.

[71]   Knipp GT, Audus KL, Soares MJ. Nutrient transport across the placenta. Adv Drug Deliv Rev 1999; 38(1): 41-58.

CHAPTER 7

Placental Disorders in Preeclampsia: Maternal and Perinatal Outcomes

Dave Lanoix[1,2], Sophie Haché[2,3], Evemie Dubé [2,3], Julie Lafond[2,3] and Cathy Vaillancourt[1,2,*]

[1]*INRS-Institut Armand-Frappier, Université du Québec, 531 blvd. des Prairies, Laval, QC, Canada, H7V 1B7;* [2]*BioMed Research Centre and* [3]*Department of Sciences Biologiques, Université du Québec à Montréal, C.P. 8888, Succursale Centre-Ville, Montreal, QC, H3C 3P8, Canada*

Abstract: Preeclampsia, a disorder of pregnancy, is a leading cause of maternal and infant illness and death affecting about 3-15 % of all pregnancies worldwide. It is characterized by high blood pressure and the presence of protein in the urine. It originates in the placenta and causes variable maternal and fetal problems. At its worst, it may threaten maternal and perinatal survival. Preeclampsia is defined as a syndrome (a pattern of clinical features) and is probably heterogeneous in its origin as it is in its presentation. To date, the only complete cure known for preeclampsia is delivery, accompanied by the removal of the placenta. As the complete etiology of preeclampsia is still unknown, researches are crucial in order to know more about this pathophysiology and to develop different treatments and prediction approaches. This chapter focuses on current knowledge and recent discoveries on preeclampsia, especially on the role of placenta in its physiopathology. The chapter also presents current knowledge concerning preeclampsia diagnosis, epidemiology, risk factors and pathogenesis with an emphasis on maternal and perinatal outcomes related to this most common cause of death for both children and mothers during pregnancy.

Keywords: Preeclampsia, placenta, fetal development, maternal hypertension, proteinuria, trophoblast, intra-uterine growth restriction (IUGR).

INTRODUCTION: EPIDEMIOLOGY AND RISK FACTORS

Preeclampsia is one of the most common pregnancy complication with a worldwide incidence of 3-15% and causes approximately 63 000 deaths annually, mainly in less developed countries [1, 2]. This disorder is the most common cause of death for both children and mothers during pregnancy and is responsible for 15% of premature births in industrialized countries. High blood pressure is relatively common in pregnancy, affecting 12-18% of all pregnancies [3]. About 50% of women with gestational hypertension will develop preeclampsia [4]. Healthy nulliparous women correspond to nearly 75% of cases where the disease is mild and the risk of pregnancy outcome is negligible [5-7]. However, the burden and frequency of preeclampsia are significantly increased with by medical conditions, such as multiparous pregnancy, chronic hypertension, pre-existing diabetes mellitus, pre-gestational thrombophilia and previous preeclampsia. Table **1** summarizes the most commons risk factors associated with increased risk of preeclampsia.

Preeclampsia is often described as a disease of first pregnancies. Indeed, risk of preeclampsia is most important in first pregnancies [34, 35] while it is decreased by pre-conception maternal sperm exposure [36, 37]. Furthermore, conception through assisted reproductive technologies using donor sperm increases the risk of preeclampsia [38, 39]. These studies suggest a major immunological and paternal factor in the pathogenesis of preeclampsia. Moreover, women who have preeclampsia during their first pregnancy have more chances of developing preeclampsia again in the next pregnancy. In fact, when preeclampsia is developed before 30 weeks of gestation during the first pregnancy, the recurrence rate may be as high as 40% in future pregnancies [3].

*Address correspondence to Cathy Vaillancourt: INRS-Institut Armand-Frappier, Université du Québec, 531 blvd. des Prairies, Laval, QC, Canada, H7V 1B7; Tel: 450-687-5010, Fax: 450-686-5389, E-mail: cathy.vaillancourt@iaf.inrs.ca

Table 1: Risk factors

Maternal risk factors
❖ Multiparous pregnancy [8-10]
❖ Chronic hypertension [11, 12]
❖ Bilateral notches [13]
❖ Pre-existing diabetes mellitus [14, 15]
❖ Previous preeclampsia [16-18]
❖ Pre-gestational thrombophilia [19, 20]
❖ Elevated or low maternal age [21, 22]
❖ Obesity and insulin resistance [23-25]
❖ Familiar history of preeclampsia [26, 27]
❖ Maternal infections [28-30]
❖ Maternal susceptibility genes [31-33]
Paternal risk factors
❖ Primipaternity [34, 35]
❖ Limited sperm exposure [36, 37]
❖ Conception after assisted reproductive technologies [38-40]

CLINICAL SYMPTOMS

Preeclampsia is an heterogeneous and systemic disease, which usually develops after 20 weeks of gestation and prior 48 h postpartum [41]. Clinical guidelines support the distinction into mild and severe preeclampsia, as well as early (before 34 weeks) and late (after 34 weeks) onset of preeclampsia [42, 43]. Typical symptoms of mild preeclampsia include systolic blood pressure (SBP) $\geq$ 140 mm Hg or diastolic blood pressure (DBP) $\geq$ 90 mm Hg and proteinuria ($\geq$ 300 mg in 24 h urine sample) [44, 45]. Generally the late onset preeclampsia shows mild symptoms and accounts for more than 80% of all cases worldwide [42]. Severe preeclampsia, which usually includes the early onset type, is described as SBP $\geq$ 160 mm Hg or DBP $\geq$ 110 mm Hg on two occasions at least 6 h apart in a woman on bed rest and proteinuria ($\geq$ 5 g in 24 h urine sample) on two random urine samples collected at least 4 h apart [42, 45].

Blood Pressure

In normotensive pregnancies, several changes in uterine blood flow are observed including a decrease in blood pressure and peripheral vascular resistance [46], an increase of maternal blood volume, cardiac output [47] and artery volume flow [48]. These changes are essential to meet metabolic demands from the placenta and to increase the flow of nutrients to the growing fetus [49]. However, preeclamptic pregnant women show impaired endothelium-dependent vasorelaxation, widespread vasoconstriction, high vascular resistance, low cardiac output [50, 51] and a decrease in utero-placental blood flow by up to 50% [52].

Hemodynamic and vascular adaptations are also altered in preeclamptic pregnancies. The parathyroid hormone related protein (PTHrP), which is one of the factors involved in this regulation, shows decreased circulating levels in preeclamptic women [53]. PTHrP plays many roles during the pregnancy, such as the relaxation of uterine arteries [54] and placental calcium transfer [55-57]. In addition, disturbances of the utero-placental renin-angiotensin system (RAS) in pregnancies complicated by preeclampsia could lead to dysfunctional bleeding and reduced utero-placental blood flow [58]. Indeed the circulating RAS plays a key role in regulating blood pressure and electrolyte balance. Furthermore, the utero-placental RAS is important for the regeneration of the endometrium after shedding, and for decidualization, implantation and placentation.

Calcium supplementation reduces blood pressure in pregnant women at risk for hypertensive disorders or with low dietary calcium intake [59-62]. Urinary calcium excretion also correlates to increase blood pressure in preeclampsia [63]. In fact, during normotensive pregnancies, the extracellular fluid volume expands. In consequence, there is a dilution of calcium and an increased glomerular filtration which causes calcium losses [63].

Proteinuria

Proteinuria is a major dysfunction of preeclampsia, defined as a urinary total protein of $\geq$ 300 mg in 24 h. Proteinuria is generally associated with glomerular endotheliosis, described as the swelling of the glomerular capillary endothelium that causes decreased glomerular perfusion and filtration rate [41, 64]. It is not permanent and recovers after delivery [65].

Proteinuria is not universally considered obligatory for the diagnosis of preeclampsia [66]. For example, the Australasian Society for the Study of Hypertension in Pregnancy (ASSHP) and the Society of Obstetric Medicine of Australia and New Zealand (SOMANZ) do not required proteinuria [67]. In this case, to be diagnosed for preeclampsia, women need to have hypertension and one of the following clinical features: renal insufficiency, pulmonary edema, liver disease, neurological problems, hematological disturbance, intra-uterine growth restriction (IUGR) or proteinuria. On the other hand, the International Society for the Study of Hypertension in Pregnancy (ISSHP) [68] and the National High Blood Pressure Education Program Working Party (NHBPEP) in United States [3] require proteinuria for the diagnosis of preeclampsia. Besides, the Canadian Hypertension Society (CHS) [69] has restrained the use of the term preeclampsia and focuses more on gestational hypertension with and without proteinuria. In general, the term "proteinuric preeclampsia" is now used in several researches and clinical trials [70]. There is another discrepancy in the definition of proteinuria, since the ISSHP [68] and the ASSHP [67] define proteinuria as > 300 mg protein in a 24 h sample or a random spot protein-to-creatinine ratio of > 30 mg/mmol, while the NHBPEP [3] requires > 300 mg protein in a 24 h specimen and the CHS [69] accepts only a 24 h sample result for diagnostic purposes. Furthermore, it was demonstrated that women with proteinuric preeclampsia used more magnesium sulfate ($MgSO_4$) and had higher blood pressure at earlier gestation than non-proteinuric preeclampsia women [66]. Proteinuria is often absent in women who develop HELLP (Hemolysis, Elevated Liver enzymes, Low Platelet count) syndrome [71], but IUGR occurs equally in proteinuric or non-proteinuric preeclampsia women [66]. Moreover, the loss of serum protein leads to a decrease of intravascular volume and increased tissue edema [72]. The maternal decreased blood volume can lead to an increase in hemoglobin concentration, which is associated to an increased risk of developing IUGR [73].

Edema

In normotensive pregnancy, the amount of maternal body fluids, mostly blood, nearly doubles in order to support the growth and development of the fetus and the placenta. Edema (*e.g.* severe swelling of the face, hands and feet), caused by fluid retention, is often associated with preeclampsia. Severe edema in preeclampsia is related to proteinuria. In fact, the loss of serum protein along with increased capillary endothelial permeability leads to a decrease in intravascular volume and increased tissue edema. Loss of proteins from the blood through the urine has an osmotic attraction toward the water contained in blood and, as a consequence, the water leaks from the blood into the body's tissues [72].

As mentioned earlier, preeclampsia is a systemic disease and edema affects many organs, including liver, brain and lungs. Acute pulmonary edema is a major cause of death in women affected by preeclampsia [74] and refers to an excessive accumulation of fluid in the pulmonary interstitial and alveolar spaces [75]. During normotensive pregnancy, physiological changes in the maternal cardiovascular system, including increased plasma blood volume, cardiac output, heart rate, capillary permeability and a decrease in plasma colloid osmotic pressure, are intensified in preeclampsia and predispose women to develop pulmonary edema [76].

PATHOGENESIS: ROLE OF THE PLACENTA

Preeclampsia has been known as the "disease of theories" since the sixties [77]. Today, the precise cause of preeclampsia still remains unknown. However, extensive research has led to major advances in the comprehension of the pathogenesis of this presumably multifactorial disease. Based on those advancements, the concept of a 2 stage development of preeclampsia has been originally proposed in 1991 by Chris Redman [78]. The first stage occurs before the appearance of clinical signs (before the 20th week of pregnancy) and is characterized by a poor placentation. The second stage (after the 20th week of pregnancy) is characterized by placental stress in response to the poor placentation, leading to the maternal syndrome of preeclampsia (hypertension, proteinuria and edema). Although the 2 stage model has been revised and challenged, it remains the most widely accepted theory to explain the development of preeclampsia [42, 79-82]. It is noteworthy to mention that Drs Redman and Sargent have recently proposed that preeclampsia could be a 4 stage disease; a maternal-fetal immune maladaptation would be the cause of the poor placentation [83, 84]. This chapter will focus on the currently accepted 2 stage model but the new 4 stage theory will be discussed.

Role of the Placenta

The central role of the placenta in preeclampsia is known for more than a hundred years [85]. The development of preeclampsia is dependent on the presence of a placenta. Furthermore, the only definitive treatment for preeclampsia is the complete removal of placental tissue. It has even been shown that a fetus is not required for the development of preeclampsia, such as in molar pregnancies [86]. Moreover, in cases of preeclampsia where only the fetus has been removed, the maternal syndrome persisted until removal of the placenta [87, 88]. Even though cases of postpartum preeclampsia have been described, they have been associated with incomplete removal of placental tissue since resection of maternal syndrome has been shown after uterine curettage [89, 90].

Important pathologic changes are observed in the preeclampsia placenta, such as insufficient utero-placental blood flow leading to placental ischemia and consequently oxidative stress. In the most severe cases of preeclampsia, these pathologic changes will lead to infarcts (for a review of placental pathologic modifications in preeclampsia, see [91]). These anatomopathological modifications are not necessarily all present in cases of preeclampsia but they are significantly more frequent [92]. Moreover, these gross anatomical or histological lesions are not useful as diagnosis criteria because they are not specific to preeclampsia [93]. For example, antiphospholipid syndrom (lupus anticoagulant antibodies) presents exactly the same placental pathology as preeclampsia but without the specific maternal syndrome [94-97]. Many attempted to make correlation between the severity of these pathologic changes and the severity of the maternal syndrome but it is still disputed [98-101]. Even if no specific pathological lesions of the preeclampsia placenta have been established, the placenta is still an essential stimulus for the development of preeclampsia. Furthermore, a poor placentation is an important predisposing factor for the development of preeclampsia while placental stress is the keystone of the maternal syndrome.

Stage 1-Poor Placentation

The abnormal development of the early placenta, the insufficient invasion and remodeling of uterine spiral arteries by extravillous cytotrophoblasts, which results in reduced maternal blood supply to the placenta, is called poor placentation. The preeclampsia syndrome was considered to be caused by poor placentation [102]. However, because poor placentation also occurs in normotensive pregnancies with small fetuses, it is more likely a powerful predisposing factor for preeclampsia rather than its origin [103-105].

In normotensive pregnancies, the formation of the chorionic villi, the structural and functional unit of the placenta, is initiated at 13 days post-conception. The core of the chorionic villi is composed of the fetal stroma and the outer epithelial layer is formed by the trophoblast. The villi are classified as anchoring (or stem) villi, promoting implantation and maintenance of early pregnancy, or as floating villi, mediating placental growth and transplacental exchanges. The subtypes of trophoblast cells present in the floating villi are the villous cytotrophoblast and the syncytiotrophoblast whereas the extravillous cytotrophoblasts are located in the anchoring villi (for a review of human placental development, see [106]). The tip of the anchoring villi is formed by a column of extravillous cytotrophoblasts. The cells from layers adjacent to the fetal stroma are proliferative extravillous cytotrophoblasts. The cells from distal layers of the column have exited the cell cycle and have acquired an invasive phenotype. Invasive extravillous cytotrophoblasts (small spindle-shaped extravillous cytotrophoblasts) will spread from the distal part of the cell column into the decidua and myometrium [107]. These highly invasive extravillous cytotrophoblasts will either invade the placental bed or terminally differentiate in large polygonal trophoblast cells [108, 109] or in multinucleated trophoblast giant cells [110]. Otherwise these cells will invade the uterine spiral arteries, acquire an endothelial-like phenotype, replace the spiral arteries endothelial cells, participate in the degradation of tunica media smooth muscle cells and terminally differentiate into endovascular extravillous cytotrophoblasts [111, 112]. The spiral arteries are thus remodeled from small and highly constricted vessels to large capacitance vessels devoid of contractile capability (Fig. **1**). This remodeling of the spiral arteries is essential to allow a proper placental perfusion to sustain fetal growth and pregnancy well-being [113].

In preeclampsia, the remodeling of uterine spiral arteries is altered. Reduced invasion of uterine spiral arteries by extravillous cytotrophoblasts in preeclampsia has been identified for the first time in 1972 [102]. Decreased number of invasive extravillous cytotrophoblasts in placental bed as well as decreased depth of invasion of these cells has been demonstrated in preeclampsia [114]. These observations correlate with the defective differentiation from proliferative to invasive extravillous cytotrophoblasts in preeclampsia [115, 116]. Moreover, increased apoptosis of extravillous cytotrophoblasts in placental bed of preeclampsia has been shown [117, 118]. Taken together, these findings support the partial invasion of the decidual segments of spiral arteries by extravillous cytotrophoblasts and the important decreased invasion of their myometrial segments [119]. In addition, spiral arteries endothelial cells are not replaced by extravillous cytotrophoblasts and smooth muscle cells are not degraded in the myometrial segments, resulting in inadequate remodeling of spiral arteries [113]. Consequently, in preeclampsia, the uterine spiral arteries remain small, contractile and high-resistance vessels, resulting in insufficient uteroplacental arterial blood flow and in poor placentation (Fig. **1**) [120, 121]. The sequence of events leading to the poor placental perfusion takes place before the 20th week of pregnancy, prior to the appearance of clinical signs. It is thus difficult to determine which mechanisms are implicated in its development. However, several factors involved in extravillous cytotrophoblasts invasion seem to be altered in preeclampsia, the most important being oxygen tension and immunologic factors.

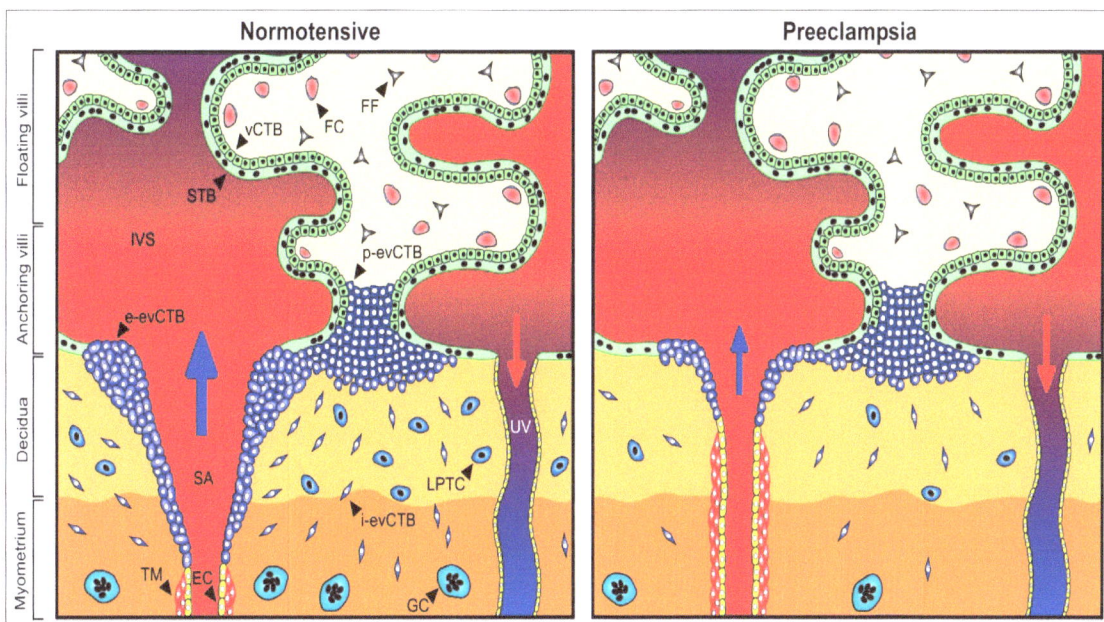

Figure 1: Placentation in normotensive and preeclamptic pregnancies. EC (endothelial cell), e-evCTB (endovascular extravillous cytotrophoblast), FC (fetal capillaries), FF (fetal fibroblast), GC (trophoblast giant cell), IVS (intervillous space), LPTC (large-polygonal trophoblast cell), i-evCTB (invasive extravillous cytotrophoblast), p-evCTB (proliferative extravillous cytotrophoblast), STB (syncytiotrophoblast), SA (uterine spiral arteries), TM (tunica media smooth muscle cell), UV (uterine vein), vCTB (villous cytotrophoblast).

Oxygen Tension

In early pregnancy, before the 10th week, there is negligible maternal blood flow to the placenta since invasive extravillous cytotrophoblasts have not yet reached and remodeled the spiral arteries. This creates a hypoxic environment that is reduced after remodeling of the spiral arteries by invasive extravillous cytotrophoblasts. Moreover, the oxygen tension is higher in the spiral arteries than in the placental bed, creating an increasing oxygen gradient that seem to act as a stimulus for extravillous cytotrophoblasts invasion and differentiation in their endovascular phenotype [122]. *In vitro*, increased oxygen tension stimulates the differentiation of extravillous cytotrophoblasts from their proliferative to their invasive phenotype [123]. Furthermore, at higher oxygen tension, extravillous cytotrophoblasts express cellular adhesion molecules similar to those of vascular endothelial cells [124]. Accordingly, decreased oxygen tension alters extravillous cytotrophoblasts differentiation and invasion, mimicking the events taking place in preeclampsia [123-125]. In addition, the hypoxia-inducible transcription factor-1α (HIF-1α) is expressed in first trimester placental explants cultured under low oxygen and its expression is decreased under increased oxygen tension [126]. Interestingly, HIF-1α expression and activity is highly up-regulated in the preeclampsia placenta [127, 128]. HIF-1α stimulates the expression of transforming growth factor-β3 (TGF-β3), an inhibitor of villous trophoblast invasion, and the antisens inhibition of HIF-1α expression inhibits invasion and TGF-β3 expression in placental explants [129]. Taken together, these findings indicate that oxygen is a master regulator of extravillous cytotrophoblasts invasion and differentiation. However, it is currently not known if an early hypoxic placenta is the cause to the altered extravillous cytotrophoblasts differentiation and invasion or if it is the consequence of the defective remodeling of the spiral arteries.

Immunologic Factors

The fetus is an allograft, carrying both maternal and paternal antigens. The immune theory of preeclampsia proposes that a maternal-fetal immune maladaptation would result in the recognition of the extravillous cytotrophoblasts (fetal) by the decidual immune cells (maternal), causing the poor placentation [39, 130]. As mentioned earlier, a recent study by the fathers of the concept of the 2 stage disease argues that preeclampsia could be a 3 stage disease, the first step being this maternal-fetal immune maladaptation [83]. The immune theory of preeclampsia relies on many epidemiological and clinical studies. Preeclampsia occurs mostly in first pregnancies [34, 35]. It suggests that the foreign fetus triggers the maternal immune system and that it could become tolerant through successive pregnancies [131, 132]. This protective effect of multiparity is lost with a new partner [36]. Moreover, a great exposition of the maternal organism to paternal antigens, through oral and vaginal sperm exposure, will result in reduced risk of preeclampsia [36, 37]. The use of barrier contraceptives (condom or diaphragm) abolishes these protective effects [133, 134]. In addition, conception through assisted reproductive technologies, using donor sperm or surgically obtained sperm, increases the risk of preeclampsia; supporting the importance of pre-conception exposure to paternal sperm [38, 39]. Overall, these studies reinforce the concept that preeclampsia could be caused by a defective maternal immunosuppressive response to induce tolerance to paternal antigens.

The most abundant leukocytes in the decidua are uterine natural killer (uNK) cells, macrophages and T lymphocytes [135]. In the first trimester of pregnancy, 30-40% of the decidual cells are leukocytes in close contact with the invading extravillous cytotrophoblasts [135]. Invasive extravillous cytotrophoblasts expressed human leukocyte antigen (HLA)-C, which can trigger a maternal immune response since it has a paternal specificity [136]. Both uNK and T lymphocytes can recognize the HLA-C [137, 138]. Moreover, uNK are the only decidual cells expressing killer immunoglobulin-like receptors (KIR), for which HLA-C is the main ligand [137]. KIR and HLA-C are both highly polymorphic genes that are genetically inherited [139]. It is noteworthy to mention that epidemiological studies show a genetic susceptibility for both men and women born from preeclamptic pregnancies to have a child from a preeclamptic pregnancy and this risk is increased in cases of both maternal and paternal familial history of preeclampsia [140, 141]. In normal pregnancies, uNK promotes extravillous cytotrophoblasts invasion and spiral arteries remodeling by chemokines, cytokines and growth factors secretion [142]. These preeclampsia-protective effects were associated with a specific polymorphic combination of KIR and HLA-C [143]. In opposition, a specific combination of KIR and HLA-C was associated with an increased risk or preeclampsia [144]. This extravillous cytotrophoblasts-uNK recognition pattern could explain the partner-specificity and genetically inherited susceptibility for preeclampsia [83]. However, the KIR-HLA-C interaction does not clarify why preeclampsia occurs mostly in first pregnancies and why the risk decreases with subsequent pregnancies with the same partner. This could be explained by T-cell memory. As mentioned, T-lymphocytes can recognize the HLA-C. T-lymphocytes memory seems stable enough to induce tolerance to paternal antigens in a second pregnancy [145]. In addition, NK cells and macrophages, both localized in the decidua, can elicit a form of immune memory [146-148]. As mentioned by Redman and Sargent, the greater risk of preeclampsia in first pregnancies, partner-specificity and genetic susceptibility could be explained by their novel immune theory of a 4 stage disease, although further experiments are required [83]. For more detailed review in immunology and preeclampsia see Chapter 5 from Saito in this eBook.

Stage 2 – Placental Oxidative Stress and the Maternal Syndrome

The final stage of preeclampsia is a maternal syndrome characterized by a new appearance of hypertension and proteinuria after 20 weeks' pregnancy and resolving after delivery. According to the 2 stage model – and supported by evidence – these clinical signs are the result of a maternal systemic inflammatory stress in response to the release of various syncytiotrophoblast factors. The release of these factors is stimulated by the placental oxidative stress secondary to the poor placentation (Fig. **2**).

Placental Oxidative Stress

There is an increased oxidative stress during normal pregnancy [149, 150]. Furthermore, the oxidative stress and resulting damages are significantly amplified in preeclampsia [151]. In addition, numerous placental oxidative stress biomarkers are increased in preeclampsia, such as TNF-α levels [152], HNE-modified proteins [153, 154], 8-isoprostane levels [155], superoxide radical's concentration [156] and protein carbonyls [157]. Accordingly, the placenta is a major source of oxidative stress in preeclampsia and several studies have shown that the generation of placental oxidative stress is a key event in its pathogenesis [79, 82, 151, 158-160].

The placental oxidative stress was suggested to be generated by reduced utero-placental arterial blood flow resulting from deficient remodeling of uterine spiral arteries and thus creating a chronically hypoxic placenta [113, 161]. However, as reported by Hung and Burton, chronic placental hypoxia – the placenta is starved of oxygen – does not seem to be the inducer of oxidative stress in preeclampsia for many reasons [162]. In sheep, chronic restriction of the uterine blood flow is responsible for reduced placental metabolism and significant decrease of placental and fetal weight [163]. It is not the case in preeclampsia [164, 165]. Moreover, in high altitude pregnancies with restrict oxygen supply to the placental bed, the placenta does not show signs of oxidative damage [166, 167]. The trophoblast is used to low oxygen tension. During first trimester, the placental oxygen concentration is far below the one at the third trimester until it rises around 12 weeks' [168]. Hung and Burton thus suggest that the placental oxidative stress occurring in preeclampsia might be induced by hypoxia-reoxygenation rather than by hypoxia alone [162]. In preeclampsia, remodeling of the uterine spiral arteries only occurs in the decidual segment of the spiral arteries and they remain mostly vasoactive (Fig. **1**). The maternal blood flow would thus enter the intervillous space at high pressure in a pulsatile manner, exposing the placenta to arbitrarily oscillating oxygen tension [169, 170]. This is supported by studies showing that hypoxia/reoxygenation generates high levels of free radicals, namely reactive nitrogen species (RNS) and reactive oxygen species (ROS) that are present in the preeclampsia placenta [171, 172]. In addition, first trimester placental explants survive well in low oxygen condition but become stressed when the oxygen tension is raised, inducing oxidative stress and apoptosis [173-175].

ROS Generation

In preeclampsia, the predominant ROS produced by the placenta are superoxide radicals ($\bullet O_2^-$) and hydrogen peroxide (H_2O_2) [156]. They are mainly generated by two intracellular sources, the xanthine dehydrogenase/xanthine oxidase (XDH/XO) pathway and the mitochondria respiratory chain.

XDH is a key enzyme in purine catabolism, catalyzing the hydroxylation of hypoxanthine to xanthine and of xanthine to urate. However, in hypoxia, XDH is irreversibly converted to XO through protease-mediated sulfhydryl oxidation [176]. Thus, cellular ATP is catalyzed to hypoxanthine and it accumulates throughout the hypoxic period. On reoxygenation, reintroduced oxygen, hypoxanthine and XO will combine to generate superoxide and hydrogen peroxide [177, 178]. Moreover, hypoxia upregulates XO activity, enhancing hypoxanthine build up and consequently ROS formation [179]. XDH/XO mRNA and protein expression as well as enzyme activity have been detected in normal term placenta [180, 181]. In preeclampsia placentas, increased protein expression of XDH/XO is shown compared to normal placentas and XDH/XO co-localizes with nitrotyrosine residues, a marker of oxidative stress [182]. In addition, XO activity is increased in preeclampsia placenta [183]. The release of XDH/XO in the circulation upon hypoxia/reoxygenation has been demonstrated in the liver and intestine [184, 185]. However, it is yet to be shown whether it is the case in the placenta. Nevertheless, maternal circulating levels of XO are higher in preeclampsia than in normal pregnancies, so it is likely it could originate from the placenta subsequently to hypoxia/reoxygenation [186, 187]. Finally, perfusion of normal human placentas with XO induces changes in oxidative stress and apoptosis-related genes expression similar to what is described in preeclampsia [188].

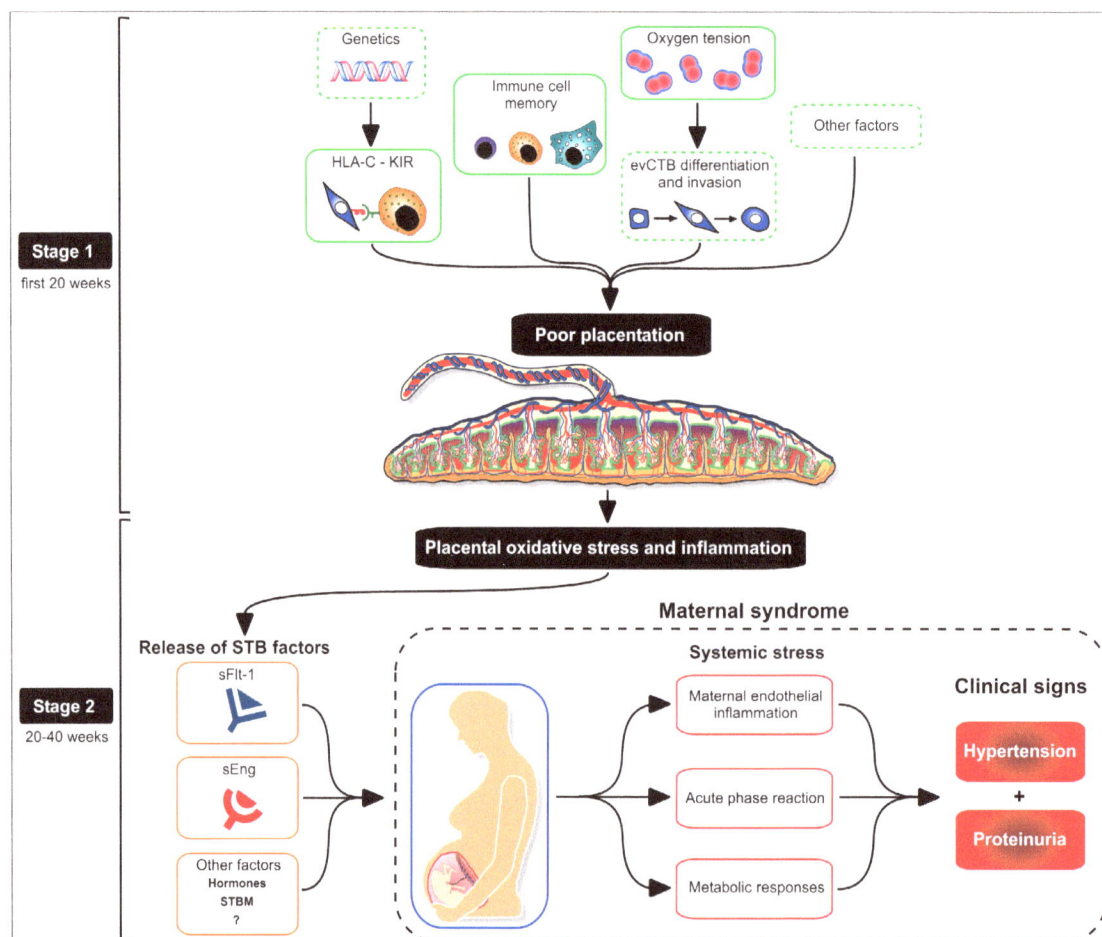

Figure 2: Summary of the pathogenesis of preeclampsia, according to the 2 stage disease theory. HLA-C (human leukocyte antigen-C), KIR (killer-cell immunoglobulin-like receptors), evCTB (extravillous cytotrophoblast), STB (syncytiotrophoblast), sFlt-1 (soluble fms-like tyrosine kinase-1), sEng (soluble endoglin), STBM (syncytiotrophoblast microparticles).

The placental mitochondria respiratory chain is another source of ROS in preeclampsia [189]. During mitochondrial oxidative phosphorylation, electrons are transferred from reduced nicotinamide adenine dinucleotide (NADH) or flavin adenine dinucleotide (FADH$_2$) to molecular oxygen (O$_2$), resulting in adenosine triphosphate (ATP) synthesis [190]. The electron transfer process generates superoxide radicals [191, 192]. In normal placenta, superoxide radical's levels are tightly regulated by the manganese superoxide dismutase (Mn-SOD), in the mitochondria, and by its isoform, the copper/zinc superoxide dismutase (Cu/Zn-SOD), in the cytoplasm [193]. The SOD catalyzes the dismutation of superoxide radicals to hydrogen peroxide and molecular oxygen [194]. However, in preeclampsia, decreased expression and activity of placental SOD are reported, resulting in increased superoxide radicals levels [160, 171, 195, 196]. The decomposition of cellular hydrogen peroxide to water and molecular oxygen is catalyzed by the catalase and the glutathione peroxidase (GPX) [197]. No difference in catalase expression and an increased catalase activity have been reported in placenta from preeclamptic compared to normal pregnancies [196]. However, the expression and activity of placental GPX are decreased in preeclampsia, reducing hydrogen peroxide elimination [160, 198-202]. Two studies have shown no difference in GPX levels between normal and preeclamptic placentas, suggesting that the GPX expression may not be correlated to its activity [203, 204]. Taken together, these findings show that preeclampsia is characterized by an increased placental ROS production and decreased placental antioxidant defense mechanisms.

Oxidative Stress Damage

Placental ROS generate broad spectrum cytotoxic effects, ranging from damaged cellular proteins and lipids to activation of cell signaling cascades leading to syncytiotrophoblast injury and ultimately cell death.

Common ROS-mediated injuries include protein carbonylation and nitrosylation as well as lipid peroxidation. Protein carbonylation is an irreversible type of protein oxidation leading to loss of protein function and to structural alterations [205]. The irreparable nature of protein carbonyls makes them markers of choice for oxidative stress damage [206]. Placentas from preeclampsia are characterized by increased levels of protein carbonyls [157, 160, 207]. Another type of oxidative-stress mediated protein alteration is the nitrosylation of protein by peroxynitrite anions. Peroxynitrite anion is the product of superoxide radical and nitric oxide interaction [208]. Peroxinitrite is a strong oxidant which, in addition to protein nitrosylation, can generates protein carbonyls, initiates lipid peroxidation, inhibits mitochondrial electron transport and nitrate tyrosine residues, thereby affecting signal transduction pathways [209-212]. Nitrotyrosine detection is used as a marker of peroxinitrite formation since they are undetectable due to their unstability [213]. Increased levels of nitrotyrosine residues are observed in placenta from preeclampsia, indicating adverse action of peroxinitrites [172, 214, 215]. Lipid peroxidation is the degradation of cellular lipids upon exposure to ROS [216]. Lipid peroxides are formed in a chain reaction which if not stop, can disturb membrane fluidity and permeability, alter ion transport, inhibit metabolic processes and injure mitochondria, inducing further ROS generation and apoptosis [217, 218]. Increased lipid peroxides have been shown in preeclamptic placentas [219-221]. An increase in lipid peroxides has been specifically demonstrated in the mitochondria and cellular membrane of the syncytiotrophoblast of preeclamptic placentas [153, 222-224]. Accordingly, syncytiotrophoblast membrane integrity alteration and mitochondrial apoptosis are observed in preeclampsia [225, 226].

ROS can regulate several cellular processes by acting as second messengers, by altering signaling pathways or by altering cellular homeostasis. In the placenta, the mitogen activated protein kinases (MAPK), the nuclear factor-κB (NF-κB) and the calcium transport are among the most significant [227, 228]. The MAPK are a family of protein kinases involved in many physiologic responses and regulatory mechanisms [229]. There are four families of MAPK, the extracellular signal-regulated kinases (ERK 1/2), the p38 kinases, the stress-activated protein kinase/c-Jun NH2-terminal kinases (SAPK/JNK) and the ERK5. ROS are known inducers of apoptosis through the p38 and SAPK/JNK pathways [230]. Hypoxia/reoxygenation activates p38 and SAPK/JNK stress pathways in villous trophoblast explants, inducing pro-inflammatory cytokines release and apoptosis [228, 231]. Moreover, increased placental activation of p38 has been reported in preeclampsia [232]. NF-κB is a dimeric transcription factor. ROS-activated NF-κB promotes the transcription of genes involved in inflammation, stress response and apoptosis, such as HIF-1α [233, 234]. Hypoxia/reoxygenation induces the NF-κB pathway in villous trophoblast explants, stimulating pro-inflammatory cytokines secretion and apoptosis [231]. Increased expression of placental NF-κB is also demonstrated in preeclampsia [235]. Calcium transport through the placenta regulates numerous cellular processes [236]. Calcium homeostasis is involved in signal transduction, neurotransmission, hormone secretion, cell-cycle regulation and mitochondrial functions [237]. Oxidative stress is a known modulator of calcium homeostasis, inducing apoptosis [238-241]. Altered placental calcium homeostasis is observed in preeclampsia [227]. A recent study suggest that altered calcium homeostasis in preeclampsia syncytiotrophoblast is secondary to oxidative stress [227]. As reviewed, ROS activate placental signaling pathways and altere cellular homeostasis, inducing placental inflammatory stress and apoptosis in preeclampsia.

The most damaging effect of ROS is cellular death. ROS-mediated cellular death can be from necrotic or apoptotic origin. Necrosis is caused by elevated ROS levels whereas apoptosis occurs at low ROS levels [228]. As discussed previously, ROS can promote apoptosis through several ways, such as peroxynitrites and lipid peroxides generation as well as signaling cascades activation. Apoptosis is a programmed and organized, ATP-dependent, cell death occurring in normal placental development which increases throughout pregnancy [242]. Necrosis is an accidental and ATP-independent cell death not taking place in normal placental development. In normal pregnancy, apoptosis controls trophoblast differentiation, syncytial fusion and villous trophoblast turnover [243, 244]. In preeclampsia, placental apoptosis is significantly increased compared to normal pregnancy [245]. Abnormal placental apoptosis is particularly taking place in the syncytiotrophoblast [225, 245, 246]. Increased syncytial necrosis is also observed in preeclampsia [247]. Consequently, villous trophoblast turnover is altered in preeclampsia [248]. Hypoxia/reoxygenation has been demonstrated to promote syncytiotrophoblast apoptosis and necrosis as well as oxidative stress *in vitro*, mimicking changes occurring in preeclampsia [174, 231, 249]. Currently, it is not known whether these apoptotic and necrotic changes are a primary pathologic event or a secondary manifestation. The 2 stage model implies that it is a secondary event taking place after altered extravillous trophoblast invasion [78, 79, 81, 82]. However, Huppertz suggest that it is the primary placental alteration which occurs in preeclampsia [42]. Nevertheless, both hypotheses agreed that oxidative stress disrupts syncytial architecture, through increased apoptosis and necrosis, and stimulates the release of factors in the maternal blood which are responsible for the systemic inflammatory response [42, 250]. Furthermore, it has been demonstrated that H/R stimulates the release of syncytiotrophoblast pro-inflammatory factors, such as tumor necrosis factor-alpha (TNF-α), cell-free DNA, soluble fms-like tyrosine kinase-1 (sFlt-1), soluble endoglin (sEng) and syncytiotrophoblast microfragments (STBM) [249, 251-254].

Release of Syncytiotrophoblast Factors

In preeclampsia, oxidative stress disrupts syncytial architecture and promotes the release of pro-inflammatory factors (Fig. 2). These syncytiotrophoblast factors include activin-A [255], cell-free fetal DNA [256], corticotrophin releasing hormone (CRH) [257], leptin [258] and TNF-α [152]. The most studied are the STBM [259], the sFlt-1 [254] and the sEng [253]. STBM are syncytial membranes shed into the maternal circulation that impair maternal endothelial cell functions and stimulate inflammation [226, 259-262]. Their levels in maternal blood are correlated with the severity of preeclampsia [263]. In preeclampsia, sFlt-1, a circulating antagonist of vascular endothelial growth factor A (VEGF-A), binds and inactivates VEGF and placental growth factor (PlGF), inducing systemic endothelial dysfunction [254]. Levels of sFlt-1 are elevated in patients with preeclampsia 2 to 5 weeks before onset of clinical symptoms [264-266]. Moreover, sFlt-1 levels are associated with the severity of the syndrome [264, 267]. The expression of sFlt-1 is regulated by HIF-1α [268]. Hypoxia/reoxygenation-induced oxidative stress increased HIF-1α and sFlt-1 expression in placental explants by a p38 and a NF-κB dependent pathway [228, 269]. sEng, a transforming growth factor-beta (TGF-β) co-receptor, interferes with TGF-β signaling, disrupting vascular homeostasis and inducing hypertension *in vivo* [253]. As for sFlt-1, sEng levels are elevated weeks before onset of clinical symptoms in patients with preeclampsia [270]. sEng expression is also regulated by HIF-1α and correlates with disease severity [253, 271]. Redman and Sargent propose that sFlt-1 and sEng are as much upregulated by hypoxia than by placental inflammatory stress since HIF-1α has been shown to be regulated by both [79]. Thus, the cocktail of pro-inflammatory syncytial factors will contribute to the development of the maternal systemic inflammatory response.

Systemic Inflammatory Response

Preeclampsia is often described as an endothelial disorder. It is true that sFlt-1 and s-Eng are powerful anti-angiogenic factors and probably constitute the primary cause of the endothelial dysfunction associated with the clinical signs of preeclampsia. Although, endothelium inflammation is involved in preeclampsia, the stress response is mostly systemic and involves other components of the inflammatory network such as acute-phase response and metabolic responses [79] (Fig. 2).

The clinical feature of preeclampsia is new onset of maternal hypertension and proteinuria resolving after delivery. The maternal hypertension results from diffuse endothelial dysfunction and the proteinuria is ascribed to glomerular endotheliosis [272, 273]. There is an increased expression of endothelial activation and endothelial dysfunction markers in preeclamptic women, including von Willebrand Factor [274], endothelin [275], vascular cell adhesion molecule (VCAM) [276], thrombomodulin [277], platelet-derived growth factor (PDGF) [278], cellular fibronectin [279] and soluble E-selectin [280]. The incubation of serum from preeclamptic women with endothelial cells results in endothelial dysfunction, suggesting that circulating factors could be responsible for the hypertension and proteinuria [253]. Therefore, in pregnant rats, elevated levels of sFlt-1 cause preeclampsia-like symptoms, including hypertension, proteinuria and glomerular endotheliosis [254]. Moreover, sEng administration amplifies sFlt-1-mediated endothelial damage in rats [253]. sFlt-1 and sEng could thus be responsible for the maternal endothelial dysfunction and the clinical feature of preeclampsia [273].

In addition to endothelium inflammation, preeclampsia is characterized by an acute-phase reaction [79, 281]. The acute-phase reaction is a complex endocrine and metabolic response triggered by a number of inflammatory cytokines mainly secreted by macrophages and monocytes at the inflammatory site [282, 283]. These cytokines stimulate the production of acute-phase proteins by hepatocytes. Acute-phase proteins are defined as positive when their plasma concentration increases and negative when it decreases by at least 25% in reaction to inflammatory disorder [284]. In preeclampsia, positive acute-phase response proteins include c-reactive protein [285], plasminogen [286], angiotensinogen [287], many proteins of the complement system [288-290] and several clotting factors [291, 292]. Negative acute-phase response proteins consist of C56 complement protein [293] and albumin [294].

Finally, various metabolic responses are activated secondary to the systemic inflammation in preeclampsia; supporting the proposition that preeclampsia is not just an endothelial dysfunction [79]. They mainly involve lipid metabolism. Hyperlipidemia is a feature of normal pregnancy but it is significantly increased in preeclampsia before onset of maternal symptoms [295]. Hypertriglyceridemia, insulin resistance, increased circulating level of free fatty acids, small density lipoproteins, and occurrence of oxidized low density lipoproteins characterize preeclampsia [296-298]. TNF-α and other pro-inflammatory factors are known inducers of hyperlipidemia, indicating that it may be mediated by syncytial factors [299, 300]. In addition to be a risk factor, obesity increases the inflammatory response in preeclampsia [23-25, 301, 302]. Adipocytes secrete numerous pro-inflammatory cytokines, including TNF-α and leptin [303, 304]. Leptin is a powerful pro-inflammatory stimulus and its secretion is significantly increased in preeclampsia [305-307].

The involvement of multiple components of the inflammatory network in the pathology of preeclampsia points toward a more systemic response than just an endothelial dysfunction.

PREDICTION, PREVENTION AND TREATMENTS

The most effective treatment for preeclampsia is delivery itself [3, 44], but it may not be possible for a premature fetus, particularly if the mother has mild disease [3]. Several factors are considered to determine the best time to deliver, including the severity of the condition, the risk of complications, how badly the fetus is affected and the chances of survival or of a premature baby. Clear indications for delivery are: severe IUGR, alarming fetal surveillance or oligohydramnios (i.e deficiency in amniotic fluid), gestational age of 38 weeks or more, maternal platelet count below 200 x 10^9/L, maternal progressive deterioration of hepatic or renal functions, placental abruption presumption and eclampsia [3]. In general, the later the baby is born, the better, with the exception of severe preeclampsia if the baby grows very inadequately because of the poorly functioning placenta.

In general, vaginal delivery is preferable, in order to avoid extra stress of cesarean delivery. In the latter case, the use of regional anesthesia is preferred because it involves less maternal risk, except in the presence of coagulopathy, where the use of regional anesthesia is generally contraindicated [3]. During labor, efforts are made to prevent seizures and to control hypertension [44]. Until the baby is born, preeclampsia symptoms can be managed and several randomized trials reported the effective use of various methods to reduce the rate or severity of preeclampsia [308]. Methods used to prevent or treat preeclampsia are resumed in Table **2**.

Table 2: Possible prevention and treatment of preeclampsia

❖	Anti-hypertensive drugs [309, 310]
❖	Low-dose aspirin (anti-platelet agent) [311, 319]
❖	Low-molecular-weight heparin (LMWH) (anti-coagulant) [312, 313]
❖	Calcium supplementation [60, 62]
❖	Antioxidant [79, 82, 173]
❖	Exercise [314, 315]

Treatments

Magnesium Sulfate (MgSO₄) and other Antihypertensive Drugs

$MgSO_4$ is an antihypertensive agent that helps to prevent eclamptic seizures in pregnant women [316, 317]. Antihypertensive drugs are given to handle or prevent worsening of the symptoms and can thus temporize over the short term to allow safe delivery with a more mature fetus [318]. $MgSO_4$ is superior to phenytoin (Dilantin) and diazepam (Valium) for the treatment of eclamptic seizures. Usually, a 6 g dose of $MgSO_4$, followed by a continuous infusion at a rate of 2 g/h is applied [316, 317]. Although $MgSO_4$ is commonly used, there is yet no study demonstrating its preventive action on preeclampsia [309, 310].

Other antihypertensive drugs are commonly used in the treatment of severe preeclampsia. The aim of antihypertensive therapy is to prevent maternal cerebrovascular complications and to lower gradually systolic pressure to 140-155 mm Hg and diastolic pressure to 90-105 mm Hg [3]. The medical treatment should be initiated in hospitals. Antihypertensive agents are indicated at a SBP of ≥ 170 mm Hg or at a DBP of ≥110 mm Hg. For high-risk women, a threshold of 160/100 mm Hg is appropriate. These measures are consistent with international guidelines [44]. Note that a rise in SBP to ≥ 160 mm Hg is more related to development of strokes in preeclampsia than a rise in DBP to ≥110 mm Hg [319]. Hydralazine (Apresoline) and labetalol (Normody, Trandate) are most commonly used, but the latter should not be used in women with asthma or congestive heart failure.

Alternative treatments exist, such as nifedipine (Procardia), a dihydropyridine calcium antagonist, and sodium nitroprusside (Nitropress), a nitric oxide donor/releaser and potent vasodilator, but significant risks are associated with their use. Use of angiotensin-converting enzyme inhibitors is contraindicated in pregnant women [3]. Usually, blood pressure normalizes after delivery but a diagnosis of chronic hypertension is made if it remains elevated at 12 weeks postpartum [3]. Some studies have shown that the use of long-acting oral antihypertensive agents in mild preeclampsia, may lead to IUGR [320, 321]. In addition, abrupt drops in blood pressure should be avoided [322].

Prevention

Many measures have been suggested to prevent preeclampsia but none are well-established [26, 44]. These measures include prophylaxis as low-dose aspirin, low molecular weight heparin, calcium supplementation, and antioxidant use.

Low-Dose Aspirin (Anti-Platelet Agent)

Prophylaxis with aspirin has been investigated in a number of studies. The underlying principle is that preeclampsia is characterized by an imbalance between vasoconstrictive and vasodilating prostaglandins, with an excess of the vasoconstrictive thromboxane. Preeclampsia involves an imbalance between prostacyclin (PGI2), an anticoagulant and vasodilator prostaglandin, and thromboxane A2 (TXA2), a pro-coagulant and vasoconstrictor prostaglandin. Aspirin, which is an inhibitor of cyclooxygenases (COX), reduces TXA2, amends the report PGI2/TXA2 and therefore tends to reestablish the physiological balance

[311]. It has been shown that low-dose aspirin inhibits thromboxane overproduction induced by preeclampsia, but has no effect on vascular prostacyclin production [323].

Some evidences support the use of low-dose aspirin in certain high-risk women, like in women with abnormal uterine artery on Doppler ultrasound examination performed in the second trimester [324]. On the other hand, aspirin therapy does not seem to be generally beneficial for pregnant women [3, 44]. Other studies observed that oral aspirin 75 to 150 mg/day reduces by 10% [325] to 17% [323] the rate of preeclampsia and by 9% [325] to 14% [323] the rate of neonatal mortality. In 2007, a meta-analysis conducted using individual data from all trials on low-dose aspirin study against placebo during pregnancy, brought together 32 217 patients [325]. Overall, results confirmed that aspirin was effective in the prevention of preeclampsia with a decreased risk of about 10%. Treatment should be started between 12 and 14 gestational weeks with a dose between 75 and 160 mg/day. Two randomized studies showed taken at bedtime, aspirin could achieve lower blood pressure values [326, 327]. Despite the large number of studies and patients involved, it remains difficult to define precisely the groups of patients for whom this treatment is indicated.

Low-Molecular-Weight Heparin (LMWH) (Anti-Coagulant)

Low-molecular-weight heparin has been proposed in the prevention of preeclampsia. In reality, there is no evidence that this treatment is effective. After a first pregnancy marked by a vascular complication, several authors have shown that the rate of preeclampsia was reduced during the next pregnancy when treated with LMWH [312, 313]. In a recent randomized trial, the use of LMWH (deltaparin, weight adjusted, 4000-6000 IU/day, on or before the 16th to 36th gestational week) lowered the incidence of preeclampsia from 23.6% to 5.5% in women with previous preeclampsia or IUGR [328]. Nevertheless, the level of evidence of these studies is questionable, in part because of the low recruitment [311].

Calcium Supplementation

Several studies have shown that calcium supplementation reduces blood pressure in pregnant women [59] at risk for hypertensive disorders or with low dietary calcium intake [60-62]. Calcium supplements probably act by relaxing either parathyroid hormone or renin release, decreasing intracellular calcium in vascular smooth muscle and consequently its contractility [60, 329]. Thus, calcium supplementation could reduce preterm labor and delivery if it reduces uterine smooth muscle contractility [330]. One of the hypotheses that could explain this relationship is that lack of calcium stimulates parathyroid hormones and release of renin, which led to an increase of intracellular calcium in smooth muscle cells and therefore to vasoconstriction. Thus, intake of calcium may also have an indirect effect on smooth muscle cells functions. Results of many studies led to recommend a calcium intake of at least 1.5 g/day, starting at 15 gestational weeks and maintained throughout pregnancy in populations with a basic calcium intake of 600 mg/day, especially in patients at high risk of preeclampsia [60]. A recent study observed that calcium homeostasis was perturbed in preeclamptic primary syncytiotrophoblast cells. In addition, they observed that the expression of many important genes for the trans-placental transfer of calcium was decreased in preeclamptic placentas. They concluded that an excess of oxidative stress and a lack of ATP level could be the cause of these perturbations [227].

Antioxidants

As discussed above, it has been proposed that oxidative stress could be a causative mechanism of the systemic inflammatory response in preeclampsia. Likewise, studies have demonstrated higher level of oxidative stress in placentas from preeclampsia pregnancies [79, 82, 151, 158-160]. Consequently, antioxidant therapy has been projected. Vitamin C is a dietary scavenger of free radicals acting in liquid phase, while vitamin E acts *in vivo* by preventing the formation of lipid peroxides. These vitamins thus protect enzymes, proteins and cells from destruction caused by oxidative stress. Preeclampsia is associated with a decrease of these antioxidants which are essential in maintaining the defenses of the organism facing oxidative stress [311]. Trials do not support the administration of vitamin C and E to prevent preeclampsia and proposed that massive and expensive trials should ceased until further research is undertaken [331-

336]. They demonstrated that the combination of 1000 mg of vitamin C and 400 IU of vitamin E did not reduce the risk of preeclampsia. A proposed explanation for the failure of vitamins to prevent or ameliorate preeclampsia is the inadequate dosage [336]. Extrapolation from animal models suggested that 10-15 g of vitamin C is required to reduce oxidative stress in humans [336].

Moreover, among its many benefits, regular physical activity has shown to enhance endogenous antioxidant defenses, which may reduce the risk of preeclampsia [314, 315]. A randomized clinical trial comparing walking versus stretching on the incidence of preeclampsia has observed that the incidence of preeclampsia was of 14.6% among walkers and of 2.6% among stretchers. Moreover, the mean level of transferrin, an antioxidant marker, was significantly higher in the stretching group. They conclude that regular stretching exercises may promote endogenous antioxidants among women at risk for preeclampsia [337]. Still, further researches with larger sample size are needed to determine optimal timing, intensity and other types of exercises that could be beneficial for pregnant woman. Antioxidant therapy is not currently undergoing but research on this alternative is promising. Novel approaches to prevent through amelioration of the oxidative stress include melatonin supplements, selenium supplements, antiperoxinitries strategies and statins [338, 339].

MATERNAL OUTCOMES

Women affected by preeclampsia who do not receive prenatal care are 7 times more likely to die from complications related to preeclampsia [350]. Black women seem to be 3 times more affected by maternal death than Caucasians. Precise reasons of racial differences remain elusive, but disparities in health status and access or quality of prenatal care [350] and vitamin D deficiency [351] are proposed.

Women who suffer from severe preeclampsia may develop serious headaches, visual blurring, acute liver pain, seizures and/or eclampsia in 0.1% of all pregnancies [340, 341], severe proteinuria from renal failure, hemolysis, thrombocytopenia, HELLP syndrome in 0.17 to 0.8% of all live births or kidney damage [342]. Besides maternal complications, the fetus can also be distressed. For instance, preeclampsia leads to IUGR in 30% of cases [308]. As mentioned earlier, proteinuria is not universally considered for the diagnosis of preeclampsia [66]. It was observed that in up to 20% of eclampsia cases [343, 344] and 5% to 15% of HELLP syndrome cases [345], proteinuria may not be present. This section will give details about brain, liver and kidney damage [103, 340], in addition to some fetal outcomes, in particular IUGR. Most common maternal and perinatal outcomes are listed in Table **3**.

Table 3: Maternal and perinatal outcomes

❖   Eclampsia (2%)
❖   HELLP syndrome
❖   Kidney damage
❖   IUGR

Eclampsia

Eclampsia complicates about 2% of preeclampsia cases [317] and is defined as the occurrence of seizures. Severe headaches or visual blurring are common signs of its onset. In general, eclamptic seizures occur after the development of hypertension and proteinuria [344], but in 20% of cases, proteinuria is absent [344]. It should also be noted that in 10-15% of cases of eclampsia, blood pressure is normal [346]

Postpartum (48 h to one month after delivery) eclamptic seizures occurs in 28% of cases [341]. Although it has been theorized that eclampsia was the linear evolvement of preeclampsia, more than one-third of women with postpartum eclampsia do not manifest signs of preeclampsia [347]. A retrospective analysis showed that eclampsia was not an evolution from preeclampsia [348].

Prevention and treatment of eclampsia is facilitated by the use of $MgSO_4$ [349], which is the anticonvulsant of choice, inexpensive and clearly more effective than others treatments [350-352]. Unfortunately, $MgSO_4$

is not available in all developing countries, characterized as system and market failures for several people [353, 354].

HELLP Syndrome

In normotensive pregnancies, the maternal blood volume expended and the platelet count can fall below 200×10^9/L. Probably due to an increased consumption and intravascular destruction, the platelet count can fall further in preeclamptic pregnancies [355]. Hemolysis, HELLP syndrome can be, in 10-20% of cases [308], a severe deviation of preeclampsia and may lead to immediate delivery to prevent development of precarious thrombocytopenia or hemolysis [356]. In about 15% of HELLP syndromes cases, patients do not present symptoms, or complain about upper right quadrant and/or epigastric pain, nausea or vomiting [357]. Women with HELLP syndrome might need intensive care because of the possible complications of hepatic encephalopathy, acute renal dysfunction, hepatic rupture and bleeding [357]. The presence of HELLP syndrome is an indication for delivery, in order to prevent detrimental thrombocytopenia or hemolysis [356]. Maternal mortality rates due to HELLP syndrome range from 1% in the US [358] to 30% in less developed countries [359].

Generally, this syndrome arises in the 2nd or 3rd trimester and the liver's condition normalizes within 2 weeks after delivery [357], but 7-30% of preeclampsia cases developed HELLP syndrome postpartum [360]. Multiparity, advanced maternal age and white ethnic origin are known risk factors [342]. In women who already experience HELLP syndrome, the risk of recurrence in subsequent pregnancies is increased [361, 362].

Endothelial dysfunction is considered central in systemic disease like PE and HELLP is characterized by microangiopathic hemolysis, which suggests endothelial damage. In many cases, HELLP is accompanied by eclampsia. It was reported that the incidence of HELLP syndrome after diagnosis of eclampsia ranges from 10.8% to 32.1% [363, 364]. Moreover, the incidence of eclampsia after HELLP syndrome diagnosis ranges from 6% to 52% [358, 365]. In presence of HELLP syndrome, endothelial dysfunction may injured blood-brain barrier and contributed to higher blood pressure in the cerebral area [319] and increased risk of dispersed intravascular coagulation which may contribute to cerebral hemorrhage. It was demonstrated that the majority of women with multiple seizures had HELLP syndrome [366]. HELLP must be described as a systemic disorder, involving the lungs [367], liver [368-370], central nervous system [368, 371]and kidney damage [359, 368].

Treatment with diuretics are not recommended because they can cause utero-placental hypoperfusion [372]. On the other hand, intravenous $MgSO_4$ with platelet, coagulation support, or both, are recommended, in particular in the presence of bleeding. If gestational age is less than 34 weeks, corticosteroids should be taken in order to promote fetal lung maturity, with no maternal benefits [373].

Kidney Damage

The kidney participates directly in the regulation of blood pressure. During normotensive pregnancies, a number of renal physiological adaptations are implemented and their sudden or progressive disappearance is part of the pathophysiological process observed in preeclampsia [374]. Renal failure during preeclampsia is defined by creatinine concentrations exceeding 90 mmol/L and urea concentrations superior to 7 mmol/L [374]. Acute renal failure may occur in about 5% severe cases of preeclampsia [308, 374], frequently complicated by pulmonary edema.

Kidneys pathologic analysis of women that suffer from preeclampsia may show infarction, necrosis and intraparenchymal hemorrhage of adrenal glands [375]. Structural changes in renal glomeruli, as vacuolization and swelling of the endothelial cells, as well as loss of the capillary space are described by the term glomerular endotheliosis, which is accompanied by subendothelial deposits of fibrin, decreasing the surface area for filtration [376]. As mentioned earlier, glomerular endotheliosis is associated with the proteinuria observed in preeclampsia cases. In some cases, trace to mild glomerular endotheliosis may occur at term in normotensive pregnancies [340].

Podocyturia, defined as urinary excretion of viable podocytes (glomerular epithelial cells), was recently observed in women with preeclampsia [377]. It was demonstrated that podocyte damage and detachment have a role in the development of proteinuria, but podocyturia seems to be confined to active disease only, when proteinuria can be present also during chronic phases of glomerular damage [378, 379]. Garovic *et al.* [377] suggested that podocyturia may contribute to proteinuria in preeclampsia since podocytes have a very restricted regenerative capacity. As a consequence, podocytes loss may lead to a disruption of the glomerular filtration barrier, generating proteinuria. On the other hand, normotensive pregnant women and women with hypertension or proteinuria in the absence of preeclampsia did not have podocyturia. Hence, podocyturia is not a direct result of all hypertensive kidney damage or a marker of proteinuria, but it appears to be a sensitive marker of renal damage and proteinuria in preeclampsia, where a positive correlation between the degree of proteinuria and podocyturia was observed [377].

Fetal Outcomes

IUGR

Besides the fact that maternal health can be affected by severe preeclampsia, fetal condition can also be altered. Fetal and neonatal complications include iatrogenic prematurity (i.e delivery intended by the doctor given the critical condition of the mother), oligohydramnios, increased risk of perinatal death and IUGR [308].

IUGR complicates about 10% to 25% of severe preeclampsia cases [308]. Similar to preeclampsia, IUGR usually appears in the 2nd or 3rd trimester of pregnancy, its underlying pathology taking place in the 1st trimester [113]. Although often interchanged, terms IUGR and "small for gestational age" (SGA) do not refer to the same condition. IUGR refers to a fetus that is at risk for adverse perinatal morbidity and mortality, while SGA fetuses can be just constitutionally small. Therefore, IUGR refers to SGA fetuses who display other signs of chronic hypoxia or malnutrition [380]. The American College of Obstetricians and Gynecologists (ACOG) suspects IUGR when fetuses have an estimated weight below the 10th percentile [44].

Preeclampsia and IUGR are pregnancy specific disorders sharing characteristics such as an abnormal placental implantation, a marked proliferation of villous cytotrophoblastic cells and a focal necrosis of the syncytiotrophoblast [381, 382], placental malperfusion secondary to abnormal implantation and deficient maternal spiral artery conversion [383, 384], decreased intrauterine artery blood flow leading to abnormal placentation and consequently decreased supply to the developing fetus [384]. The decreased blood volume seen in preeclampsia can lead to an increased in maternal hemoglobin concentration and is associated with an increases risk of IUGR [355].

A recent study provides strong evidences for the relation between preeclampsia and IUGR [382] but others have different hypotheses. Newhouse *et al.* [384] suggested that normotensive IUGR and IUGR with preeclampsia are two distinct pathologies with a unique impact on trophoblast function. Mari *et al.* [385] demonstrated that fetal cardiovascular changes (Doppler wavelength) observed in patients with preeclampsia differed from those seen in normotensive IUGR patients. Lorenzi *et al.* [381] described preeclampsia as a maternal syndrome, while IUGR affects mostly the fetus, suggesting that preeclampsia and preeclampsia associated with IUGR could be considered as two pathologies with different origins (maternal/placental-fetal). Huppertz proposed that not the same trophoblast cells would be altered in PE and IUGR [42]. PE would be caused by altered release of villous trophoblast factors while IUGR would result from failure of extravillous trophoblast to transform maternal spiral arteries. This however remains to be shown. A recent study showed evidences of greater maternal vascular compromise of the placental in preeclampsia cases compared to IUGR [383]. However, a recent review exposed links between those pathologies [386]. A few years ago, Rasmussen *et al.* [382] demonstrated that women who have had a growth-restricted infant without preeclampsia are more likely to have preeclampsia in subsequent pregnancies. This indicates the similarity between IUGR and preeclampsia. It was also shown that critical maternal complications are more frequent in preeclampsia patients with IUGR compared to preeclampsia patients without IUGR; the smaller the fetus, the more severe the maternal complications [387].

In general, IUGR appear as a complication of severe preeclampsia but in some cases, preeclampsia is described as an outcome of IUGR. In fact, it was reported that patients with IUGR tend to have higher blood pressure than women with normal growth fetuses [388] and that elevated maternal blood pressure is associated with decreased birth weight in normotensive pregnancies [389]. Results obtained from Tranquilli and Giannubilo suggest that IUGR is a step toward preeclampsia [388]. These two conditions may be very closely linked [390]. IUGR has been considered one of the symptoms resulting from impaired uteroplacental blood flow and it was suggested that preeclampsia should be considered as the clinical syndrome [308]. Additionally, as in preeclampsia, it has recently been suggested that the use of 1st trimester biochemical markers in combination with Doppler screening is promising for the early detection of IUGR [391].

Growth restriction is now documented as a major risk factor for premature atherosclerosis [392]. In addition, IUGR has been associated with low bone mass in infancy and increased risk for osteoporosis development in the adult [393]. With respect to maternal-fetal transfer of nutrients, there is growing evidence that limited intrauterine growth due to inadequate maternal-fetal nutritional exchange is associated with lower bone mass in infants [394], children [395] and elderly men [396].

CONCLUSION

In conclusion, concerning long-term prognosis, women with severe preeclampsia have significant higher risks of developing cardiovascular disease afterwards. A meta-analysis has observed a relative risk of 3.7 for hypertension (14 years of follow up), 2.16 for ischemic heart disease (11.7 years), 1.81 for stroke (10.4 years) and 1.49 for maternal death (14.5 years) [397].

REFERENCES

[1]   WHO. The World Health Report 2005-make every mother and child count. World Health Organization 2005.
[2]   World Health Report: Make every mother and child count. Geneva, Switzerland: World Health Organization 2005.
[3]   Report of the National High Blood Pressure Education Program Working Group on High Blood Pressure in Pregnancy. Am J Obstet Gynecol 2000; 183(1): S1-S22.
[4]   Chandiramani M, Shennan A. Hypertensive disorders of pregnancy: a UK-based perspective. Curr Opin Obstet Gynecol 2008; 20(2): 96-101.
[5]   WHO. World Health Organization survey. World Health Organization 2003.
[6]   Saftlas AF, Levine RJ, Klebanoff MA, *et al.* Abortion, changed paternity, and risk of preeclampsia in nulliparous women. Am J Epidemiol 2003; 157(12): 1108-1114.
[7]   Hauth JC, Ewell MG, Levine RJ, *et al.* Pregnancy outcomes in healthy nulliparas who developed hypertension. Calcium for Preeclampsia Prevention Study Group. Obstet Gynecol 2000; 95(1): 24-28.
[8]   Sibai BM, Hauth J, Caritis S, *et al.* Hypertensive disorders in twin versus singleton gestations. National Institute of Child Health and Human Development Network of Maternal-Fetal Medicine Units. Am J Obstet Gynecol 2000; 182(4): 938-942.
[9]   Wen SW, Demissie K, Yang Q, Walker MC. Maternal morbidity and obstetric complications in triplet pregnancies and quadruplet and higher-order multiple pregnancies. Am J Obstet Gynecol 2004; 191(1): 254-258.
[10]   Chen YY, Wu ML, Kao MH, Su TH, Chen CP. Perinatal outcome of recurrent pre-eclampsia versus pre-eclampsia in nulliparas. J Obstet Gynaecol Res 2009; 35(6): 1042-1046.
[11]   Sibai BM. Chronic hypertension in pregnancy. Obstet Gynecol 2002; 100(2): 369-377.
[12]   Marik PE. Hypertensive disorders of pregnancy. Postgrad Med 2009; 121(2): 69-76.
[13]   Rath W, Fischer T. The diagnosis and treatment of hypertensive disorders of pregnancy: new findings for antenatal and inpatient care. Dtsch Arztebl Int 2009; 106(45): 733-738.
[14]   Howarth C, Gazis A, James D. Associations of Type 1 diabetes mellitus, maternal vascular disease and complications of pregnancy. Diabet Med 2007; 24(11): 1229-1234.
[15]   Peticca P, Keely EJ, Walker MC, Yang Q, Bottomley J. Pregnancy outcomes in diabetes subtypes: how do they compare? A province-based study of Ontario, 2005-2006. J Obstet Gynaecol Can 2009; 31(6): 487-496.
[16]   McDonald SD, Best C, Lam K. The recurrence risk of severe *de novo* pre-eclampsia in singleton pregnancies: a population-based cohort. BJOG 2009; 116(12): 1578-1584.

[17] Lykke JA, Paidas MJ, Langhoff-Roos J. Recurring complications in second pregnancy. Obstet Gynecol 2009; 113(6): 1217-1224.

[18] Hernandez-Diaz S, Toh S, Cnattingius S. Risk of pre-eclampsia in first and subsequent pregnancies: prospective cohort study. BMJ 2009; 338: b2255.

[19] Kahn SR, Platt R, McNamara H, *et al.* Inherited thrombophilia and preeclampsia within a multicenter cohort: the Montreal Preeclampsia Study. Am J Obstet Gynecol 2009; 200(2): 151 e1-9; discussion e1-5.

[20] Kupferminc MJ. Thrombophilia and pregnancy. Obstet Gynecol 2005; 48(2): 406-415.

[21] Jahromi BN, Husseini Z. Pregnancy outcome at maternal age 40 and older. Taiwan J Obstet Gynecol 2008; 47(3): 318-21.

[22] Najati N, Gojazadeh M. Maternal and neonatal complications in mothers aged under 18 years. Patient Prefer Adherence 2010; 21(4): 219-22.

[23] Bodnar LM, Ness RB, Harger GF, Roberts JM. Inflammation and triglycerides partially mediate the effect of prepregnancy body mass index on the risk of preeclampsia. Am J Epidemiol 2005; 162(12): 1198-206.

[24] Bodnar LM, Ness RB, Markovic N, Roberts JM. The risk of preeclampsia rises with increasing prepregnancy body mass index. Ann Epidemiol 2005; 15(7): 475-82.

[25] Walsh SW. Obesity: a risk factor for preeclampsia. Trends Endocrinol Metab 2007; 18(10): 365-70.

[26] Dekker G, Sibai B. Primary, secondary, and tertiary prevention of pre-eclampsia. Lancet 2001; 357(9251): 209-215.

[27] Lie RT. Intergenerational exchange and perinatal risks: a note on interpretation of generational recurrence risks. Paediatr Perinat Epidemiol 2007; 21(Suppl 1): 13-8.

[28] Horton AL, Boggess KA, Moss KL, Beck J, Offenbacher S. Periodontal disease, oxidative stress, and risk for preeclampsia. J Periodontol 2010; 81(2) :199-204.

[29] Pouliot SH, Xiong X, Harville E, *et al.* Maternal dengue and pregnancy outcomes: a systematic review. Obstet Gynecol Surv 2010; 65(2): 107-118.

[30] Nguyen G, Garcia RT, Nguyen N, Trinh H, Keeffe EB, Nguyen MH. Clinical course of hepatitis B virus infection during pregnancy. Aliment Pharmacol Ther 2009; 29(7): 755-764.

[31] Ciarmela P, Boschi S, Bloise E, *et al.* Polymorphisms of FAS and FAS ligand genes in preeclamptic women. Eur J Obstet Gynecol Reprod Biol 2010; 148(2): 144-146.

[32] Zusterzeel PL, Peters WH, Burton GJ, Visser W, Roelofs HM, Steegers EA. Susceptibility to pre-eclampsia is associated with multiple genetic polymorphisms in maternal biotransformation enzymes. Gynecol Obstet Invest 2007; 63(4): 209-213.

[33] Nilsson E, Salonen Ros H, Cnattingius S, Lichtenstein P. The importance of genetic and environmental effects for pre-eclampsia and gestational hypertension: a family study. BJOG 2004; 111(3): 200-206.

[34] Campbell DM, MacGillivray I, Carr-Hill R. Pre-eclampsia in second pregnancy. Br J Obstet Gynaecol 1985; 92(2): 131-40.

[35] Skjaerven R, Wilcox AJ, Lie RT. The interval between pregnancies and the risk of preeclampsia. N Engl J Med 2002; 346(1): 33-38.

[36] Dekker G. The partner's role in the etiology of preeclampsia. J Reprod Immunol 2002; 57(1-2): 203-215.

[37] Robillard PY, Hulsey TC. Association of pregnancy-induced-hypertension, pre-eclampsia, and eclampsia with duration of sexual cohabitation before conception. Lancet 1996; 347(9001): 619.

[38] Salha O, Sharma V, Dada T, *et al.* The influence of donated gametes on the incidence of hypertensive disorders of pregnancy. Hum Reprod 1999; 14(9): 2268-2273.

[39] Wang JX, Knottnerus AM, Schuit G, Norman RJ, Chan A, Dekker GA. Surgically obtained sperm, and risk of gestational hypertension and pre-eclampsia. Lancet 2002; 359(9307): 673-674.

[40] Chen XK, Wen SW, Bottomley J, Smith GN, Leader A, Walker MC. *In vitro* fertilization is associated with an increased risk for preeclampsia. Hypertens Pregnancy 2009; 28(1): 1-12.

[41] Sibai BM, Stella CL. Diagnosis and management of atypical preeclampsia-eclampsia. Am J Obstet Gynecol 2009; 200(5): 481 e1-7.

[42] Huppertz B. Placental origins of preeclampsia: challenging the current hypothesis. Hypertension 2008; 51(4): 970-975.

[43] von Dadelszen P, Magee LA, Roberts JM. Subclassification of preeclampsia. Hypertens Pregnancy 2003; 22(2): 143-148.

[44] ACOG practice bulletin. Diagnosis and management of preeclampsia and eclampsia. Number 33, January 2002. American College of Obstetricians and Gynecologists. Int J Gynaecol Obstet 2002; 77(1): 67-75.

[45] Wagner LK. Diagnosis and management of preeclampsia. Am Fam Physician 2004; 70(12): 2317-2324.

[46]   Roberts JM, Gammill HS. Preeclampsia: recent insights. Hypertension 2005; 46(6): 1243-1249.

[47]   Rockwell LC, Vargas E, Moore LG. Human physiological adaptation to pregnancy: inter-and intraspecific perspectives. Am J Hum Biol 2003; 15(3): 330-341.

[48]   Thaler I, Manor D, Itskovitz J, *et al.* Changes in uterine blood flow during human pregnancy. Am J Obstet Gynecol 1990; 162(1): 121-125.

[49]   Kliman HJ. Uteroplacental blood flow. The story of decidualization, menstruation, and trophoblast invasion. Am J Pathol 2000; 157(6): 1759-1768.

[50]   Khan F, Belch JJ, MacLeod M, Mires G. Changes in endothelial function precede the clinical disease in women in whom preeclampsia develops. Hypertension 2005; 46(5): 1123-1128.

[51]   Easterling TR. The maternal hemodynamics of preeclampsia. Clin Obstet Gynecol 1992; 35(2): 375-386.

[52]   Lunell NO, Nylund LE, Lewander R, Sarby B. Uteroplacental blood flow in pre-eclampsia measurements with indium-113m and a computer-linked gamma camera. Clin Exp Hypertens B 1982; 1(1): 105-117.

[53]   Halhali A, Wimalawansa SJ, Berentsen V, Avila E, Thota CS, Larrea F. Calcitonin gene-and parathyroid hormone-related peptides in preeclampsia: effects of magnesium sulfate. Obstet Gynecol 2001; 97(6): 893-897.

[54]   Meziani F, Van Overloop B, Schneider F, Gairard A. Parathyroid hormone-related protein-induced relaxation of rat uterine arteries: influence of the endothelium during gestation. J Soc Gynecol Investig 2005; 12(1): 14-19.

[55]   Maioli E, Fortino V, Pacini A. Parathyroid Hormone-Related Protein in Preeclampsia: A Linkage Between Maternal and Fetal Failures. Biol Reprod 2004; 71(6): 1779-1784.

[56]   Kovacs CS. PTHrP gene knock out mouse have placental calcium transport severely impaired. J Bone Miner Res 1995; 10(S1): 73.

[57]   Kovacs CS, Lanske B, Hunzelman JL, Guo J, Karaplis AC, Kronenberg HM. Parathyroid hormone-related peptide (PTHrP) regulates fetal-placental calcium transport through a receptor distinct from the PTH/PTHrP receptor. Proc Natl Acad Sci U S A 1996; 93(26): 15233-15238.

[58]   Nielsen AH, Schauser KH, Poulsen K. Current topic: the uteroplacental renin-angiotensin system. Placenta 2000; 21(5-6): 468-477.

[59]   Carroli G, Duley L, Belizan JM, Villar J. Calcium supplementation during pregnancy: a systematic review of randomised controlled trials. Br J Obstet Gynaecol 1994; 101(9): 753-758.

[60]   Hofmeyr GJ, Duley L, Atallah A. Dietary calcium supplementation for prevention of pre-eclampsia and related problems: a systematic review and commentary. BJOG 2007; 114(8): 933-943.

[61]   Gillman MW, Hood MY, Moore LL, Nguyen US, Singer MR, Andon MB. Effect of calcium supplementation on blood pressure in children. J Pediatr 1995; 127(2): 186-192.

[62]   Atallah AN, Hofmeyr GJ, Duley L. Calcium supplementation during pregnancy for preventing hypertensive disorders and related problems. Cochrane Database Syst Rev 2002; (1): CD001059.

[63]   Nielsen TF, Rylander R. Urinary calcium and magnesium excretion relates to increase in blood pressure during pregnancy. Arch Gynecol Obstet 2011; 283(3): 443-447.

[64]   Fisher KA, Luger A, Spargo BH, Lindheimer MD. Hypertension in pregnancy: clinical-pathological correlations and remote prognosis. Medicine (Baltimore) 1981; 60(4): 267-76.

[65]   Gartner HV, Sammoun A, Wehrmann M, Grossmann T, Junghans R, Weihing C. Preeclamptic nephropathy--an endothelial lesion. A morphological study with a review of the literature. Eur J Obstet Gynecol Reprod Biol 1998; 77(1): 11-27.

[66]   Thornton CE, Makris A, Ogle RF, Tooher JM, Hennessy A. The Role of Proteinuria in Defining Preeclampsia-Clinical Outcomes for Women and Babies. Clin Exp Pharmacol Physiol 2010; 37(4): 466-470.

[67]   Brown MA, Hague WM, Higgins J, *et al.* The detection, investigation and management of hypertension in pregnancy: executive summary. Aust N Z J Obstet Gynaecol 2000; 40(2): 133-138.

[68]   Brown MA, Lindheimer MD, de Swiet M, Van Assche A, Moutquin JM. The classification and diagnosis of the hypertensive disorders of pregnancy: statement from the International Society for the Study of Hypertension in Pregnancy (ISSHP). Hypertens Pregnancy 2002; 20(1): ix-xiv.

[69]   Helewa ME, Burrows RF, Smith J, Williams K, Brain P, Rabkin SW. Report of the Canadian Hypertension Society Consensus Conference: 1. Definitions, evaluation and classification of hypertensive disorders in pregnancy. CMAJ 1997; 157(6): 715-25.

[70]   Higgins JR, de Swiet M. Blood-pressure measurement and classification in pregnancy. Lancet 2001; 357(9250): 131-135.

[71]   Audibert F, Friedman SA, Frangieh AY, Sibai BM. Clinical utility of strict diagnostic criteria for the HELLP (hemolysis, elevated liver enzymes, and low platelets) syndrome. Am J Obstet Gynecol 1996; 175(2): 460-464.

[72]   Brown MA, Zammit VC, Lowe SA. Capillary permeability and extracellular fluid volumes in pregnancy-induced hypertension. Clin Sci (Lond) 1989; 77(6): 599-604.

[73]   Robillard PY, Dekker GA, Hulsey TC. Revisiting the epidemiological standard of preeclampsia: primigravidity or primipaternity? Eur J Obstet Gynecol Reprod Biol 1999; 84(1): 37-41.

[74]   Sibai BM, Mabie BC, Harvey CJ, Gonzalez AR. Pulmonary edema in severe preeclampsia-eclampsia: analysis of thirty-seven consecutive cases. Am J Obstet Gynecol 1987; 156(5): 1174-1179.

[75]   Bauer ST, Cleary KL. Cardiopulmonary complications of pre-eclampsia. Semin Perinatol 2009; 33(3): 158-165.

[76]   Zlatnik MG. Pulmonary edema: etiology and treatment. Semin Perinatol 1997; 21(4): 298-306.

[77]   Jeffcoate TN. Pre-eclampsia and eclampsia: the disease of theories. Proc R Soc Med 1966; 59(5): 397-404.

[78]   Redman CW. Current topic: pre-eclampsia and the placenta. Placenta 1991; 12(4): 301-308.

[79]   Redman CW, Sargent IL. Placental stress and pre-eclampsia: a revised view. Placenta 2009; 30(Suppl A): S38-42.

[80]   Roberts JM, Hubel CA. The two stage model of preeclampsia: variations on the theme. Placenta 2009;30(Suppl A): S32-37.

[81]   Redman CW, Sargent IL. Latest advances in understanding preeclampsia. Science 2005; 308(5728): 1592-1594.

[82]   Roberts JM, Hubel CA. Is oxidative stress the link in the two-stage model of pre-eclampsia? Lancet 1999; 354(9181): 788-789.

[83]   Redman CW, Sargent IL. Immunology of Pre-Eclampsia. Am J Reprod Immunol 2010; 63(6): 534-543

[84]   Redman CW. Preeclampsia: a multi-stress disorder. Rev Med Interne 2011; (32 Suppl 1): S41-4.

[85]   Eardley H. Recent Work on the Etiology of Eclampsia. BJOG 1909; 16(6): 384-400.

[86]   Chun D, Braga C, Chow C, Lok L. Clinical Observations on Some Aspects of Hydatidiform Moles. J Obstet Gynaecol Br Commonw 1964; 71: 180-184.

[87]   Shembrey MA, Noble AD. An instructive case of abdominal pregnancy. Aust N Z J Obstet Gynaecol 1995; 35(2): 220-221.

[88]   Piering WF, Garancis JG, Becker CG, Beres JA, Lemann J, Jr. Preeclampsia related to a functioning extrauterine placenta: report of a case and 25-year follow-up. Am J Kidney Dis 1993; 21(3): 310-313.

[89]   Matthys LA, Coppage KH, Lambers DS, Barton JR, Sibai BM. Delayed postpartum preeclampsia: an experience of 151 cases. Am J Obstet Gynecol 2004; 190(5): 1464-1466.

[90]   Matsuo K, Kooshesh S, Dinc M, Sun CC, Kimura T, Baschat AA. Late postpartum eclampsia: report of two cases managed by uterine curettage and review of the literature. Am J Perinatol 2007; 24(4): 257-266.

[91]   Benirschke K, Kaufmann P, Baergen RN. Pathology of the human placenta. 5th ed. New York: Springer; 2006; pp. 584-656.

[92]   Moldenhauer JS, Stanek J, Warshak C, Khoury J, Sibai B. The frequency and severity of placental findings in women with preeclampsia are gestational age dependent. Am J Obstet Gynecol 2003; 189(4): 1173-1177.

[93]   Wynn RM. The placenta in preeclampsia. Obstet Gynecol Annu 1977; 6: 191.

[94]   Salafia CM, Cowchock FS. Placental pathology and antiphospholipid antibodies: a descriptive study. Am J Perinatol 1997; 14(8): 435-441.

[95]   Salafia CM, Parke AL. Placental pathology in systemic lupus erythematosus and phospholipid antibody syndrome. Rheum Dis Clin North Am 1997; 23(1): 85-97.

[96]   Magid MS, Kaplan C, Sammaritano LR, Peterson M, Druzin ML, Lockshin MD. Placental pathology in systemic lupus erythematosus: a prospective study. Am J Obstet Gynecol 1998; 179(1): 226-234.

[97]   Sebire NJ, Backos M, El Gaddal S, Goldin RD, Regan L. Placental pathology, antiphospholipid antibodies, and pregnancy outcome in recurrent miscarriage patients. Obstet Gynecol 2003; 101(2): 258-263.

[98]   Salafia CM, Pezzullo JC, Ghidini A, Lopez-Zeno JA, Whittington SS. Clinical correlations of patterns of placental pathology in preterm pre-eclampsia. Placenta 1998; 19(1): 67-72.

[99]   Muller G, Philippe E, Lefakis P, *et al.* Placental lesions in gestosis. Anatomo-clinical study. Gynecol Obstet (Paris) 1971; 70(3): 309-315.

[100] Schuhmann R, Geier G. Histomorphologic placenta findings in pregnancy toxemias. Contribution to the morphology of placenta insufficiency. Arch Gynakol 1972; 213(1): 31-47.

[101] Holzl M, Luthje D, Seck-Ebersbach K. [Aterations of the placenta in EPH-gestosis morphological findings and degree of severity of the disease (author's transl)] Arch Gynakol 1974; 217(3): 315-334.

[102] Brosens IA, Robertson WB, Dixon HG. The role of the spiral arteries in the pathogenesis of preeclampsia. Obstet Gynecol Annu 1972; 1: 177-191.

[103] Redman CW, Sacks GP, Sargent IL. Preeclampsia: an excessive maternal inflammatory response to pregnancy. Am J Obstet Gynecol 1999; 180(2 Pt 1): 499-506.

[104] De Wolf F, Brosens I, Renaer M. Fetal growth retardation and the maternal arterial supply of the human placenta in the absence of sustained hypertension. Br J Obstet Gynaecol 1980; 87(8): 678-685.

[105] Gerretsen G, Huisjes HJ, Elema JD. Morphological changes of the spiral arteries in the placental bed in relation to pre-eclampsia and fetal growth retardation. Br J Obstet Gynaecol 1981; 88(9): 876-881.

[106] Benirschke K, Kaufmann P, Baergen RN. Pathology of the human placenta. 5th ed. New York: Springer: 2006; pp. 42-120.

[107] Aplin JD. Implantation, trophoblast differentiation and haemochorial placentation: mechanistic evidence *in vivo* and *in vitro*. J cell sci 1991; 99 (Pt 4): 681-692.

[108] Kemp B, Kertschanska S, Kadyrov M, Rath W, Kaufmann P, Huppertz B. Invasive depth of extravillous trophoblast correlates with cellular phenotype: a comparison of intra-and extrauterine implantation sites. Histochem Cell Biol 2002; 117(5): 401-414.

[109] Zybina TG, Frank HG, Biesterfeld S, Kaufmann P. Genome multiplication of extravillous trophoblast cells in human placenta in the course of differentiation and invasion into endometrium and myometrium. II. Mechanisms of polyploidization. Tsitologiia 2004; 46(7): 640-648.

[110] Winterhager E, Kaufmann P, Gruemmer R. Cell-cell-communication during placental development and possible implications for trophoblast proliferation and differentiation. Placenta 2000; 21(Suppl A): S61-68.

[111] Pijnenborg R, Bland JM, Robertson WB, Brosens I. Uteroplacental arterial changes related to interstitial trophoblast migration in early human pregnancy. Placenta 1983; 4(4): 397-413.

[112] Pijnenborg R, Bland JM, Robertson WB, Dixon G, Brosens I. The pattern of interstitial trophoblastic invasion of the myometrium in early human pregnancy. Placenta 1981; 2(4): 303-316.

[113] Kaufmann P, Black S, Huppertz B. Endovascular trophoblast invasion: implications for the pathogenesis of intrauterine growth retardation and preeclampsia. Biol Reprod 2003; 69(1): 1-7.

[114] Kadyrov M, Kingdom JC, Huppertz B. Divergent trophoblast invasion and apoptosis in placental bed spiral arteries from pregnancies complicated by maternal anemia and early-onset preeclampsia/intrauterine growth restriction. Am J Obstet Gynecol 2006; 194(2): 557-563.

[115] Lim KH, Zhou Y, Janatpour M, *et al.* Human cytotrophoblast differentiation/invasion is abnormal in pre-eclampsia. Am J Pathol 1997; 151(6): 1809-1818.

[116] Redline RW, Patterson P. Pre-eclampsia is associated with an excess of proliferative immature intermediate trophoblast. Human pathology 1995; 26(6): 594-600.

[117] DiFederico E, Genbacev O, Fisher SJ. Preeclampsia is associated with widespread apoptosis of placental cytotrophoblasts within the uterine wall. Am J Pathol 1999; 155(1): 293-301.

[118] Genbacev O, DiFederico E, McMaster M, Fisher SJ. Invasive cytotrophoblast apoptosis in pre-eclampsia. Hum Reprod 1999; 14(Suppl 2): 59-66.

[119] Meekins JW, Pijnenborg R, Hanssens M, McFadyen IR, van Asshe A. A study of placental bed spiral arteries and trophoblast invasion in normal and severe pre-eclamptic pregnancies. Br J Obstet Gynaecol 1994; 101(8): 669-674.

[120] Harrington K, Goldfrad C, Carpenter RG, Campbell S. Transvaginal uterine and umbilical artery Doppler examination of 12-16 weeks and the subsequent development of pre-eclampsia and intrauterine growth retardation. Ultrasound Obstet Gynecol 1997; 9(2): 94-100.

[121] Papageorghiou AT, Yu CK, Cicero S, Bower S, Nicolaides KH. Second-trimester uterine artery Doppler screening in unselected populations: a review. J Matern Fetal Neonatal Med 2002; 12(2): 78-88.

[122] Rodesch F, Simon P, Donner C, Jauniaux E. Oxygen measurements in endometrial and trophoblastic tissues during early pregnancy. Obstet Gynecol. 1992;80(2):283-235.

[123] Genbacev O, Zhou Y, Ludlow JW, Fisher SJ. Regulation of human placental development by oxygen tension. Science 1997; 277(5332): 1669-1672.

[124] Zhou Y, Genbacev O, Damsky CH, Fisher SJ. Oxygen regulates human cytotrophoblast differentiation and invasion: implications for endovascular invasion in normal pregnancy and in pre-eclampsia. J Reprod Immunol 1998; 39(1-2): 197-213.

[125] Genbacev O, Joslin R, Damsky CH, Polliotti BM, Fisher SJ. Hypoxia alters early gestation human cytotrophoblast differentiation/invasion *in vitro* and models the placental defects that occur in preeclampsia. The Journal of clinical investigation 1996; 97(2): 540-550.

[126] Caniggia I, Mostachfi H, Winter J, *et al.* Hypoxia-inducible factor-1 mediates the biological effects of oxygen on human trophoblast differentiation through TGFbeta(3). The Journal of clinical investigation 2000; 105(5):577-587.

[127] Rajakumar A, Whitelock KA, Weissfeld LA, Daftary AR, Markovic N, Conrad KP. Selective overexpression of the hypoxia-inducible transcription factor, HIF-2alpha, in placentas from women with preeclampsia. Biol Reprod 2001; 64(2): 499-506.

[128] Rajakumar A, Brandon HM, Daftary A, Ness R, Conrad KP. Evidence for the functional activity of hypoxia-inducible transcription factors overexpressed in preeclamptic placentae. Placenta 2004; 25(10): 763-769.

[129] Caniggia I, Grisaru-Gravnosky S, Kuliszewsky M, Post M, Lye SJ. Inhibition of TGF-beta 3 restores the invasive capability of extravillous trophoblasts in preeclamptic pregnancies. The Journal of clinical investigation 1999; 103(12): 1641-1650.

[130] Dekker G, Robillard PY. The birth interval hypothesis-does it really indicate the end of the primipaternity hypothesis. J Reprod Immunol 2003; 59(2): 245-251.

[131] Xia Y, Kellems RE. Is preeclampsia an autoimmune disease? Clin Immunol 2009; 133(1): 1-12.

[132] Billington WD. The immunological problem of pregnancy: 50 years with the hope of progress. A tribute to Peter Medawar. J Reprod Immunol 2003; 60(1): 1-11.

[133] Klonoff-Cohen HS, Savitz DA, Cefalo RC, McCann MF. An epidemiologic study of contraception and preeclampsia. JAMA 1989; 262(22): 3143-3147.

[134] Einarsson JI, Sangi-Haghpeykar H, Gardner MO. Sperm exposure and development of preeclampsia. Am J Obstet Gynecol 2003; 188(5): 1241-1243.

[135] Bulmer JN, Morrison L, Longfellow M, Ritson A, Pace D. Granulated lymphocytes in human endometrium: histochemical and immunohistochemical studies. Hum Reprod 1991; 6(6): 791-798.

[136] King A, Burrows TD, Hiby SE, *et al.* Surface expression of HLA-C antigen by human extravillous trophoblast. Placenta 2000; 21(4): 376-387.

[137] Verma S, King A, Loke YW. Expression of killer cell inhibitory receptors on human uterine natural killer cells. Eur J Immunol 1997; 27(4): 979-983.

[138] Lewis BJ, Croker S, Newton DJ, Lennon GP, Johnson PM, Christmas SE. Natural killer cell receptor expression by human first trimester decidual granular leukocytes and T-lymphocytes. Am J Reprod Immunol 2002; 48(2): 103-109.

[139] Parham P. MHC class I molecules and KIRs in human history, health and survival. Nat Rev Immunol 2005; 5(3): 201-214.

[140] Esplin MS, Fausett MB, Fraser A, *et al.* Paternal and maternal components of the predisposition to preeclampsia. N Engl J Med 2001; 344(12): 867-872.

[141] Mogren I, Hogberg U, Winkvist A, Stenlund H. Familial occurrence of preeclampsia. Epidemiology 1999; 10(5): 518-522.

[142] Engert S, Rieger L, Kapp M, Becker JC, Dietl J, Kammerer U. Profiling chemokines, cytokines and growth factors in human early pregnancy decidua by protein array. Am J Reprod Immunol 2007; 58(2): 129-137.

[143] Moffett A, Hiby SE. How Does the maternal immune system contribute to the development of pre-eclampsia? Placenta 2007; 28(Suppl A): S51-56.

[144] Hiby SE, Walker JJ, O'Shaughnessy K M, *et al.* Combinations of maternal KIR and fetal HLA-C genes influence the risk of preeclampsia and reproductive success. J Exp Med 2004; 200(8): 957-965.

[145] Komatsu N, Mariotti-Ferrandiz ME, Wang Y, Malissen B, Waldmann H, Hori S. Heterogeneity of natural Foxp3+ T cells: a committed regulatory T-cell lineage and an uncommitted minor population retaining plasticity. Proc Natl Acad Sci USA 2009; 106(6): 1903-1908.

[146] Sun JC, Beilke JN, Lanier LL. Adaptive immune features of natural killer cells. Nature 2009; 457(7229): 557-561.

[147] Sun JC, Lanier LL. Natural killer cells remember: an evolutionary bridge between innate and adaptive immunity? Eur J Immunol 2009; 39(8): 2059-2064.

[148] Foster SL, Hargreaves DC, Medzhitov R. Gene-specific control of inflammation by TLR-induced chromatin modifications. Nature 2007; 447(7147): 972-978.

[149] Little RE, Gladen BC. Levels of lipid peroxides in uncomplicated pregnancy: a review of the literature. Reprod Toxicol 1999; 13(5): 347-352.

[150] Hung TH, Lo LM, Chiu TH, *et al.* A longitudinal study of oxidative stress and antioxidant status in women with uncomplicated pregnancies throughout gestation. Reprod Sci 2010; 17(4): 401-409.

[151] Hubel CA. Oxidative stress in the pathogenesis of preeclampsia. Proc Soc Exp Biol Med 1999; 222(3): 222-235.

[152] Wang Y, Walsh SW. TNF alpha concentrations and mRNA expression are increased in preeclamptic placentas. J Reprod Immunol 1996; 32(2): 157-169.

[153] Morikawa S, Kurauchi O, Tanaka M, *et al.* Increased mitochondrial damage by lipid peroxidation in trophoblast cells of preeclamptic placentas. Biochem Mol Biol Int 1997; 41(4): 767-775.

[154]   Shibata E, Nanri H, Ejima K, *et al.* Enhancement of mitochondrial oxidative stress and up-regulation of antioxidant protein peroxiredoxin III/SP-22 in the mitochondria of human pre-eclamptic placentae. Placenta 2003; 24(6): 698-705.

[155]   Walsh SW, Vaughan JE, Wang Y, Roberts LJ, 2nd. Placental isoprostane is significantly increased in preeclampsia. FASEB J 2000; 14(10): 1289-1296.

[156]   Sikkema JM, van Rijn BB, Franx A, *et al.* Placental superoxide is increased in pre-eclampsia. Placenta 2001; 22(4): 304-308.

[157]   Zusterzeel PL, Rutten H, Roelofs HM, Peters WH, Steegers EA. Protein carbonyls in decidua and placenta of pre-eclamptic women as markers for oxidative stress. Placenta 2001; 22(2-3): 213-219.

[158]   Burton GJ, Jauniaux E. Placental oxidative stress: from miscarriage to preeclampsia. Journal of the Society for Gynecologic Investigation 2004; 11(6): 342-52.

[159]   Redman CW, Sargent IL. Placental debris, oxidative stress and pre-eclampsia. Placenta 2000; 21(7): 597-602.

[160]   Vanderlelie J, Venardos K, Clifton VL, Gude NM, Clarke FM, Perkins AV. Increased biological oxidation and reduced anti-oxidant enzyme activity in pre-eclamptic placentae. Placenta 2005; 26(1): 53-58.

[161]   Burton GJ, Caniggia I. Hypoxia: implications for implantation to delivery-a workshop report. Placenta 2001; 22(Suppl A): S63-65.

[162]   Hung TH, Burton GJ. Hypoxia and reoxygenation: a possible mechanism for placental oxidative stress in preeclampsia. Taiwan J Obstet Gynecol 2006; 45(3): 189-200.

[163]   Lang U, Baker RS, Khoury J, Clark KE. Effects of chronic reduction in uterine blood flow on fetal and placental growth in the sheep. Am J Physiol Regul Integr Comp Physiol 2000; 279(1): R53-59.

[164]   Bloxam DL, Bullen BE, Walters BN, Lao TT. Placental glycolysis and energy metabolism in preeclampsia. Am J Obstet Gynecol 1987; 157(1): 97-101.

[165]   Xiong X, Demianczuk NN, Buekens P, Saunders LD. Association of preeclampsia with high birth weight for age. Am J Obstet Gynecol 2000; 183(1): 148-155.

[166]   Espinoza J, Sebire NJ, McAuliffe F, Krampl E, Nicolaides KH. Placental villus morphology in relation to maternal hypoxia at high altitude. Placenta 2001; 22(6): 606-608.

[167]   Reshetnikova OS, Burton GJ, Milovanov AP. Effects of hypobaric hypoxia on the fetoplacental unit: the morphometric diffusing capacity of the villous membrane at high altitude. Am J Obstet Gynecol 1994; 171(6): 1560-1565.

[168]   Jauniaux E, Watson AL, Hempstock J, Bao YP, Skepper JN, Burton GJ. Onset of maternal arterial blood flow and placental oxidative stress. A possible factor in human early pregnancy failure. Am J Pathol 2000; 157(6): 2111-2122.

[169]   Jauniaux E, Jurkovic D, Campbell S. Current topic: *in vivo* investigation of the placental circulations by Doppler echography. Placenta 1995; 16(4): 323-331.

[170]   Jauniaux E, Ramsay B, Campbell S. Ultrasonographic investigation of placental morphologic characteristics and size during the second trimester of pregnancy. Am J Obstet Gynecol 1994; 170(1 Pt 1): 130-137.

[171]   Wang Y, Walsh SW. Increased superoxide generation is associated with decreased superoxide dismutase activity and mRNA expression in placental trophoblast cells in pre-eclampsia. Placenta 2001; 22(2-3): 206-212.

[172]   Myatt L, Rosenfield RB, Eis AL, Brockman DE, Greer I, Lyall F. Nitrotyrosine residues in placenta. Evidence of peroxynitrite formation and action. Hypertension 1996; 28(3): 488-493.

[173]   Hung TH, Skepper JN, Burton GJ. *In vitro* ischemia-reperfusion injury in term human placenta as a model for oxidative stress in pathological pregnancies. Am J Pathol 2001; 159(3): 1031-1043.

[174]   Hung TH, Skepper JN, Charnock-Jones DS, Burton GJ. Hypoxia-reoxygenation: a potent inducer of apoptotic changes in the human placenta and possible etiological factor in preeclampsia. Circ Res 2002; 90(12): 1274-1281.

[175]   Watson AL, Skepper JN, Jauniaux E, Burton GJ. Susceptibility of human placental syncytiotrophoblastic mitochondria to oxygen-mediated damage in relation to gestational age. J Clin Endocrinol Metab 1998; 83(5): 1697-1705.

[176]   Harrison R. Structure and function of xanthine oxidoreductase: where are we now? Free Radic Biol Med 2002; 33(6): 774-797.

[177]   Granger DN, Hollwarth ME, Parks DA. Ischemia-reperfusion injury: role of oxygen-derived free radicals. Acta Physiol Scand Suppl 1986; 548: 47-63.

[178]   McCord JM. Oxygen-derived free radicals in postischemic tissue injury. N Engl J Med 1985; 312(3): 159-163.

[179]   Nishino T, Nakanishi S, Okamoto K, *et al.* Conversion of xanthine dehydrogenase into oxidase and its role in reperfusion injury. Biochem Soc Trans 1997; 25(3): 783-786.

[180] Many A, Westerhausen-Larson A, Kanbour-Shakir A, Roberts JM. Xanthine oxidase/dehydrogenase is present in human placenta. Placenta 1996; 17(5-6): 361-365.

[181] Telfer JF, Thomson AJ, Cameron IT, Greer IA, Norman JE. Expression of superoxide dismutase and xanthine oxidase in myometrium, fetal membranes and placenta during normal human pregnancy and parturition. Hum Reprod 1997; 12(10): 2306-2312.

[182] Many A, Hubel CA, Fisher SJ, Roberts JM, Zhou Y. Invasive cytotrophoblasts manifest evidence of oxidative stress in preeclampsia. Am J Pathol 2000; 156(1): 321-331.

[183] Many A, Hubel CA, Roberts JM. Hyperuricemia and xanthine oxidase in preeclampsia, revisited. Am J Obstet Gynecol 1996; 174(1 Pt 1): 288-291.

[184] Muller MJ, Vollmar B, Friedl HP, Menger MD. Xanthine oxidase and superoxide radicals in portal triad crossclamping-induced microvascular reperfusion injury of the liver. Free Radic Biol Med 1996; 21(2): 189-197.

[185] Tan S, Gelman S, Wheat JK, Parks DA. Circulating xanthine oxidase in human ischemia reperfusion. South Med J 1995; 88(4): 479-482.

[186] Yildirim A, Altinkaynak K, Aksoy H, Sahin YN, Akcay F. Plasma xanthine oxidase, superoxide dismutase and glutathione peroxidase activities and uric acid levels in severe and mild pre-eclampsia. Cell Biochem Funct 2004; 22(4): 213-217.

[187] Karabulut AB, Kafkasli A, Burak F, Gozukara EM. Maternal and fetal plasma adenosine deaminase, xanthine oxidase and malondialdehyde levels in pre-eclampsia. Cell Biochem Funct 2005; 23(4): 279-283.

[188] Centlow M, Junus K, Nystrom H, *et al.* Perfusion of the human placenta with red blood cells and xanthine oxidase mimics preeclampsia *in-vitro*. Z Geburtshilfe Neonatol 2009; 213(3): 89-95.

[189] Wang Y, Walsh SW. Placental mitochondria as a source of oxidative stress in pre-eclampsia. Placenta 1998; 19(8): 581-586.

[190] Brown GC. Control of respiration and ATP synthesis in mammalian mitochondria and cells. Biochem J 1992; 284(Pt 1): 1-13.

[191] Pitkanen S, Robinson BH. Mitochondrial complex I deficiency leads to increased production of superoxide radicals and induction of superoxide dismutase. The Journal of clinical investigation 1996; 98(2): 345-351.

[192] Jezek P, Hlavata L. Mitochondria in homeostasis of reactive oxygen species in cell, tissues, and organism. Int J Biochem Cell Biol 2005; 37(12): 2478-2503.

[193] Weisiger RA, Fridovich I. Mitochondrial superoxide simutase. Site of synthesis and intramitochondrial localization. J Biol Chem 1973; 248(13): 4793-4796.

[194] McCord JM, Keele BB, Jr., Fridovich I. An enzyme-based theory of obligate anaerobiosis: the physiological function of superoxide dismutase. Proc Natl Acad Sci USA 1971; 68(5): 1024-1027.

[195] Wiktor H, Kankofer M. Superoxide dismutase activity in normal and preeclamptic placentas. Ginekol Pol 1998; 69(12): 915-918.

[196] Wang Y, Walsh SW. Antioxidant activities and mRNA expression of superoxide dismutase, catalase, and glutathione peroxidase in normal and preeclamptic placentas. J Soc Gynecol Investig 1996; 3(4): 179-184.

[197] Hochstein P, Utley H. Hydrogen peroxide detoxication by glutathione peroxidase and catalase in rat liver homogenates. Mol Pharmacol 1968; 4(6): 574-579.

[198] Madazli R, Benian A, Aydin S, Uzun H, Tolun N. The plasma and placental levels of malondialdehyde, glutathione and superoxide dismutase in pre-eclampsia. J Obstet Gynaecol 2002; 22(5): 477-480.

[199] Poranen AK, Ekblad U, Uotila P, Ahotupa M. Lipid peroxidation and antioxidants in normal and pre-eclamptic pregnancies. Placenta 1996; 17(7): 401-405.

[200] Mistry HD, Kurlak LO, Williams PJ, Ramsay MM, Symonds ME, Pipkin FB. Differential expression and distribution of placental glutathione peroxidases 1, 3 and 4 in normal and preeclamptic pregnancy. Placenta 2010; 31(5): 401-408.

[201] Atamer Y, Kocyigit Y, Yokus B, Atamer A, Erden AC. Lipid peroxidation, antioxidant defense, status of trace metals and leptin levels in preeclampsia. Eur J Obstet Gynecol Reprod Biol 2005; 119(1): 60-66.

[202] Walsh SW, Wang Y. Deficient glutathione peroxidase activity in preeclampsia is associated with increased placental production of thromboxane and lipid peroxides. Am J Obstet Gynecol 1993; 169(6): 1456-1461.

[203] Vanderlelie J, Gude N, Perkins AV. Antioxidant gene expression in preeclamptic placentae: a preliminary investigation. Placenta 2008; 29(6): 519-522.

[204] Funai EF, MacKenzie A, Kadner SS, Roque H, Lee MJ, Kuczynski E. Glutathione peroxidase levels throughout normal pregnancy and in pre-eclampsia. J Matern Fetal Neonatal Med 2002; 12(5): 322-326.

[205] Levine RL. Oxidative modification of glutamine synthetase. I. Inactivation is due to loss of one histidine residue. J Biol Chem 1983; 258(19): 11823-11827.

[206]   Levine RL. Carbonyl modified proteins in cellular regulation, aging, and disease. Free Radic Biol Med 2002; 32(9): 790-796.

[207]   Padmini E, Lavanya S, Uthra V. Preeclamptic placental stress and over expression of mitochondrial HSP70. Clin Chem Lab Med 2009; 47(9): 1073-1080.

[208]   Beckman JS, Chen J, Ischiropoulos H, Crow JP. Oxidative chemistry of peroxynitrite. Methods Enzymol 1994; 233: 229-240.

[209]   Ischiropoulos H, al-Mehdi AB. Peroxynitrite-mediated oxidative protein modifications. FEBS Lett 1995; 364(3): 279-282.

[210]   Radi R, Rodriguez M, Castro L, Telleri R. Inhibition of mitochondrial electron transport by peroxynitrite. Arch Biochem Biophys 1994; 308(1): 89-95.

[211]   Radi R, Beckman JS, Bush KM, Freeman BA. Peroxynitrite-induced membrane lipid peroxidation: the cytotoxic potential of superoxide and nitric oxide. Arch Biochem Biophys 1991; 288(2): 481-417.

[212]   Ischiropoulos H, Zhu L, Chen J, *et al.* Peroxynitrite-mediated tyrosine nitration catalyzed by superoxide dismutase. Arch Biochem Biophys 1992; 298(2): 431-437.

[213]   Pacher P, Beckman JS, Liaudet L. Nitric oxide and peroxynitrite in health and disease. Physiol Rev 2007; 87(1): 315-424.

[214]   Kossenjans W, Eis A, Sahay R, Brockman D, Myatt L. Role of peroxynitrite in altered fetal-placental vascular reactivity in diabetes or preeclampsia. Am J Physiol Heart Circ Physiol 2000; 278(4): H1311-1319.

[215]   Webster RP, Brockman D, Myatt L. Nitration of p38 MAPK in the placenta: association of nitration with reduced catalytic activity of p38 MAPK in pre-eclampsia. Mol Hum Reprod 2006; 12(11): 677-685.

[216]   Catala A. An overview of lipid peroxidation with emphasis in outer segments of photoreceptors and the chemiluminescence assay. Int J Biochem Cell Biol 2006; 38(9): 1482-1495.

[217]   Nigam S, Schewe T. Phospholipase A(2)s and lipid peroxidation. Biochim Biophys Acta 2000; 1488(1-2): 167-181.

[218]   Green DR, Reed JC. Mitochondria and apoptosis. Science 1998; 281(5381): 1309-12.

[219]   Wang Y, Walsh SW, Kay HH. Placental lipid peroxides and thromboxane are increased and prostacyclin is decreased in women with preeclampsia. Am J Obstet Gynecol 1992; 167(4 Pt 1): 946-949.

[220]   Borekci B, Aksoy H, Toker A, Ozkan A. Placental tissue cyclo-oxygenase 1 and 2 in pre-eclamptic and normal pregnancy. Int J Gynaecol Obstet 2006; 95(2): 127-131.

[221]   Biri A, Bozkurt N, Gunaydin G, Korucuoglu U, Durak I, Kavutcu M. Antioxidant enzyme activities and lipid peroxidation in preeclampsia. Int J Gynaecol Obstet 2007; 96(3): 196-197.

[222]   Walsh SW, Wang Y. Trophoblast and placental villous core production of lipid peroxides, thromboxane, and prostacyclin in preeclampsia. J Clin Endocrinol Metab 1995; 80(6): 1888-1893.

[223]   Borrego-Diaz E, Rosales JC, Proverbio T, *et al.* Effect of placental hypoxia on the plasma membrane Ca-ATPase (PMCA) activity and the level of lipid peroxidation of syncytiotrophoblast and red blood cell ghosts. Placenta 2008; 29(1): 44-50.

[224]   Walsh SW, Wang Y, Jesse R. Placental Production of Lipid Peroxides, Thromboxane, And Prostacyclin in Preeclampsia. Hypertension in Pregnancy 1996; 15(1): 101-111.

[225]   Ishihara N, Matsuo H, Murakoshi H, Laoag-Fernandez JB, Samoto T, Maruo T. Increased apoptosis in the syncytiotrophoblast in human term placentas complicated by either preeclampsia or intrauterine growth retardation. Am J Obstet Gynecol 2002; 186(1): 158-166.

[226]   Knight M, Redman CW, Linton EA, Sargent IL. Shedding of syncytiotrophoblast microvilli into the maternal circulation in pre-eclamptic pregnancies. Br J Obstet Gynaecol 1998; 105(6): 632-640.

[227]   Hache S, Takser L, Lebellego F, *et al.* Alteration of calcium homeostasis in primary preeclamptic syncytiotrophoblasts: effect on calcium exchange in placenta. J Cell Mol Med 2011; 15(3): 654-667.

[228]   Cindrova-Davies T. Gabor Than Award Lecture 2008: pre-eclampsia-from placental oxidative stress to maternal endothelial dysfunction. Placenta 2009; 30(Suppl A): S55-65.

[229]   Chen Z, Gibson TB, Robinson F, *et al.* MAP kinases. Chem Rev 2001; 101(8): 2449-2476.

[230]   Matsuzawa A, Ichijo H. Stress-responsive protein kinases in redox-regulated apoptosis signaling. Antioxid Redox Signal 2005; 7(3-4): 472-481.

[231]   Cindrova-Davies T, Spasic-Boskovic O, Jauniaux E, Charnock-Jones DS, Burton GJ. Nuclear factor-kappa B, p38, and stress-activated protein kinase mitogen-activated protein kinase signaling pathways regulate proinflammatory cytokines and apoptosis in human placental explants in response to oxidative stress: effects of antioxidant vitamins. Am J Pathol 2007; 170(5): 1511-1520.

[232]   Shin JK, Jeong YT, Jo HC, *et al.* Increased interaction between heat shock protein 27 and mitogen-activated protein kinase (p38 and extracellular signal-regulated kinase) in pre-eclamptic placentas. J Obstet Gynaecol Res 2009; 35(5): 888-894.

[233]   Jung Y, Isaacs JS, Lee S, Trepel J, Liu ZG, Neckers L. Hypoxia-inducible factor induction by tumour necrosis factor in normoxic cells requires receptor-interacting protein-dependent nuclear factor kappa B activation. Biochem J 2003; 370(Pt 3): 1011-1017.

[234]   Schreck R, Albermann K, Baeuerle PA. Nuclear factor kappa B: an oxidative stress-responsive transcription factor of eukaryotic cells [Review] Free Radic Res Commun 1992; 17(4): 221-237.

[235]   Aban M, Cinel L, Arslan M, *et al.* Expression of nuclear factor-kappa B and placental apoptosis in pregnancies complicated with intrauterine growth restriction and preeclampsia: an immunohistochemical study. Tohoku J Exp Med 2004; 204(3): 195-202.

[236]   Belkacemi L, Bedard I, Simoneau L, Lafond J. Calcium channels, transporters and exchangers in placenta: a review. Cell Calcium 2005; 37(1): 1-8.

[237]   Peacock M. Calcium metabolism in health and disease. Clin J Am Soc Nephrol 2010; (Suppl 1): S23-30.

[238]   Mattson MP, Chan SL. Calcium orchestrates apoptosis. Nat Cell Biol 2003; 5(12): 1041-1043.

[239]   Smaili S, Hirata H, Ureshino R, *et al.* Calcium and cell death signaling in neurodegeneration and aging. An Acad Bras Cienc 2009; 81(3): 467-475.

[240]   Hool LC. The L-type Ca(2+) channel as a potential mediator of pathology during alterations in cellular redox state. Heart Lung Circ 2009; 18(1): 3-10.

[241]   Droge W, Schipper HM. Oxidative stress and aberrant signaling in aging and cognitive decline. Aging Cell 2007; 6(3): 361-370.

[242]   Smith SC, Baker PN, Symonds EM. Placental apoptosis in normal human pregnancy. Am J Obstet Gynecol 1997; 177(1): 57-65.

[243]   Huppertz B, Frank HG, Reister F, Kingdom J, Korr H, Kaufmann P. Apoptosis cascade progresses during turnover of human trophoblast: analysis of villous cytotrophoblast and syncytial fragments *in vitro.* Lab Invest 1999; 79(12): 1687-1702.

[244]   Levy R, Nelson DM. To be, or not to be, that is the question. Apoptosis in human trophoblast. Placenta 2000; 21(1): 1-13.

[245]   Allaire AD, Ballenger KA, Wells SR, McMahon MJ, Lessey BA. Placental apoptosis in preeclampsia. Obstet Gynecol 2000; 96(2): 271-276.

[246]   Leung DN, Smith SC, To KF, Sahota DS, Baker PN. Increased placental apoptosis in pregnancies complicated by preeclampsia. Am J Obstet Gynecol 2001; 184(6): 1249-1250.

[247]   Jones CJ, Fox H. An ultrastructural and ultrahistochemical study of the human placenta in maternal pre-eclampsia. Placenta 1980; 1(1): 61-76.

[248]   Huppertz B, Kingdom JC. Apoptosis in the trophoblast--role of apoptosis in placental morphogenesis. J Soc Gynecol Investig 2004; 11(6): 353-362.

[249]   Huppertz B, Kingdom J, Caniggia I, *et al.* Hypoxia favours necrotic versus apoptotic shedding of placental syncytiotrophoblast into the maternal circulation. Placenta 2003; 24(2-3): 181-190.

[250]   Redman CWG, Sargent IL, Roberts JM, *et al.* Immunology of Normal Pregnancy and Preeclampsia. Chesley's Hypertensive Disorders in Pregnancy. 3rd ed. San Diego: Academic Press 2009; pp. 129-142.

[251]   Tjoa ML, Cindrova-Davies T, Spasic-Boskovic O, Bianchi DW, Burton GJ. Trophoblastic oxidative stress and the release of cell-free feto-placental DNA. Am J Pathol 2006; 169(2): 400-404.

[252]   Hung TH, Charnock-Jones DS, Skepper JN, Burton GJ. Secretion of tumor necrosis factor-alpha from human placental tissues induced by hypoxia-reoxygenation causes endothelial cell activation *in vitro*: a potential mediator of the inflammatory response in preeclampsia. Am J Pathol 2004; 164(3): 1049-1061.

[253]   Venkatesha S, Toporsian M, Lam C, *et al.* Soluble endoglin contributes to the pathogenesis of preeclampsia. Nat Med 2006; 12(6): 642-649.

[254]   Maynard SE, Min JY, Merchan J, *et al.* Excess placental soluble fms-like tyrosine kinase 1 (sFlt1) may contribute to endothelial dysfunction, hypertension, and proteinuria in preeclampsia. J Clin Invest 2003; 111(5): 649-658.

[255]   Muttukrishna S, Knight PG, Groome NP, Redman CW, Ledger WL. Activin A and inhibin A as possible endocrine markers for pre-eclampsia. Lancet 1997; 349(9061): 1285-1258.

[256]   Lo YM, Leung TN, Tein MS, *et al.* Quantitative abnormalities of fetal DNA in maternal serum in preeclampsia. Clin Chem 1999; 45(2): 184-188.

[257] Perkins AV, Linton EA, Eben F, Simpson J, Wolfe CD, Redman CW. Corticotrophin-releasing hormone and corticotrophin-releasing hormone binding protein in normal and pre-eclamptic human pregnancies. Br J Obstet Gynaecol 1995; 102(2): 118-122.

[258] Mise H, Sagawa N, Matsumoto T, *et al.* Augmented placental production of leptin in preeclampsia: possible involvement of placental hypoxia. J Clin Endocrinol Metab 1998; 83(9): 3225-3229.

[259] Redman CW, Sargent IL. Circulating microparticles in normal pregnancy and pre-eclampsia. Placenta 2008; 29(Suppl A): S73-77.

[260] Aly AS, Khandelwal M, Zhao J, Mehmet AH, Sammel MD, Parry S. Neutrophils are stimulated by syncytiotrophoblast microvillous membranes to generate superoxide radicals in women with preeclampsia. Am J Obstet Gynecol 2004; 190(1): 252-258.

[261] Lok CA, Van Der Post JA, Sargent IL, *et al.* Changes in microparticle numbers and cellular origin during pregnancy and preeclampsia. Hypertens Pregnancy 2008; 27(4): 344-360.

[262] Cockell AP, Learmont JG, Smarason AK, Redman CW, Sargent IL, Poston L. Human placental syncytiotrophoblast microvillous membranes impair maternal vascular endothelial function. Br J Obstet Gynaecol 1997; 104(2): 235-240.

[263] Johansen M, Redman CW, Wilkins T, Sargent IL. Trophoblast deportation in human pregnancy--its relevance for pre-eclampsia. Placenta 1999; 20(7): 531-539.

[264] Levine RJ, Maynard SE, Qian C, *et al.* Circulating angiogenic factors and the risk of preeclampsia. N Engl J Med 2004; 350(7): 672-683.

[265] Hertig A, Berkane N, Lefevre G, *et al.* Maternal serum sFlt1 concentration is an early and reliable predictive marker of preeclampsia. Clin Chem 2004; 50(9): 1702-1703.

[266] Wathen KA, Tuutti E, Stenman UH, *et al.* Maternal serum-soluble vascular endothelial growth factor receptor-1 in early pregnancy ending in preeclampsia or intrauterine growth retardation. J Clin Endocrinol Metab 2006; 91(1): 180-184.

[267] Chaiworapongsa T, Romero R, Espinoza J, *et al.* Evidence supporting a role for blockade of the vascular endothelial growth factor system in the pathophysiology of preeclampsia. Young Investigator Award. Am J Obstet Gynecol 2004; 190(6): 1541-1547

[268] Nevo O, Soleymanlou N, Wu Y, *et al.* Increased expression of sFlt-1 in *in vivo* and *in vitro* models of human placental hypoxia is mediated by HIF-1. Am J Physiol Regul Integr Comp Physiol 2006; 291(4): R1085-1093.

[269] Gu Y, Lewis DF, Wang Y. Placental productions and expressions of soluble endoglin, soluble fms-like tyrosine kinase receptor-1, and placental growth factor in normal and preeclamptic pregnancies. J Clin Endocrinol Metab 2008; 93(1): 260-266.

[270] Levine RJ, Lam C, Qian C, *et al.* Soluble endoglin and other circulating antiangiogenic factors in preeclampsia. N Engl J Med 2006; 355(10): 992-1005.

[271] Sanchez-Elsner T, Botella LM, Velasco B, Langa C, Bernabeu C. Endoglin expression is regulated by transcriptional cooperation between the hypoxia and transforming growth factor-beta pathways. J Biol Chem 2002; 277(46): 43799-43808.

[272] Gaber LW, Spargo BH, Lindheimer MD. Renal pathology in pre-eclampsia. Baillieres Clin Obstet Gynaecol 1994; 8(2): 443-468.

[273] Roberts JM, Taylor RN, Musci TJ, Rodgers GM, Hubel CA, McLaughlin MK. Preeclampsia: an endothelial cell disorder. Am J Obstet Gynecol 1989; 161(5): 1200-4.

[274] Deng L, Bremme K, Hansson LO, Blomback M. Plasma levels of von Willebrand factor and fibronectin as markers of persisting endothelial damage in preeclampsia. Obstet Gynecol 1994; 84(6): 941-945.

[275] Clark BA, Halvorson L, Sachs B, Epstein FH. Plasma endothelin levels in preeclampsia: elevation and correlation with uric acid levels and renal impairment. Am J Obstet Gynecol 1992; 166(3): 962-968.

[276] Lyall F, Greer IA, Boswell F, Macara LM, Walker JJ, Kingdom JC. The cell adhesion molecule, VCAM-1, is selectively elevated in serum in pre-eclampsia: does this indicate the mechanism of leucocyte activation? Br J Obstet Gynaecol 1994; 101(6): 485-487.

[277] Minakami H, Takahashi T, Izumi A, Tamada T. Increased levels of plasma thrombomodulin in preeclampsia. Gynecol Obstet Invest 1993; 36(4): 208-210.

[278] Roberts JM, Taylor RN, Goldfien A. Clinical and biochemical evidence of endothelial cell dysfunction in the pregnancy syndrome preeclampsia. Am J Hypertens 1991; 4(8): 700-708.

[279] Friedman SA, Schiff E, Emeis JJ, Dekker GA, Sibai BM. Biochemical corroboration of endothelial involvement in severe preeclampsia. Am J Obstet Gynecol 1995; 172(1Pt 1): 202-203.

[280] Austgulen R, Lien E, Vince G, Redman CW. Increased maternal plasma levels of soluble adhesion molecules (ICAM-1, VCAM-1, E-selectin) in preeclampsia. Eur J Obstet Gynecol Reprod Biol 1997; 71(1): 53-58.

[281] Redman CWG, Sargent IL. Preeclampsia and the systemic inflammatory response. Seminars in Nephrology 2004; 24(6): 565-570.

[282] Gabay C, Kushner I. Acute-phase proteins and other systemic responses to inflammation. N Engl J Med 1999; 340(6): 448-454.

[283] Ruminy P, Gangneux C, Claeyssens S, Scotte M, Daveau M, Salier JP. Gene transcription in hepatocytes during the acute phase of a systemic inflammation: from transcription factors to target genes. Inflamm Res 2001; 50(8): 383-390.

[284] Morley JJ, Kushner I. Serum C-reactive protein levels in disease. Ann N Y Acad Sci 1982; 389: 406-418.

[285] Mihu D, Costin N, Mihu CM, Blaga LD, Pop RB. C-reactive protein, marker for evaluation of systemic inflammatory response in preeclampsia. Rev Med Chir Soc Med Nat Iasi 2008; 112(4): 1019-1025.

[286] Belo L, Santos-Silva A, Rumley A, *et al.* Elevated tissue plasminogen activator as a potential marker of endothelial dysfunction in pre-eclampsia: correlation with proteinuria. BJOG 2002; 109(11): 1250-1255.

[287] Morgan T, Craven C, Nelson L, Lalouel JM, Ward K. Angiotensinogen T235 expression is elevated in decidual spiral arteries. J Clin Invest 1997; 100(6): 1406-1415.

[288] von Versen-Hoeynck FM, Hubel CA, Gallaher MJ, Gammill HS, Powers RW. Plasma levels of inflammatory markers neopterin, sialic acid, and C-reactive protein in pregnancy and preeclampsia. Am J Hypertens 2009; 22(6): 687-692.

[289] Derzsy Z, Prohaszka Z, Rigo J, Jr., Fust G, Molvarec A. Activation of the complement system in normal pregnancy and preeclampsia. Mol Immunol 2010; 47(7-8): 1500-1506.

[290] Lynch AM, Salmon JE. Dysregulated complement activation as a common pathway of injury in preeclampsia and other pregnancy complications. Placenta 2010; 31(7): 561-567.

[291] Lox CD, Dorsett MM, Hampton RM. Observations on clotting activity during pre-eclampsia. Clin Exp Hypertens B 1983; 2(2): 179-190.

[292] Auer J, Camoin L, Guillonneau F, *et al.* Serum profile in preeclampsia and intra-uterine growth restriction revealed by iTRAQ technology. J Proteomics 2010; 73(5): 1004-1017.

[293] Johansen KA, Williams JH, Stark JM. Acute-phase C56-forming ability and concentrations of complement components in normotensive and hypertensive pregnancies. Br J Obstet Gynaecol 1981; 88(5): 504-512.

[294] Margarson MP, Soni N. Serum albumin: touchstone or totem? Anaesthesia 1998; 53(8): 789-803.

[295] Lorentzen B, Endresen MJ, Clausen T, Henriksen T. Fasting serum free fatty acids and triglycerides are increased before 20 weeks of gestation in women who later develop preeclampsia. Hypertension in Pregnancy 1994; 13(1): 103-109.

[296] Hubel CA, McLaughlin MK, Evans RW, Hauth BA, Sims CJ, Roberts JM. Fasting serum triglycerides, free fatty acids, and malondialdehyde are increased in preeclampsia, are positively correlated, and decrease within 48 hours post partum. Am J Obstet Gynecol 1996; 174(3): 975-982.

[297] Ogura K, Miyatake T, Fukui O, Nakamura T, Kameda T, Yoshino G. Low-density lipoprotein particle diameter in normal pregnancy and preeclampsia. J Atheroscler Thromb 2002; 9(1): 42-47.

[298] Qiu C, Phung TT, Vadachkoria S, Muy-Rivera M, Sanchez SE, Williams MA. Oxidized low-density lipoprotein (Oxidized LDL) and the risk of preeclampsia. Physiol Res 2006; 55(5): 491-500.

[299] Harris HW, Gosnell JE, Kumwenda ZL. The lipemia of sepsis: triglyceride-rich lipoproteins as agents of innate immunity. J Endotoxin Res 2000; 6(6): 421-30.

[300] Sethi JK, Hotamisligil GS. The role of TNF alpha in adipocyte metabolism. Semin Cell Dev Biol 1999; 10(1):19-29.

[301] Stepan H, Philipp A, Reiche M, *et al.* Serum levels of the adipokine lipocalin-2 are increased in preeclampsia. J Endocrinol Invest 2010; 33(9): 626-632.

[302] Fasshauer M, Seeger J, Waldeyer T, *et al.* Serum levels of the adipokine adipocyte fatty acid-binding protein are increased in preeclampsia. Am J Hypertens 2008; 21(5): 582-586.

[303] Wozniak SE, Gee LL, Wachtel MS, Frezza EE. Adipose tissue: the new endocrine organ? A review article. Dig Dis Sci 2009; 54(9): 1847-1856.

[304] Fantuzzi G. Adipose tissue, adipokines, and inflammation. J Allergy Clin Immunol 2005; 115(5): 911-919.

[305] Martinez-Abundis E, Gonzalez-Ortiz M, Pascoe-Gonzalez S. Serum leptin levels and the severity of preeclampsia. Arch Gynecol Obstet 2000; 264(2): 71-73.

[306] Matarese G, Moschos S, Mantzoros CS. Leptin in immunology. J Immunol 2005; 174(6): 3137-3142.

[307] Iikuni N, Lam QL, Lu L, Matarese G, La Cava A. Leptin and Inflammation. Curr Immunol Rev 2008 1;4(2): 70-79.

[308] Sibai B, Dekker G, Kupferminc M. Pre-eclampsia. Lancet 2005; 365(9461): 785-99.

[309] Scott JR. Magnesium sulfate for mild preeclampsia. Obstet Gynecol 2003; 101(2): 213.

[310] Livingston JC, Livingston LW, Ramsey R, Mabie BC, Sibai BM. Magnesium sulfate in women with mild preeclampsia: a randomized controlled trial. Obstet Gynecol 2003; 101(2): 217-220.

[311] Deruelle P, Girard JM, Coutty N, Subtil D. Prevention of preeclampsia. Ann Fr Anesth Reanim 2010; 29(3): e31-35.

[312] Sergio F, Maria Clara D, Gabriella F, *et al.* Prophylaxis of recurrent preeclampsia: low-molecular-weight heparin plus low-dose aspirin versus low-dose aspirin alone. Hypertens Pregnancy 2006; 25(2): 115-127.

[313] Alguel G, Vormittag R, Simanek R, *et al.* Preeclampsia and pregnancy loss in women with a history of venous thromboembolism and prophylactic low-molecular-weight heparin (LMWH) during pregnancy. Thromb Haemost 2006; 96(3): 28525-28529.

[314] Sorensen TK, Williams MA, Lee IM, Dashow EE, Thompson ML, Luthy DA. Recreational physical activity during pregnancy and risk of preeclampsia. Hypertension 2003; 41(6): 1273-1280.

[315] Yeo S, Davidge ST. Possible beneficial effect of exercise, by reducing oxidative stress, on the incidence of preeclampsia. J Womens Health Gend Based Med 2001; 10(10): 983-989.

[316] Witlin AG, Sibai BM. Magnesium sulfate therapy in preeclampsia and eclampsia. Obstet Gynecol 1998; 92(5): 883-889.

[317] Altman D, Carroli G, Duley L, *et al.* Do women with pre-eclampsia, and their babies, benefit from magnesium sulphate? The Magpie Trial: a randomised placebo-controlled trial. Lancet 2002; 359(9321): 1877-1890.

[318] Grill S, Rusterholz C, Zanetti-Dallenbach R, *et al.* Potential markers of preeclampsia--a review. Reprod Biol Endocrinol 2009; 7: 70.

[319] Martin JN, Jr., Thigpen BD, Moore RC, Rose CH, Cushman J, May W. Stroke and severe preeclampsia and eclampsia: a paradigm shift focusing on systolic blood pressure. Obstet Gynecol 2005; 105(2): 246-254.

[320] Magee LA, Duley L. Oral beta-blockers for mild to moderate hypertension during pregnancy. Cochrane Database Syst Rev 2003; (3): CD002863.

[321] Abalos E, Duley L, Steyn DW, Henderson-Smart DJ. Antihypertensive drug therapy for mild to moderate hypertension during pregnancy. Cochrane Database Syst Rev 2007; (1): CD002252.

[322] Sibai BM. Hypertensive disorders of pregnancy: the United States perspective. Curr Opin Obstet Gynecol 2008; 20(2): 102-106.

[323] Duley L, Henderson-Smart DJ, Meher S, King JF. Antiplatelet agents for preventing pre-eclampsia and its complications. Cochrane Database Syst Rev 2007; (2): CD004659.

[324] Coomarasamy A, Papaioannou S, Gee H, Khan KS. Aspirin for the prevention of preeclampsia in women with abnormal uterine artery Doppler: a meta-analysis. Obstet Gynecol 2001; 98(5Pt1): 861-866.

[325] Askie LM, Duley L, Henderson-Smart DJ, Stewart LA. Antiplatelet agents for prevention of pre-eclampsia: a meta-analysis of individual patient data. Lancet 2007; 369(9575): 1791-1798.

[326] Hermida RC, Ayala DE, Calvo C, *et al.* Administration time-dependent effects of aspirin on blood pressure in untreated hypertensive patients. Hypertension 2003; 41(6): 1259-1267.

[327] Hermida RC, Ayala DE, Iglesias M, *et al.* Time-dependent effects of low-dose aspirin administration on blood pressure in pregnant women. Hypertension 1997; 30(3 Pt 2): 589-595.

[328] Rey E, Garneau P, David M, *et al.* Dalteparin for the prevention of recurrence of placental-mediated complications of pregnancy in women without thrombophilia: a pilot randomized controlled trial. J Thromb Haemost 2009; 7(1): 58-64.

[329] Belizan JM, Villar J, Repke J. The relationship between calcium intake and pregnancy-induced hypertension: up-to-date evidence. Am J Obstet Gynecol 1988; 158(4): 898-902.

[330] Villar J, Repke JT. Calcium supplementation during pregnancy may reduce preterm delivery in high-risk populations. Am J Obstet Gynecol 1990; 163(4 Pt 1): 1124-1131.

[331] Rumbold AR, Crowther CA, Haslam RR, Dekker GA, Robinson JS. Vitamins C and E and the risks of preeclampsia and perinatal complications. N Engl J Med 2006; 354(17): 1796-1806.

[332] Poston L, Briley AL, Seed PT, Kelly FJ, Shennan AH. Vitamin C and vitamin E in pregnant women at risk for pre-eclampsia (VIP trial): randomised placebo-controlled trial. Lancet 2006; 367(9517): 1145-1154.

[333] Talaulikar VS, Manyonda IT. Vitamin C as an antioxidant supplement in women's health: a myth in need of urgent burial. Eur J Obstet Gynecol Reprod Biol 2011; 157(1): 10-13.

[334] Rossi AC, Mullin PM. Prevention of pre-eclampsia with low-dose aspirin or vitamins C and E in women at high or low risk: a systematic review with meta-analysis. Eur J Obstet Gynecol Reprod Biol 2011; 158(1): 9-16.

[335] Kalpdev A, Saha SC, Dhawan V. Vitamin C and E Supplementation Does Not Reduce the Risk of Superimposed PE in Pregnancy. Hypertens Pregnancy 2011; 30(4): 447-56

[336] Talaulikar V, Manyonda I. The myth of vitamins C and E for the prevention of preeclampsia: just when will the penny drop? Am J Obstet Gynecol 2010; 203(6): e7-8.

[337] Yeo S, Davidge S, Ronis DL, Antonakos CL, Hayashi R, O'Leary S. A comparison of walking versus stretching exercises to reduce the incidence of preeclampsia: a randomized clinical trial. Hypertens Pregnancy 2008; 27(2): 113-130.

[338] Aversa S, Pellegrino S, Barberi I, Reiter RJ, Gitto E. Potential utility of melatonin as an antioxidant during pregnancy and in the perinatal period. J Matern Fetal Neonatal Med 2011 [May 11 Epub ahead of print]

[339] Poston L, Igosheva N, Mistry HD, et al. Role of oxidative stress and antioxidant supplementation in pregnancy disorders. Am J Clin Nutr 2011; 94(6): 198; 0S-5S

[340] Young BC, Levine RJ, Karumanchi SA. Pathogenesis of preeclampsia. Annu Rev Pathol 2010; 5: 173-192.

[341] Karumanchi SA, Lindheimer MD. Advances in the understanding of eclampsia. Curr Hypertens Rep 2008; 10(4): 305-312.

[342] Williams KP, Wilson S. Ethnic variation in the incidence of HELLP syndrome in a hypertensive pregnant population. J Perinat Med 1997; 25(6): 498-501.

[343] Douglas KA, Redman CW. Eclampsia in the United Kingdom. BMJ 1994; 309(6966): 1395-1400.

[344] Noraihan MN, Sharda P, Jammal AB. Report of 50 cases of eclampsia. J Obstet Gynaecol Res. 2005;31(4):302-309.

[345] Airoldi J, Weinstein L. Clinical significance of proteinuria in pregnancy. Obstet Gynecol Surv 2007; 62(2): 117-124.

[346] Sibai BM. Diagnosis, controversies, and management of the syndrome of hemolysis, elevated liver enzymes, and low platelet count. Obstet Gynecol 2004; 103(5 Pt 1): 981-91.

[347] Sibai BM. Diagnosis, prevention, and management of eclampsia. Obstet Gynecol 2005; 105(2): 402-410.

[348] Katz VL, Farmer R, Kuller JA. Preeclampsia into eclampsia: toward a new paradigm. Am J Obstet Gynecol 2000; 182(6): 1389-1396.

[349] Sheth SS, Chalmers I. Magnesium for preventing and treating eclampsia: time for international action. Lancet 2002; 359(9321): 1872-1873.

[350] Duley L, Gulmezoglu AM. Magnesium sulphate versus lytic cocktail for eclampsia. Cochrane Database Syst Rev 2001; (1): CD002960.

[351] Duley L, Henderson-Smart D. Magnesium sulphate versus phenytoin for eclampsia. Cochrane Database Syst Rev 2003; (4): CD000128.

[352] Duley L, Henderson-Smart D. Magnesium sulphate versus diazepam for eclampsia. Cochrane Database Syst Rev 2003; (4): CD000127.

[353] Aaserud M, Lewin S, Innvaer S, et al. Translating research into policy and practice in developing countries: a case study of magnesium sulphate for pre-eclampsia. BMC Health Serv Res 2005; 1: 5-68.

[354] Sevene E, Lewin S, Mariano A, et al. System and market failures: the unavailability of magnesium sulphate for the treatment of eclampsia and pre-eclampsia in Mozambique and Zimbabwe. BMJ 2005; 331(7519): 765-769.

[355] Brown MA, Buddle ML. Hypertension in pregnancy: maternal and fetal outcomes according to laboratory and clinical features. Med J Aust 1996; 165(7): 360-365.

[356] Sibai BM, Ramadan MK, Usta I, Salama M, Mercer BM, Friedman SA. Maternal morbidity and mortality in 442 pregnancies with hemolysis, elevated liver enzymes, and low platelets (HELLP syndrome). Am J Obstet Gynecol 1993; 169(4): 1000-1006.

[357] Joshi D, James A, Quaglia A, Westbrook RH, Heneghan MA. Liver disease in pregnancy. Lancet 2010; 375(9714): 594-605.

[358] Haddad B, Barton JR, Livingston JC, Chahine R, Sibai BM. Risk factors for adverse maternal outcomes among women with HELLP (hemolysis, elevated liver enzymes, and low platelet count) syndrome. Am J Obstet Gynecol 2000; 183(2): 444-448.

[359] Osmanagaoglu MA, Osmanagaoglu S, Ulusoy H, Bozkaya H. Maternal outcome in HELLP syndrome requiring intensive care management in a Turkish hospital. Sao Paulo Med J 2006; 124(2): 85-89.

[360] Martin JN, Jr., Rose CH, Briery CM. Understanding and managing HELLP syndrome: the integral role of aggressive glucocorticoids for mother and child. Am J Obstet Gynecol 2006; 195(4): 914-934.

[361] Sibai BM, Ramadan MK, Chari RS, Friedman SA. Pregnancies complicated by HELLP syndrome (hemolysis, elevated liver enzymes, and low platelets): subsequent pregnancy outcome and long-term prognosis. Am J Obstet Gynecol 1995; 172(1 Pt 1): 125-129.

[362] Sullivan CA, Magann EF, Perry KG, Jr., Roberts WE, Blake PG, Martin JN, Jr. The recurrence risk of the syndrome of hemolysis, elevated liver enzymes, and low platelets (HELLP) in subsequent gestations. Am J Obstet Gynecol 1994; 171(4): 940-943.

[363] Mattar F, Sibai BM. Eclampsia. VIII. Risk factors for maternal morbidity. Am J Obstet Gynecol 2000; 182(2): 307-312.

[364] Martin JN, Jr., Rinehart BK, May WL, Magann EF, Terrone DA, Blake PG. The spectrum of severe preeclampsia: comparative analysis by HELLP (hemolysis, elevated liver enzyme levels, and low platelet count) syndrome classification. Am J Obstet Gynecol 1999; 180(6 Pt 1): 1373-1384.

[365] Cavkaytar S, Ugurlu EN, Karaer A, Tapisiz OL, Danisman N. Are clinical symptoms more predictive than laboratory parameters for adverse maternal outcome in HELLP syndrome? Acta Obstet Gynecol Scand 2007; 86(6): 648-651.

[366] Zeeman GG, Fleckenstein JL, Twickler DM, Cunningham FG. Cerebral infarction in eclampsia. Am J Obstet Gynecol 2004; 190(3): 714-720.

[367] Zeidman LA, Videnovic A, Bernstein LP, Pellar CA. Lethal pontine hemorrhage in postpartum syndrome of hemolysis, elevated liver enzyme levels, and low platelet count. Arch Neurol 2005; 62(7): 1150-1153.

[368] Isler CM, Rinehart BK, Terrone DA, Martin RW, Magann EF, Martin JN, Jr. Maternal mortality associated with HELLP (hemolysis, elevated liver enzymes, and low platelets) syndrome. Am J Obstet Gynecol 1999; 181(4): 924-928.

[369] Araujo AC, Leao MD, Nobrega MH, *et al.* Characteristics and treatment of hepatic rupture caused by HELLP syndrome. Am J Obstet Gynecol 2006; 195(1): 129-133.

[370] Reck T, Bussenius-Kammerer M, Ott R, Muller V, Beinder E, Hohenberger W. Surgical treatment of HELLP syndrome-associated liver rupture--an update. Eur J Obstet Gynecol Reprod Biol 2001; 99(1): 57-65.

[371] Miguil M, Chekairi A. Eclampsia, study of 342 cases. Hypertens Pregnancy 2008; 27(2): 103-111.

[372] Sibai BM, Caritis S, Hauth J. What we have learned about preeclampsia. Semin Perinatol 2003; 27(3): 239-246.

[373] Fonseca JE, Mendez F, Catano C, Arias F. Dexamethasone treatment does not improve the outcome of women with HELLP syndrome: a double-blind, placebo-controlled, randomized clinical trial. Am J Obstet Gynecol 2005; 193(5): 1591-1598.

[374] Moulin B, Hertig A, Rondeau E. Kidney and preeclampsia. Ann Fr Anesth Reanim 2010; 29(4): e83-90.

[375] Roberts JM, Lain KY. Recent Insights into the pathogenesis of pre-eclampsia. Placenta 2002; 23(5): 359-372.

[376] Lafayette RA, Druzin M, Sibley R, *et al.* Nature of glomerular dysfunction in pre-eclampsia. Kidney Int 1998; 54(4): 1240-1249.

[377] Garovic VD, Wagner SJ, Turner ST, *et al.* Urinary podocyte excretion as a marker for preeclampsia. Am J Obstet Gynecol 2007; 196(4): 320. e1-7.

[378] Yu D, Petermann A, Kunter U, Rong S, Shankland SJ, Floege J. Urinary podocyte loss is a more specific marker of ongoing glomerular damage than proteinuria. J Am Soc Nephrol 2005; 16(6): 1733-41.

[379] Nakamura T, Ushiyama C, Suzuki S, *et al.* Urinary podocytes for the assessment of disease activity in lupus nephritis. Am J Med Sci 2000; 320(2): 112-6.

[380] Harkness UF, Mari G. Diagnosis and management of intrauterine growth restriction. Clin Perinatol 2004; 31(4): 743-764.

[381] Lorenzi T, Marzioni D, Giannubilo S, *et al.* Expression patterns of two serine protease HtrA1 forms in human placentas complicated by preeclampsia with and without intrauterine growth restriction. Placenta 2009; 30(1): 35-40.

[382] Rasmussen S, Irgens LM. History of fetal growth restriction is more strongly associated with severe rather than milder pregnancy-induced hypertension. Hypertension 2008; 51(4): 1231-1238.

[383] Burton G.J, Cindrova-Davies T, Charnock-Jones D.S. Placental Endoplasmic Reticulum Stress and Oxidative Stress in the Pathophysiology of Unexplained Intrauterine Growth Restriction and Early Onset Preeclampsia. Placenta 2009; (30 Suppl A): S43-48.

[384] Newhouse SM, Davidge ST, Winkler-Lowen B, Demianczuk N, Guilbert LJ. *In vitro* differentiation of villous trophoblasts from pregnancies complicated by intrauterine growth restriction with and without pre-eclampsia. Placenta 2007; 28(10): 999-1003.

[385] Mari G, Hanif F, Kruger M. Sequence of cardiovascular changes in IUGR in pregnancies with and without preeclampsia. Prenat Diagn 2008; 28(5): 377-383.

[386] Roberts JM, Catov JM. Preeclampsia more than 1 disease: or is it? Hypertension 2008; 51(4): 989-990.

[387] Shear RM, Rinfret D, Leduc L. Should we offer expectant management in cases of severe preterm preeclampsia with fetal growth restriction? Am J Obstet Gynecol 2005; 192(4): 1119-1125.

[388] Tranquilli AL, Giannubilo SR. Blood pressure is elevated in normotensive pregnant women with intrauterine growth restriction. Eur J Obstet Gynecol Reprod Biol 2005; 122(1): 45-48.

[389] Churchill D, Perry IJ, Beevers DG. Ambulatory blood pressure in pregnancy and fetal growth. Lancet 1997; 349(9044): 7-10.

[390] Mitani M, Matsuda Y, Makino Y, Akizawa Y, Ohta H. Clinical features of fetal growth restriction complicated later by preeclampsia. J Obstet Gynaecol Res 2009; 35(5): 882-887.

[391] Zhong Y, Tuuli M, Odibo AO. First-trimester assessment of placenta function and the prediction of preeclampsia and intrauterine growth restriction. Prenat Diagn 2010; 30(4): 293-308.

[392] Hack M, Flannery DJ, Schluchter M, Cartar L, Borawski E, Klein N. Outcomes in young adulthood for very-low-birth-weight infants. N Engl J Med 2002; 346(3): 149-157.

[393] Briana DD, Gourgiotis D, Boutsikou M, *et al.* Perinatal bone turnover in term pregnancies: the influence of intrauterine growth restriction. Bone 2008; 42(2): 307-313.

[394] Chunga Vega F, Gomez de Tejada MJ, Gonzalez Hachero J, Perez Cano R, Coronel Rodriguez C. Low bone mineral density in small for gestational age infants: correlation with cord blood zinc concentrations. Arch Dis Child Fetal Neonatal Ed 1996; 75(2): F126-129.

[395] Helin I, Landin LA, Nilsson BE. Bone mineral content in preterm infants at age 4 to 16. Acta Paediatr Scand 1985; 74(2): 264-267.

[396] Fall C, Hindmarsh P, Dennison E, Kellingray S, Barker D, Cooper C. Programming of growth hormone secretion and bone mineral density in elderly men: a hypothesis. J Clin Endocrinol Metab 1998; 83(1): 135-139.

[397] Bellamy L, Casas JP, Hingorani AD, Williams DJ. Pre-eclampsia and risk of cardiovascular disease and cancer in later life: systematic review and meta-analysis. BMJ 2007; 335(7627): 974.

CHAPTER 8

Epigenetic Regulation of Pregnancy Outcome

Jeffrey M. Craig[1], Ji-Hoon Eric Joo[1], Boris Novakovic[2] and Richard Saffery[2,*]

[1]*Early Life Epigenetics and* [2]*Cancer, Disease and Developmental Epigenetics, Murdoch Childrens Research Institute, Royal Children's Hospital; and Department of Paediatrics, University of Melbourne, Melbourne, Victoria 3052, Australia*

Abstract: Epigenetic modifications regulate the expression of all genes, including those showing dynamic profile associated with cell differentiation and growth. Numerous lines of evidence have confirmed that epigenetic profile is sensitive to a variety of environmental and genetic factors, and that epigenetic mechanisms underpin most environmentally-mediated changes to gene expression. The dynamic process of epigenetic remodeling associated with early human development *in utero* is thought to be a particularly sensitive period for environmental perturbation and it is therefore not surprising that a variety of adverse pregnancy outcomes are now believed to involve some epigenetic disruption in the developing pregnancy (embryo, fetus, placenta). This chapter summarizes our current understanding of epigenetic mechanisms and the emerging evidence for a link between epigenetic change and pregnancy outcome.

Keywords: Epigenetics, DNA methylation, placenta, fetal programming, imprinting.

EPIGENETIC MECHANISMS

Epigenetics refers to the "structural adaptations of chromosomal regions so as to register, signal, or perpetuate altered activity states" [1]. This definition encompasses changes to gene expression that are mitotically and/or meiotically heritable independently of changes in DNA sequence [2]. Epigenetic change regulates the alterations in gene expression accompanying cell differentiation and is the mechanism underpinning most environmentally-mediated changes to gene expression. Recent studies have also identified highly-dynamic epigenetic regulation, with specific modifications being established and removed within a single cell-cycle or in terminally-differentiated cells (reviewed in [1]).

Primary and secondary epigenetic marks include changes to nucleotides and DNA-associated proteins. These marks in turn attract macromolecular complexes that together determine the higher order structure and function of a genomic region, whether at the level of a gene promoter, whole chromosome, or the entire genome. Higher order epigenetic state encompasses the degree of DNA compaction, replication timing and spatial positioning within the cell nucleus. The result is the highly-coordinated control of genomic activities such as gene expression (or the potential for gene expression), DNA replication and cell division. The most readily assayable epigenetic modification, and the most widely studied, is DNA methylation. Unlike other epigenetic modifications, the ability to measure DNA methylation is largely independent of the method of sample handling and storage.

DNA Methylation

The DNA double helix is a ladder-like molecule where each side, the backbone, is made up of alternating phosphate and sugar molecules. The "rungs", attached to the sugar molecules, comprise the four nucleotides of DNA linked with hydrogen bonds as base pairs: adenine (A) with thymine (T), guanine (G) with cytosine (C). In somatic cells, DNA is methylated only at 5th carbon of cytosine residues (^{5me}C) within the dinucleotide CpG, 'p' designating the phosphate part of the DNA backbone (Fig. **1**). CpG islands are regions of DNA that contain a high density of CpG sites and are usually unmethylated [3]. In many cases, these are located in the control region (promoter) of genes or in association with repetitive DNA elements

Address correspondence to Richard Saffery: Cancer, Disease and Developmental Epigenetics, Murdoch Childrens Research Institute, Royal Children's Hospital; and Department of Paediatrics, University of Melbourne, Melbourne, Victoria 3052, Australia; Tel: 61-3-83416341, Fax: 61-3-93481391, E-Mail: Richard.saffery@mcri.edu.au

Julie Lafond and Cathy Vaillancourt (Eds)

[4]. In general, low levels of DNA methylation (hypomethylation) are associated with higher gene activity, and high levels of methylation (hypermethylation) with gene silencing [5].Repeat-associated CpG islands generally exist in a methylated state [4]. Recent genome-wide studies of methylation distribution in human cells have revealed that CpG sites located in non-regulatory gene regions or intergenic locations also tend to be methylated (reviewed in [6]). Very recently, an alternative form of modified cytosine, 5-hydroxymethylcytosine (^{5hme}C), within CpG dinucleotides, has also been described. This appears limited to pluripotent stem cells and Purkinje neurons and little is currently known about its regulation and function in development [7, 8].

The Interplay of Higher-Order Epigenetic Factors

Methylation and hydroxy-methylation of the CpG DNA dinucleotide are the only known examples of primary epigenetic modification of the underlying DNA sequence in eukaryotes. Other primary epigenetic marks include changes to histone proteins, around which DNA is packaged and "functional" non-protein coding ribonucleic acids (ncRNAs) (Fig. **1**). The interested reader is referred elsewhere for a detailed account of these mechanisms [9, 10]. At present, studying histone proteins modifications and nc-RNAs is generally more technically challenging than studying DNA methylation due to the specific sample handling requirements necessary to maintain the integrity of such epigenetic markers prior to analysis.

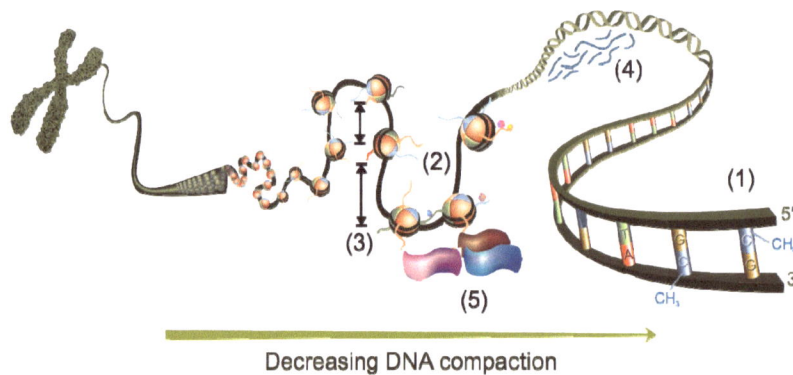

Decreasing DNA compaction

Figure 1: Epigenetic mechanisms. Genomic DNA within eukaryotic cells does not exist in isolation. Rather, it undergoes many levels of compaction that regulate accessibility to transcription factors and determine the overall 'activity state' of specific genomic regions. Epigenetic modifications play an important role in this process. These include: (1) symmetrical DNA methylation of cytosine residues within CpG dinucleotides on both strands of DNA, (2) packaging of DNA into nucleosomes comprising canonical histones (or histone variants) subject to extensive covalent modification, primarily at the 5' amino terminal tails, (3) variable nucleosome positioning/spacing, (4) incorporation of non-coding RNAs (into chromatin), (5) association of chromatin remodeling complexes with underlying DNA, amongst others.

The 'Epigenetic Cycle' and Development

Given the complexity of mammalian development, which involves the production of many thousands of specialized cell types, it is not surprising that there is no single epigenetic equivalent of the genome (the epigenome) of an individual. Rather, each cell type within an individual has its own epigenome that differs in a manner inversely related to the difference, both temporal and functional, from that of all other cell types in the same individual [11, 12]. Achieving this complexity requires the establishment of a 'blank slate' in the very early embryo that can be selectively re-written ('programmed') as progenitor cells give rise to heterogeneous daughter cells as part of various developmental cascades, producing different cell types and ultimately tissues within an individual.

To establish this blank slate, genome-wide DNA demethylation occurs twice during mammalian development [13]. The first demethylation event occurs during the generation of germ cells in both males and females. During these events, nearly all methylation marks that govern gene expression, including imprinted genes, are erased, and new marks (imprints) are established in the gametes in a sex-specific manner [14, 15]. Non-imprinted genes largely remain unmethylated at this stage. Following fertilization, gene-specific methylation marks of both the maternal and paternal genomes are extensively erased (Fig. **2**). Lineage-specific marks are then re-established from the blastocyst stage onwards [16]. Demethylation of the paternal pronuclear genome appears to be an active process, whereas the maternal genome is passively demethylated with each cell division. Imprinted genes escape this second wave of demethylation to retain their parent-of-origin methylation profile. At present, the extent of each wave of demethylation remains unclear; with some evidence for non-imprinted genes escaping erasure of methylation during gametogenesis [17-20].

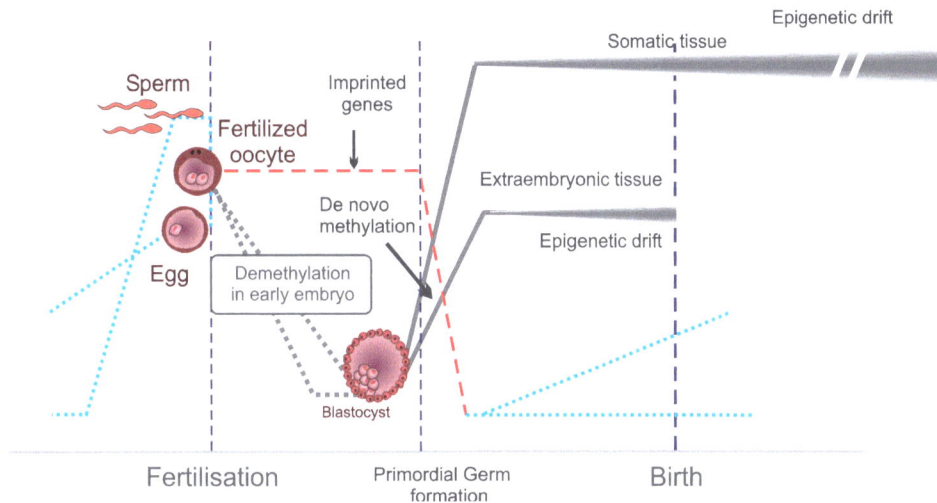

Figure 2: The mammalian DNA methylation cycle. Genomic DNA methylation is highly dynamic during early embryogenesis. Following fertilisation both the paternal and maternal genomes undergo extensive demethylation. Imprinted genes escape this process. Following blastocyst formation, extraembryonic and embryonic cells undergo remethylation in a tissue/cell lineage specific manner. Extraembryonic tissues (including the placenta) remain hypomethylated relative to embryonic cell lineages. Primordial germ cells undergo a second wave of demethylation that is followed by a 'resetting' of imprinting-associated methylated regions in a parent of origin-specific manner. During pregnancy and postnatally, the resulting epigenome is sensitive to environmentally-mediated epigenetic drift that occurs throughout the life course.

INTRAUTERINE ENVIRONMENT AND THE DEVELOPING EPIGENOME

Introduction

Mammalian development is driven by epigenetic change. However, epigenetic marks are reversible and can be influenced by factors originating outside the gene, the cell, and even the body. During embryonic development, rapid, genome-scale epigenetic changes occur as cells divide at a rate faster than at almost any other time during the life course. It is likely that this results in a higher rate of epigenetic error of stochastic and environmental origin.

Fetal Programming

The term 'fetal programming' was first coined by Koldovsky in 1979 [21] to describe the long term effect of intrauterine environment on offspring. This idea was developed by Barker and colleagues in the early 1990s in response to an observed negative association between death from cardiovascular diseases in adults and birth weight in a UK cohort [22-24]. The 'fetal programmin' hypothesis (as it is now known), is supported by a large number of studies in animals and fewer, largely epidemiological studies in humans [23-34]. According to this hypothesis, individuals born outside the normal weight range are more susceptible to diseases that fall under the umbrella of metabolic syndrome (such as type 2 Diabetes Mellitus and glucose impairment) and cardiovascular disease in later life. This susceptibility is believed to be 'programmed' *in utero* by the maternal environment *e.g.* maternal nutrition, maternal body composition and levels of stress hormones [29, 30, 35-37]. It has been proposed that fetal exposure to an inadequate intrauterine environment can result in a permanent adaptation of the developing fetus, potentially involving altered tissue physiology, hormone production, and glucose and lipid metabolism [38]. The molecular mechanism(s) underlying this phenomenon are largely speculative but are not predicted to be encoded in DNA (Fig. **3**).

Not surprisingly, changes in epigenetic profile have recently emerged as prime candidates for the environmentally-mediated molecular changes underpinning fetal programming. The most studied maternal environments in this regard are diet, stress, assisted reproductive technologies, alcohol, smoking, exposure to endocrine disruptors, toxins and drugs, each of which is discussed below. All have been shown to induce epigenetic change in offspring, and, in some cases, subsequent generations. However, it is promising to note that induced epigenetic marks found in offspring are potentially reversible by appropriate dietary or pharmacologic interventions [39, 40].

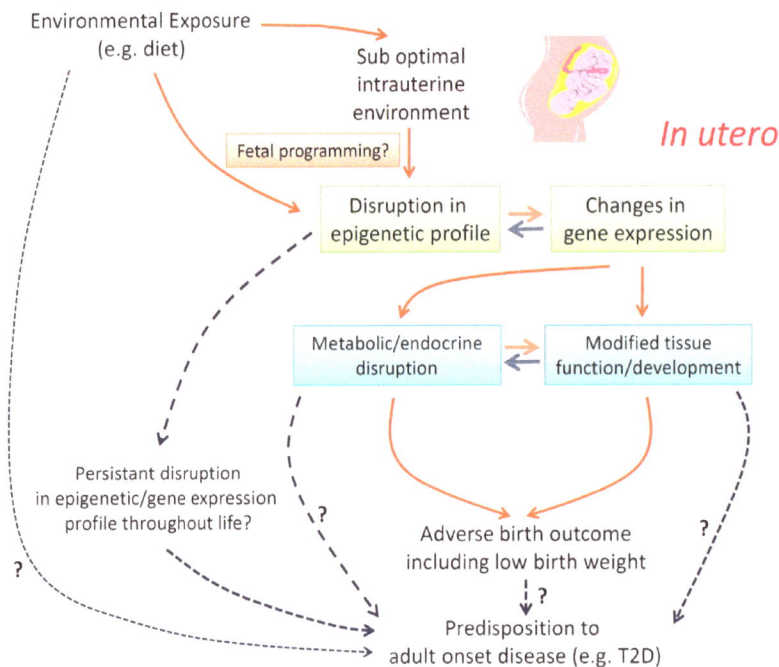

Figure 3: Model for fetal programming in response to adverse environmental exposures: An epigenetic perspective.

Diet

The universal methyl donor for all transmethylation reactions (including DNA methylation) is S-adenosylmethionine (SAM), produced as a result of one-carbon (folate) metabolism in all cells. This pathway utilizes several substrates and cofactors obtained exclusively from dietary sources, and involves a large number of enzymatic reactions [41]. Evidence from both animal and human studies suggests that the effects of folate deficiency on DNA methylation are very complex, being cell type-and target organ-dependent, and are gene and site specific [42, 43]. Both circumstantial and direct evidence exists for a link between disruption in the folate pathway, changes in DNA methylation, altered gene expression, and disease predisposition. Animal studies have shown that prenatal feeding of a methyl-supplemented diet can increase DNA methylation and decrease expression of genes in offspring [44-49], while limiting folate supply in humans, results in increasing levels of homocysteine and reduced DNA methylation [50-52]. Reducing levels of nutrients reaching the fetus, either by maternal low protein diet [45, 53, 54] or bilateral uterine artery ligation [55], results in a lower level of methylation, both at a global [55] and gene-specific level [45, 53, 54]. As folate supplementation can reverse such changes [45, 54], this suggests that optimal folate intake during pregnancy is essential for correct establishment of the developing neonatal epigenome.

Human studies are difficult for obvious reasons, but have taken advantage of events such as the Dutch famine, which occurred during the Second World War. One study found that individuals exposed to the famine at the time of conception had less methylation at the imprinted Insulin-Like Growth Factor-2 (*IGF2*) gene than unexposed siblings [56]. However, when the same investigators examined a set of genes that were a mixture of imprinted and non-imprinted genes in the same subjects, they found that some genes showed an increase in methylation and some a decrease [57]. It is therefore likely that the results of dietary restriction in humans are more complex than in rodents. Indeed, sex and exposure timing (early *vs.* late gestation) may also influence methylation levels in offspring [57]. Periconceptional folic acid supplementation (>400 ug/day) has also been directly correlated with increased methylation of the imprinted IGF2 gene in offspring at 18 months of age [58].

Stress

Response to stress occurs primarily through the hypothalamo-pituitary-adrenocortical (HPA) axis. Such responses are advantageous in adult life but, if occurring during pregnancy, can induce a long-lasting hyper-activation of the HPA-based stress response in exposed offspring [59]. In humans, maternal depression (and its associated stress) in the third trimester of gestation is associated with a small but significant increase in DNA methylation of the glucocorticoid receptor gene, central to the HPA axis, accompanied by an increased stress response in the offspring at three months of age [60]. These effects were very similar to those observed in rodent offspring whose mothers exhibited low levels of postnatal maternal care [61]. Evidence for systemic effects of stress on epigenetic marks comes from rodent models that revealed altered expression of genes involved in maintenance of DNA methylation and other epigenetic pathways [62].

Assisted Reproduction

Assisted reproductive technologies (ART) include *in vitro* fertilisation (IVF), a subtype of which is intracytoplasmic sperm injection (ICSI). These technologies involve subjecting eggs and sperm to environments that they do not normally experience. These include ovarian stimulation *via* hormone injection/ingestion, *in vitro* culture, puncturing of the egg's zona pellucida (ICSI), and, in some cases, freezing and thawing of embryos. Rodent studies show that many of these ART-associated environments can each independently disrupt gene expression and epigenetic marks [63-69], but some evidence does not support such a link [70]. Most human studies have focused on imprinted genes because of their role in fetal growth, with some supporting an effect of assisted reproduction on epigenetic profile [63, 71], while others report little or no effect [72]. Genome-wide DNA methylation profiling has also produced evidence for alterations of epigenetic profile in ART-derived children [73], although no differences between ICSI and non-ICSI IVF were found [74]. As there is also some evidence that ART may result in a higher proportion of human imprinting disorders [75] and developmental delay [76], more research is needed in this area.

Alcohol

Alcohol consumption is the leading preventable cause of birth defects and mental retardation [77]. Fetal Alcohol Spectrum Disorder (FASD) is an umbrella term to describe a number of adverse outcomes thought to be associated with pregnancy alcohol exposure. The most severe end of the spectrum is fetal alcohol syndrome (FAS), which is associated with chronic heavy alcohol use or frequent intermittent heavy alcohol use [78]. Alcohol can disrupt folate (one-carbon) metabolism, which can directly influence levels of available SAM needed for DNA methylation (reviewed in [79]). Rodent studies have demonstrated alcohol-induced changes to DNA methylation at a global level [80] and at specific genes [81], including imprinted genes [82, 83]. Furthermore, exposure of cultured embryos to moderate levels of alcohol has been associated with significant changes in methylation to 84 genes, including imprinted genes [84]. There is a growing body of evidence that offspring not directly exposed to alcohol in pregnancy may nevertheless be born with developmental abnormalities if their father or mother consumed alcohol prior to conception [85]; indeed, disrupted methylation at multiple imprinted loci was observed in sperm from heavy alcohol consumers [86].

Smoking

Maternal smoking in pregnancy is associated with early-onset wheezing and reduced lung function in the offspring [87, 88]. The effects of smoking on health can also be passed to grandchildren, as evidenced from studies where grandmothers but not mothers have smoked [89]. Smoking disrupts DNA methylation of cancer-associated genes in humans and mice [90-93], which most likely occurs through disruption of the activity of the enzymes that add, remove and maintain methylated DNA [92, 94]. Furthermore, children exposed to maternal tobacco smoke *in utero* may develop aberrant DNA methylation on a global and gene-specific scale [95]. The trans-generational effects of smoking exposure could be explained by induction of epigenetic change of developing gametes within a fetus, with these faulty marks potentially passed on to the grandchild. Precedents for such intergenerational transmission of exposures have been described in some rodent models (see [46] and below).

Endocrine Disruptors

Endocrine disruptors are chemicals that interfere with the function of hormones by mimicking, blocking, or disrupting their synthesis, transport, or elimination. Recent data suggest that such agents can have potentially serious effects on the developing epigenome that may be transmissible for multiple generations (reviewed in [96]). Hormones ultimately influence gene expression *via* epigenetic mechanisms; therefore, endocrine disruption may have epigenetic consequences. Prenatal exposure to the banned synthetic estrogen diethylstilbestrol (DES) has been shown to increase the risk of cervical and vaginal cancer and pregnancy-related problems in women, and testicular abnormalities in men [97]. Prenatal exposure to DES in a rodent model caused hypermethylation and long-term altered expression of the developmental transcription factor *Hoxa10*, potentially *via* the induction of aberrant epigenetic regulation of DNA methylation enzymes [98]. Bisphenol A (BPA) is a currently-used constituent of several important plastics and plastic additives. In rodents, intrauterine exposure to BPA is associated with higher body mass, altered reproductive function, increasing cancer risk, and specific DNA methylation changes including the *Hoxa10* gene [39, 99]. Genistein is an estrogen-like polyphenol found in soybeans and has been shown to decrease DNA methylation rodents exposed *in utero* [100]. Postnatal genistein exposure can disrupt the DNA methylation status of several genes [101]. Vinclozolin (a fungicide) and methoxychlor (a pesticide) can act *in utero* on developing germ cells to decrease fertility and induce aberrant DNA methylation both in male [102, 103] and female offspring [104]. These effects can last for several generations [102].

Pollution, Pathogens and other Adverse Environmental Exposures

Examining the relationship between exposures to the ultrafine particulate matter found in pollution and epigenetic disruption in humans is an emerging area of research. Limited data implicate such exposure to changes in methylation in maternal and fetal DNA, possibly associated with altered inflammatory response pathways [90, 91, 105]. Postnatal exposure to heavy metals such as nickel, cadmium, chromium, arsenic and lead has been associated with an altered epigenetic profile in rodent studies [106]. Additionally, lead has been linked to long-term alterations in DNA methylation status in adult males and to disruption of DNA methylation profile after prenatal exposure [107]. Similar results were obtained after prenatal exposure to polychlorinated biphenyls (PCBs), methylmercury [108] and cocaine [109]. The broad ranging effects of exposure to viral, bacterial and other pathogens on the epigenome are also becoming clear, with infective pathogens influencing or mimicking mechanisms involved in DNA methylation [110-114] and histone modification [115, 116].

PLACENTAL EPIGENETICS

Introduction

As the 'gateway' to the fetus, the placenta is subject to myriad environmental factors, each with the potential to alter placental epigenetic and gene expression profiles. This can have direct consequences for the developing fetus and possibly for longer term health. As a result, interest in placental epigenetics, and changes occurring in placenta-associated disease, has intensified over recent years.

The placenta regulates the rate of transfer of nutrients and gas from the mother to the fetus, waste removal from the fetal circulation, and protection of the fetus from a potentially adverse maternal immune response. Beyond these principal roles in feto-maternal exchange, the placenta is also a major endocrine organ, with the syncytiotrophoblast layer producing many hormones important for healthy embryo development [117], and several enzymes that regulate various aspects of pregnancy development. The placenta is also a critical regulator of fetal programming, a concept arising out of fetal programming hypothesis discussed above.

Emerging evidence suggests that the placenta requires a coordinated series of locus-specific epigenetic modifications for precise regulation of gene expression at key points during development (reviewed in [118]). Disruption of placental methylation is linked to aberrant placental function in both *in vitro* and in animal model systems [119-123], but equivalent data in humans is lacking. These issues will be discussed below.

Global Hypomethylation Including Specific Repeat Analysis

The separation of the extraembryonic cell lineage from the embryo proper at the blastocyst stage coincides with completion of a wave of demethylation of maternal and paternally-derived genomes [13]. Following this demethylation event is a period of remethylation in both the inner cell mass and the trophectoderm (Fig. **2**). However, there is evidence that the mechanisms responsible for the re-establishment of global DNA methylation levels differ between the two lineages [124]. Early work by Gama-Sosa and colleagues revealed that the human placenta exhibits a lower overall level of methylation compared to somatic tissue [125, 126]. The level of methylation seen in placenta is comparable to that seen in sperm and most human tumors and cancers [125-127]. The human genome is primarily composed of transposable (mobile) elements (TEs), which make up more than 50% of the genome. Therefore, in order to dissect where exactly DNA methylation is lost in the placenta, studies have concentrated on repetitive DNA. There are several different types of repetitive DNA elements in the mammalian genome, including short and long interspersed elements (SINEs and LINEs), satellite repeats and human endogenous retroviral elements (HERVs) [128]. These elements highly methylated in somatic lineages in order to prevent their movement in the genome and to prevent ectopic homologous recombination. Studies have suggested that placental hypomethylation is primarily due to a loss of methylation at specific repeat families [125, 129-131], while others do not show decreasing methylation [125]. Specific reduction in methylation has also been reported for the placental inactive X-chromosome relative to somatic counterparts [132].

Imprinting

Genomic imprinting is the phenomenon whereby one allele of a gene is silenced in a parent-of-origin manner. Silencing is usually controlled by DNA methylation at the differentially methylated region (DMR) of the gene, often at or near the promoter region. In humans, most imprinted genes occur in clusters, potentially allowing for the control of several genes by one DMR, sometimes referred to as an imprinting control region (ICR) [133]. Most imprinted genes are linked to fetal growth, and the most popular theory to explain the origin and evolution of imprinted genes is the 'parental-offspring conflict' theory, which states that paternally-imprinted (maternally expressed) genes repress, while maternally-imprinted (paternally expressed) genes promote, the use of maternal resources for fetal growth [134]. The male benefits from having larger, stronger offspring at the expense of the female and her future offspring to other males, while the female must conserve energy in order to allocate equal resources to her present, as well as future offspring.

Due to its role in feto-maternal interactions, the placenta is at the center of 'parent-offspring conflict' theory. Therefore, imprinted genes in the placenta have been the most studied genes to date. Evolutionary studies suggest that imprinting evolved with viviparity (live birth) [135, 136]. Eutherian mammals possess more imprinted genes than marsupials, which have a much shorter gestation period, which suggests that the length of gestation puts selective pressure on the placenta to drive the imprinting of growth-related genes [137]. In support of this hypothesis, a recent study found elevated levels of expression of the imprinted gene *Phlda2* in mice led to lower glycogen storage levels [138]. This finding, coupled with the lack of imprinting of the *Phlda2* in marsupials strongly implicates imprinting of this gene in increased nutrient supply in later pregnancy.

While studies have shown that correct placental imprinting is essential for proper embryo development, it is not known to what extent placental imprinting is disrupted by disease or environmental factors. Such disruption has been associated with intra-uterine growth restriction IUGR; [139, 140] and small for gestational age (SGA) babies [141], although, a recent study showed no such effect [142]. Assisted reproductive technologies [143], spontaneous pregnancy loss [144] and alcohol consumption during pregnancy [85] have all been linked with aberrant imprinting. However, data in this area are often conflicting (*e.g.* [145]).

Unique Gene-Specific Profile of Methylation

The placenta expresses a unique repertoire of genes compared to normal somatic tissues. Furthermore, different regions of the placenta show different expression patterns, in some cases due to cell composition, and in some due to the function of the cells in that part of the placenta [146]. Since DNA methylation is implicated in the silencing of a wide range of genes, it is not surprising that the placenta also possesses a unique repertoire of DNA methylation marks [147, 148]. An interesting emerging pattern is wide-spread hypermethylation at promoter regions of tumor suppressor genes, usually observed only in human cancers [149, 150]. These hypermethylated promoters include several negative-inhibitors of canonical Wnt/b-catenin signalling (*APC, EN1, SFRP2* and *WIF1*) [151-153] and a negative regulator of Ras-signalling (*RASSF1*) [154]. It is hypothesized that silencing of tumor suppressor genes by hypermethylation in the placenta contributes to the invasive properties of trophoblasts [150]. Along with global hypomethylation, these findings highlight the similarities between the epigenetic profile of the placenta and human cancers.

Cryptic Promoters Arising from Altered Epigenetic State

Transposable elements (TEs) or 'jumping DNA' make up more than 50%, and possibly up to 75% of the genome [128]. It is likely that DNA methylation evolved as a mechanism to prevent the potentially harmful movement of these sequences. However a subset of TEs, the HERVs, although lacking the capacity to 'jump', contain long terminal repeats (LTRs) that are capable of driving transcription of closely-linked genes [155]. Lower global methylation levels in the placenta relative to somatic tissues such as blood [130], has resulted in the unmasking of many LTRs, allowing them to drive the expression of nearby genes [156] in a placenta-specific manner. The extent to which TE-driven placenta-specific transcripts contribute to the function of this tissue is not completely understood, but the unique repertoire of potentially novel gene transcripts may explain some of the abundant differences in expression profile between the human placenta and somatic tissues.

DISRUPTION OF EPIGENETIC PROFILE IN PRE-ECLAMPSIA, INTRAUTERINE GROWTH RESTRICTION, AND PREMATURITY– IS THERE A LINK ?

Pre-Eclampsia

Pre-eclampsia (PE), characterized by maternal proteinuria and hypertension, affects up to 10% of pregnancies and is the single most important cause of maternal death (>50,000 per annum worldwide) and antenatal morbidity [157]. Moreover, the incidence of PE appears to be rising [158]. Women with PE are at increased risk of cardiovascular disease [159, 160]. Risks for the baby include prematurity and IUGR [161], the latter linked to chronic diseases of adulthood such as heart disease, hypertension and diabetes [162]. Many causes have been proposed for this disease [163], including abnormal maternal immune response [164], chromosomal abnormalities [165-167], and inability to respond to an increasing oxygen concentration [168]. Of critical importance is emerging data which suggests that disruption of the normal pattern of epigenetic modifications, particularly DNA methylation, in the placenta may be associated with trophoblast abnormalities seen in PE. However, the existing studies are significantly limited by both their small sample size and by the examination of tissues collected at birth rather than earlier in pregnancy [169, 170]. It is imperative that these limitations be overcome so the role of epigenetic regulation in PE can be ascertained.

Imprinting Disruption and Pre-Eclampsia

Despite some evidence for a genetic contribution to PE risk in specific populations [171], extensive attempts to identify risk genes have proven unsuccessful (*e.g.* [172]), primarily due to the potential for both fetal and maternal genetic contributions to risk, and their likely interaction with environmental factors. Molecular techniques have facilitated an understanding of networks that govern placental development (*e.g.* [173]; reviewed in [146]), with recent studies examining both gene expression profile and the role of epigenetic modification in this process [118, 149, 173]. Three recent studies have reported specific changes in gene expression in CVS tissue of women who later develop PE [174-176]. However, to date, no consistent changes have been detected, possibly reflecting inherent problems in controlling transient factors likely to influence RNA expression independent of PE phenotype.

Disruptions of imprinting have also been reported in placental diseases, such as PE and IUGR. These include reports of higher variation at imprinting-associated DMRs, suggesting a lower level of ICR control in these diseases [140], as well as loss of imprinting (LOI), a common finding in human cancers [170, 177]. Furthermore, Yu *et al.* [170] detected very low levels of imprinted *H19* expression in choriocarcinoma. Their findings implicate the role of *H19* in limiting placental invasion, with low expression in highly invasive choriocarcinoma, monoallelic expression in normal human placenta, and high biallelic expression in PE. However, LOI is not uncommon in normal human placenta, with recent studies showing biallelic expression of several imprinted genes in term placenta [178]. Furthermore, higher rates of LOI have been identified in the first trimester relative to term placentas, suggesting that imprinting is a dynamic process during placental development [179]. It has also been suggested that disruption in imprinting is a response to a poor intrauterine environment. Bourque *et al.* [180] observed a decrease in methylation at the *H19/IGF2* ICR-1 in IUGR, but not hypertensive IUGR (IUGR + PE). This finding suggests that the loss of methylation at ICR1 in IUGR, leading to repression of *IGF2*, and subsequent reduction in fetal size, is a response to poor placental development observed in IUGR. The failure of the placenta to respond to poor invasion, by reducing *IGF2* expression, results in a more serious disease – hypertensive IUGR [180].

The recent application of genome-scale epigenetic analysis to PE placental tissue collected at birth highlights the complexity of epigenetic disruption associated with the disorder. Analysis of ~1,500 methylation sites revealed highly variable methylation between different placentas independent of disease state, although some instances of altered methylation linked to PE were identified [148]. A more focused study by the same group using the same platform identified specific changes in DNA methylation of many genes, notably the tissue inhibitor of matrix metalloprotease *TIMP-3* in placentas of early-onset form of PE. No compelling evidence for similar changes in late onset PE or IUGR were noted in this study [181].

EPIGENETIC CONTRIBUTIONS TO PREGNANCY-ASSOCIATED DIABETES AND MATERNAL OBESITY – WHAT IS THE EVIDENCE?

Maternal Body Mass, Obesity and Pregnancy Outcome

Maternal malnutrition was most likely a major cause of faulty fetal programming until the mid-twentieth century [26, 27, 33, 182, 183]. Although the effect of under-nutrition on fetal programming has been studied extensively, this is less relevant in society today, as populations have become more obese in both developed and many developing countries. The rate of obesity is reaching epidemic proportions and is a major health concern, particularly as it is the major risk factor for metabolic syndrome [184]. Pregnancy is in itself a compromised condition resulting in insulin resistance increase of 40-50% and altered hormone levels [185]. Maternal obesity amplifies the risk of short-term obstetric complications such as PE and hypertension by 2 to 3 fold, thromboembolic complications by more than 2 fold, and gestational diabetes by 4 to 9 fold [186-189].

Maternal obesity also has adverse effects on offspring in both the short and long term. Many studies have shown a strong correlation between maternal obesity and fetal overgrowth or macrosomia [187, 190-194]. It is also evident that macrosomic infants and large for gestational age infants are more likely to become progressively overweight or obese in childhood and later life [191, 195, 196]. Furthermore, studies have reported an increased risk of coronary heart disease, type 2 diabetes and adult adiposity on the offspring of obese mothers [28, 197-200]. Similar findings are abundant in animal studies, with one such study looking at the consequence of obesity in mice induced by high energy diet from 6 weeks prior to mating to the end of pregnancy. Offspring from these mothers exhibited rapid weight gain in early life and increased fat pad mass at 6 months of age when compared to controls. Adult offspring also had increases rates of hypertension, insulin impairment, and altered expression levels in *PPARγ, β2AR, β3AR* and *11-βHSD1* genes which are involved in lipolysis, adipocyte differentiation and adipogenesis [201].

Gestational Diabetes and Pregnancy Outcome

The development of gestational diabetes can be influenced by multiple factors such as maternal age and genotype [202, 203]. However, maternal obesity is still the major risk factor [188]. In addition, gestationally-diabetic mothers, themselves, are more likely to develop type 2 diabetes in later life [188, 204]. Gestational diabetes can also have similar fetal outcomes; offspring of gestational diabetic mothers are 3 to 4 times more likely to be large for gestational age than the offspring of non-diabetic mothers [205, 206] and this fetal overgrowth is closely associated with child-and adult-hood obesity and metabolic disease [197]. Gestational diabetes exposes the fetus to a hyperinsulinemic environment and impaired glucose levels. Maternal glucose can cross the placenta to the fetus, however, maternal insulin cannot. This exposes the fetus to a high glucose environment and can induce an over-secretion of fetal insulin [191]. Thus the high glucose environment or impaired fetal hormone production may be a possible cause for faulty fetal programming.

The Role of Epigenetic Factors in Maternal Obesity-and Diabetes-Associated Fetal Reprogramming

Given the proven link between intrauterine environment and epigenetic profile, it is not surprising that evidence is emerging for a link between maternal obesity and diabetes and epigenetic change. One potential direct link may be through increased lipid levels themselves, which can act as transcriptional activators and signaling molecules. Fetal exposure to excess lipid levels may epigenetically regulate genes involved in lipid sensing and metabolism in the developing offspring (reviewed in [207]).

Indirect evidence supporting the role of environmentally-induced epigenetic mechanisms in obesity-induced fetal programming comes from studies involving surgical intervention using laparoscopic gastric (LAP) banding. These studies generally reported positive outcomes of such weight-limiting surgery, including a decreased risk of gestational diabetes, PE and weight gain in mothers, and a decreased rate of fetal overgrowth in offspring [208-211].

Evidence for a link also comes from twin studies. Monozygotic (MZ) twin pairs are generally assumed to have identical DNA sequences and, as such, any phenotypic discordance are likely due (at least in part) to environmentally mediated epigenetic change. The majority of twin pairs show some degree of birth weight discordance, and although MZ twin pairs have a far greater genetic similarity than dizygotic (DZ) twin pairs, the level of birth weight discordance is not greater in DZ pairs [212]. Studies have reported that the twin of lower birth weight is more likely to develop type 2 diabetes in adulthood [213]. Similar studies of the relationship between high birth weight and body size in adulthood have shown a more complex relationship between the two [214, 215]. A study of a small population of siblings who were born before or after mothers' diagnoses with diabetes showed that individuals who were exposed to a diabetic environment *in utero* have an increase chance of developing obesity and type 2 diabetes in later life [216].

Data directly implicating a role for epigenetic change in the mediation of maternal obesity-or diabetes-induced fetal programming is currently only available from animal studies. A study of Japanese macaques reported altered levels of hepatic histone modifications and changes in expression of stress-related genes in offspring of high fat fed mothers [217]. These offspring were also found to be more susceptible to liver disease in later life. A mouse study identified decreased levels of micro RNAs (miRNAs; small nc-RNAs that function epigenetically by regulating messenger RNA) in offspring of mothers fed a high fat diet [218]. A high energy diet during perinatal period in mice has been linked to altered DNA methylation of promoter region of the insulin receptor gene [219].

Even fewer studies have focused on gestational diabetes. A mouse model of chemically-induced gestational diabetes is associated with changes to gene expression and DNA methylation at the imprinted *H19/Igf2* locus [220]. However, unlike humans, pups were born low for gestational age. Clearly, more research in both animals and humans is needed to delineate the effects of maternal obesity and the related condition of gestational diabetes on the epigenetic reprogramming of offspring. A better understanding of these mechanisms could pave the way to intervention strategies aimed at preventing or reversing induced epigenetic change in offspring, prior to later onset of adverse health outcomes.

HARNESSING EPIGENETIC BIOMARKERS FOR EARLY DIAGNOSIS OF PREGNANCY-ASSOCIATED MATERNAL AND FETAL DISEASE

DNA Methylation to Detect Trisomies

Diagnosis of fetal trisomies, following implantation, is currently performed by collecting placental tissue through chorionic villous sampling (CVS). This technique is invasive, and as a result represents a risk to both the mother and the fetus [221]. The presence of fetal DNA in maternal plasma during pregnancy has provided a safe alternative to invasive prenatal testing. Measuring DNA methylation levels at specific loci in maternal blood allows the discrimination between maternal and fetal DNA. Many thousands of differentially-methylated regions have been identified between placenta and peripheral blood [222], including specific sites on chromosomes 13, 18 and 21 [223]. It is speculated that increasing levels of such methylation in maternal blood may be indicative of fetal trisomy. For example, a higher methylation level of a gene on chromosome 21 (*HLCS*) has been shown to be an effective method of diagnosing Down syndrome [224, 225]. These methods are currently being improved to allow detection of minute amounts of fetal DNA in a mixture of maternal DNA [226].

DNA Methylation to Detect Pre-Eclampsia and IUGR

Diagnosis of placental disease is usually not made until late pregnancy, at which point management of the disease is limited and the only treatment is usually delivery. As a result, there is a need for early detection methods of placental disease [227-230]. Currently, prognostic markers for placental diseases, such as PE and IUGR are based on measuring gene expression or serum levels of specific biomarkers in maternal plasma [228, 229, 231, 232]. However, there is evidence for variability in both markers, even in the absence of pregnancy-associated disease. Recently, higher levels of fetal DNA in maternal plasma have been linked to PE, due to a higher frequency of cell death associated with this disease [227]. Analysis of aberrant DNA methylation marks may allow placental disorders to be detected as early as the first trimester [233, 234], potentially facilitating development of novel interventions to prevent overt disease.

The utility of specific targets as epigenetic biomarkers is still under investigation. Due to the recent findings of hypermethylation of tumour suppressor genes in human placenta, these genes have been the main focus as potential markers *e.g. RASSF1* and *SERPINB5* [233] and *SERPINA3* [234]. The major challenge in this field is to identify methylation marks that have a high association with disease and can be quantified in minute amounts in a mixed population of DNA.

REFERENCES

[1]   Bird A. Perceptions of epigenetics. Nature 2007 May 24; 447(7143): 396-8.

[2]   Riggs AD. Epigenetic mechanisms of gene regulation. In: Russo VEA, Eds. Epigenetic mechanismns of gene regulation. Cold Spring Harbor, New York: Cold Spring Harbor Laboratory Press 1996; p. 1.

[3]   Gardiner-Garden M, Frommer M. CpG islands in vertebrate genomes. J Mol Biol 1987; 196(2): 261-82.

[4]   Yoder JA, Walsh CP, Bestor TH. Cytosine methylation and the ecology of intragenomic parasites. Trends Genet 1997; 13(8): 335-40.

[5]   Klose RJ, Bird AP. Genomic DNA methylation: the mark and its mediators. Trends Biochem Sci 2006; 31(2): 89-97.

[6]   Suzuki MM, Bird A. DNA methylation landscapes: provocative insights from epigenomics. Nature reviews 2008; 9(6): 465-76.

[7]   Tahiliani M, Koh KP, Shen Y, *et al.* Conversion of 5-methylcytosine to 5-hydroxymethylcytosine in mammalian DNA by MLL partner TET1. Science 2009; 324(5929): 930-935.

[8]   Kriaucionis S, Heintz N. The nuclear DNA base 5-hydroxymethylcytosine is present in Purkinje neurons and the brain. Science 2009; 324(5929): 929-930.

[9]   van Vliet J, Oates NA, Whitelaw E. Epigenetic mechanisms in the context of complex diseases. Cell Mol Life Sci 2007; 64(12): 1531-8.

[10]   Saetrom P, Snove O, Jr., Rossi JJ. Epigenetics and microRNAs. Pediatr Res 2007; 61(5 Pt 2): 17R-23R.

[11]   Fernandez AF, Assenov Y, Martin-Subero J, *et al.* A DNA methylation fingerprint of 1,628 human samples. Genome research 2011 [July 12 Epub ahead of print]

[12]   Yuen RK, Neumann SM, Fok AK, *et al.* Extensive epigenetic reprogramming in human somatic tissues between fetus and adult. Epigenetics Chromatin 2011; 4(1): 7.

[13]   Monk M, Boubelik M, Lehnert S. Temporal and regional changes in DNA methylation in the embryonic, extraembryonic and germ cell lineages during mouse embryo development. Development 1987; 99(3): 371-82.

[14]   Feil R. Epigenetic asymmetry in the zygote and mammalian development. The International journal of developmental biology 2009; 53(2-3): 191-201.

[15]   Jirtle RL, Skinner MK. Environmental epigenomics and disease susceptibility. Nature reviews 2007; 8(4): 253-62.

[16]   Okada Y, Yamagata K, Hong K, Wakayama T, Zhang Y. A role for the elongator complex in zygotic paternal genome demethylation. Nature 2010; 463(7280): 554-8.

[17]   Fan S, Zhang X. CpG island methylation pattern in different human tissues and its correlation with gene expression. Biochem Biophys Res Commun 2009; 383(4): 421-5.

[18]   Flanagan JM, Popendikyte V, Pozdniakovaite N, *et al.* Intra-and interindividual epigenetic variation in human germ cells. Am J Hum Genet 2006; 79(1): 67-84.

[19]   Rakyan VK, Chong S, Champ ME, *et al.* Transgenerational inheritance of epigenetic states at the murine Axin(Fu) allele occurs after maternal and paternal transmission. Proc Natl Acad Sci U S A 2003; 100(5): 2538-43.

[20]   Trasler JM. Epigenetics in spermatogenesis. Mol Cell Endocrinol 2009; 306(1-2): 33-6.

[21]   Koldovsky O. Development of sucrase activity: effect of maternal hormonal status and fetal programming of jejuno-ileal differences. Ciba Found Symp 1979; 18(70): 147-68.

[22]   Barker DJ, Osmond C, Simmonds SJ, Wield GA. The relation of small head circumference and thinness at birth to death from cardiovascular disease in adult life. BMJ 1993; 306(6875): 422-6.

[23]   Barker DJ. The fetal and infant origins of adult disease. Bmj. 1990;301(6761):1111.

[24]   Osmond C, Barker DJ. Ischaemic heart disease in England and Wales around the year 2000. J Epidemiol Community Health 1991; 45(1): 71-2.

[25]   Barker DJ, Fall CH. Fetal and infant origins of cardiovascular disease. Arch Dis Child 1993; 68(6): 797-9.

[26]   Barker DJ, Gluckman PD, Godfrey KM, Harding JE, Owens JA, Robinson JS. Fetal nutrition and cardiovascular disease in adult life. Lancet 1993; 341(8850): 938-41.

[27]   Barker DJ. Fetal origins of coronary heart disease. Br Heart J 1993; 69(3): 195-6.

[28]   Rich-Edwards JW, Kleinman K, Michels KB, *et al.* Longitudinal study of birth weight and adult body mass index in predicting risk of coronary heart disease and stroke in women. BMJ 2005; 330(7500): 1115.

[29]   Roseboom TJ, van der Meulen JH, Ravelli AC, Osmond C, Barker DJ, Bleker OP. Effects of prenatal exposure to the Dutch famine on adult disease in later life: an overview. Twin Res 2001; 4(5): 293-8.

[30]   Roseboom TJ. The fetal origins hypothesis. Twin Res 2001; 4(5): iii.

[31]   Roseboom TJ, van der Meulen JH, van Montfrans GA, *et al.* Maternal nutrition during gestation and blood pressure in later life. J Hypertens 2001; 19(1): 29-34.

[32]   McMillen IC, Robinson JS. Developmental origins of the metabolic syndrome: prediction, plasticity, and programming. Physiological reviews 2005; 85(2): 571-633.

[33]   Stein AD, Zybert PA, Lumey LH. Acute undernutrition is not associated with excess of females at birth in humans: the Dutch hunger winter. Proc Biol Sci 2004; 271 (Suppl 4): S138-41.

[34]   Stein AD, Zybert PA, van de Bor M, Lumey LH. Intrauterine famine exposure and body proportions at birth: the Dutch Hunger Winter. Int J Epidemiol 2004; 33(4): 831-6.

[35]   Langley-Evans SC. Nutritional programming of disease: unravelling the mechanism. J Anat 2009; 215(1): 36-51.

[36]   Symonds ME, Budge H. Nutritional models of the developmental programming of adult health and disease. Proc Nutr Soc 2009; 68(2): 173-8.

[37]   Martin-Gronert MS, Ozanne SE. Mechanisms linking suboptimal early nutrition and increased risk of type 2 diabetes and obesity. J Nutr 2010; 140(3): 662-6.

[38]   Symonds ME, Sebert SP, Hyatt MA, Budge H. Nutritional programming of the metabolic syndrome. Nat Rev Endocrinol 2009; 5(11): 604-10.

[39]   Dolinoy DC, Huang D, Jirtle RL. Maternal nutrient supplementation counteracts bisphenol A-induced DNA hypomethylation in early development. Proc Natl Acad Sci USA 2007; 104(32): 13056-61.

[40]   Weaver IC, Champagne FA, Brown SE, *et al.* Reversal of maternal programming of stress responses in adult offspring through methyl supplementation: altering epigenetic marking later in life. J Neurosci 2005; 25(47): 11045-54.

[41]   Davis CD, Uthus EO. DNA methylation, cancer susceptibility, and nutrient interactions. Exp Biol Med (Maywood) 2004; 229(10): 988-95.

[42]   Kim YI. Folate and DNA methylation: a mechanistic link between folate deficiency and colorectal cancer? Cancer Epidemiol Biomarkers Prev. 2004;13(4):511-9.

[43]   Jhaveri MS, Wagner C, Trepel JB. Impact of extracellular folate levels on global gene expression. Mol Pharmacol. 2001;60(6):1288-95.

[44]   Cooney CA, Dave AA, Wolff GL. Maternal methyl supplements in mice affect epigenetic variation and DNA methylation of offspring. J Nutr 2002; 132(Suppl 8): 2393S-400S.

[45]   Lillycrop KA, Phillips ES, Jackson AA, Hanson MA, Burdge GC. Dietary protein restriction of pregnant rats induces and folic acid supplementation prevents epigenetic modification of hepatic gene expression in the offspring. J Nutr 2005; 135(6): 1382-6.

[46]   Cropley JE, Suter CM, Beckman KB, Martin DI. Germ-line epigenetic modification of the murine A vy allele by nutritional supplementation. Proc Natl Acad Sci U S A 2006; 103(46): 17308-12.

[47]   Cropley JE, Suter CM, Martin DI. Methyl donors change the germline epigenetic state of the A(vy) allele. Faseb J 2007; 21(12): 3021; author reply-2.

[48]   Waterland RA, Jirtle RL. Early nutrition, epigenetic changes at transposons and imprinted genes, and enhanced susceptibility to adult chronic diseases. Nutrition 2004; 20(1): 63-8.

[49]   Wolff GL, Kodell RL, Moore SR, Cooney CA. Maternal epigenetics and methyl supplements affect agouti gene expression in Avy/a mice. Faseb J 1998; 12(11): 949-57.

[50]   Muskiet FA. The importance of (early) folate status to primary and secondary coronary artery disease prevention. Reprod Toxicol 2005; 20(3): 403-10.

[51]   Jacob RA, Gretz DM, Taylor PC, *et al.* Moderate folate depletion increases plasma homocysteine and decreases lymphocyte DNA methylation in postmenopausal women. J Nutr 1998; 128(7): 1204-12.

[52]   Rampersaud GC, Kauwell GP, Hutson AD, Cerda JJ, Bailey LB. Genomic DNA methylation decreases in response to moderate folate depletion in elderly women. Am J Clin Nutr 2000; 72(4): 998-1003.

[53]   Burdge GC, Slater-Jefferies J, Torrens C, Phillips ES, Hanson MA, Lillycrop KA. Dietary protein restriction of pregnant rats in the F0 generation induces altered methylation of hepatic gene promoters in the adult male offspring in the F1 and F2 generations. Br J Nutr 2007; 97(3): 435-9.

[54]   Lillycrop KA. Dietary protein restriction in the pregnant ratinduces altered epigenetic regulation of the glucocorticoid receptor and PPARain the heart of the offspring which is prevented by folic acid. Proc Nutr Soc 2006; 65: 65A.

[55]   MacLennan NK, James SJ, Melnyk S, *et al.* Uteroplacental insufficiency alters DNA methylation, one-carbon metabolism, and histone acetylation in IUGR rats. Physiol Genomics 2004; 18(1): 43-50.

[56]   Heijmans BT, Tobi EW, Stein AD, *et al.* Persistent epigenetic differences associated with prenatal exposure to famine in humans. Proc Natl Acad Sci U S A 2008; 105(44): 17046-9.

[57]   Tobi EW, Lumey LH, Talens RP, *et al.* DNA methylation differences after exposure to prenatal famine are common and timing-and sex-specific. Hum Mol Genet 2009; 18(21): 4046-53.

[58]   Steegers-Theunissen RP, Obermann-Borst SA, Kremer D, *et al.* Periconceptional maternal folic acid use of 400 microg per day is related to increased methylation of the IGF2 gene in the very young child. PLoS One 2009; 4(11): e7845.

[59]   Darnaudery M, Maccari S. Epigenetic programming of the stress response in male and female rats by prenatal restraint stress. Brain Res Rev 2008; 57(2): 571-85.

[60]   Oberlander TF, Weinberg J, Papsdorf M, Grunau R, Misri S, Devlin AM. Prenatal exposure to maternal depression, neonatal methylation of human glucocorticoid receptor gene (NR3C1) and infant cortisol stress responses. Epigenetics 2008; 3(2): 97-106.

[61]   Weaver IC, Cervoni N, Champagne FA, *et al.* Epigenetic programming by maternal behavior. Nat Neurosci 2004; 7(8): 847-54.

[62]   Gheorghe CP, Goyal R, Mittal A, Longo LD. Gene expression in the placenta: maternal stress and epigenetic responses. The International journal of developmental biology 2010; 54(2-3): 507-23.

[63]   Le Bouc Y, Rossignol S, Azzi S, Steunou V, Netchine I, Gicquel C. Epigenetics, genomic imprinting and assisted reproductive technology. Ann Endocrinol (Paris) 2010; 194(2): 287-297, discussion 297-300.

[64]   Menezo Y, Elder K, Benkhalifa M, Dale B. DNA methylation and gene expression in IVF. Reproductive biomedicine online 2010; 20(6): 709-10.

[65]   Peters DD, Lepikhov K, Rodenacker K, *et al.* Effect of IVF and laser zona dissection on DNA methylation pattern of mouse zygotes. Mamm Genome 2009; 20(9-10): 664-73.

[66]   Fauque P, Jouannet P, Lesaffre C, *et al.* Assisted Reproductive Technology affects developmental kinetics, H19 Imprinting Control Region methylation and H19 gene expression in individual mouse embryos. BMC Dev Biol 2007; 7:116.

[67]   Fortier AL, Lopes FL, Darricarrere N, Martel J, Trasler JM. Superovulation alters the expression of imprinted genes in the midgestation mouse placenta. Hum Mol Genet 2008; 17(11): 1653-65.

[68]   Li T, Vu TH, Ulaner GA, *et al.* IVF results in *de novo* DNA methylation and histone methylation at an Igf2-H19 imprinting epigenetic switch. Mol Hum Reprod 2005; 11(9): 631-40.

[69]   Market-Velker BA, Zhang L, Magri LS, Bonvissuto AC, Mann MR. Dual effects of superovulation: loss of maternal and paternal imprinted methylation in a dose-dependent manner. Hum Mol Genet 2010; 19(1): 36-51.

[70]   Fulka H, Fulka J, Jr. No differences in the DNA methylation pattern in mouse zygotes produced *in vivo*, *in vitro*, or by intracytoplasmic sperm injection. Fertil Steril 2006; 86(5): 1534-6.

[71]   Gomes MV, Huber J, Ferriani RA, Amaral Neto AM, Ramos ES. Abnormal methylation at the KvDMR1 imprinting control region in clinically normal children conceived by assisted reproductive technologies. Mol Hum Reprod 2009; 15(8): 471-7.

[72]   Tierling S, Souren NY, Gries J, *et al.* Assisted reproductive technologies do not enhance the variability of DNA methylation imprints in human. J Med Genet 2010; 47(6): 371-6.

[73]   Katari S, Turan N, Bibikova M, *et al.* DNA methylation and gene expression differences in children conceived *in vitro* or *in vivo*. Hum Mol Genet 2009; 18(20): 3769-78.

[74]   Santos F, Hyslop L, Stojkovic P, *et al.* Evaluation of epigenetic marks in human embryos derived from IVF and ICSI. Hum Reprod 2010; 25(9): 2387-95.

[75]   Lim D, Bowdin SC, Tee L, *et al.* Clinical and molecular genetic features of Beckwith-Wiedemann syndrome associated with assisted reproductive technologies. Hum Reprod 2009; 24(3): 741-7.

[76]   Palermo GD, Neri QV, Takeuchi T, Squires J, Moy F, Rosenwaks Z. Genetic and epigenetic characteristics of ICSI children. Reproductive biomedicine online 2008; 17(6): 820-33.

[77]   Abel EL, Hannigan JH. Maternal risk factors in fetal alcohol syndrome: provocative and permissive influences. Neurotoxicol Teratol 1995; 17(4): 445-62.

[78]   O'Leary CM. Fetal alcohol syndrome: diagnosis, epidemiology, and developmental outcomes. J Paediatr Child Health 2004; 40(1-2) :2-7.

[79]   Hamid A, Kaur J. Long-term alcohol ingestion alters the folate-binding kinetics in intestinal brush border membrane in experimental alcoholism. Alcohol (Fayetteville, NY) 2007; 41(6): 441-6.

[80]   Garro AJ, McBeth DL, Lima V, Lieber CS. Ethanol consumption inhibits fetal DNA methylation in mice: implications for the fetal alcohol syndrome. Alcohol Clin Exp Res 1991; 15(3): 395-8.

[81]   Kaminen-Ahola N, Ahola A, Maga M, *et al.* Maternal ethanol consumption alters the epigenotype and the phenotype of offspring in a mouse model. PLoS genetics 2010; 6(1): e1000811.

[82]   Rosenberg MJ, Wolff CR, El-Emawy A, Staples MC, Perrone-Bizzozero NI, Savage DD. Effects of moderate drinking during pregnancy on placental gene expression. Alcohol 2010; 44(7-8): 673-90.

[83]   Sittig LJ, Dennis K, Andrus BM, Varga K, Herzing LB, Redei EE, Eds. Ethanol in utero alters imprinting of iodothyronine deiodinase III. Proceedings of The Endocrine Society's Annual Meeting; 2009 June 10-13; Washington, USA 2009; p.1-757

[84]   Liu Y, Balaraman Y, Wang G, Nephew KP, Zhou FC. Alcohol exposure alters DNA methylation profiles in mouse embryos at early neurulation. Epigenetics 2009; 4(7): 500-11.

[85]   Haycock PC, Ramsay M. Exposure of Mouse Embryos to Ethanol During Preimplantation Development: Effect on DNA Methylation in the H19 Imprinting Control Region. Biol Reprod 2009; 81(4): 618-27.

[86]   Ouko LA, Shantikumar K, Knezovich J, Haycock P, Schnugh DJ, Ramsay M. Effect of alcohol consumption on CpG methylation in the differentially methylated regions of H19 and IG-DMR in male gametes: implications for fetal alcohol spectrum disorders. Alcohol Clin Exp Res 2009; 33(9): 1615-27.

[87]   Bisgaard H, Loland L, Holst KK, Pipper CB. Prenatal determinants of neonatal lung function in high-risk newborns. J Allergy Clin Immunol 2009; 123(3): 651-7, 7 e1-4.

[88]   Magnusson LL, Olesen AB, Wennborg H, Olsen J. Wheezing, asthma, hayfever, and atopic eczema in childhood following exposure to tobacco smoke in fetal life. Clin Exp Allergy 2005; 35(12): 1550-6.

[89]   Li YF, Langholz B, Salam MT, Gilliland FD. Maternal and grandmaternal smoking patterns are associated with early childhood asthma. Chest 2005; 127(4): 1232-41.

[90]   Belinsky SA, Snow SS, Nikula KJ, Finch GL, Tellez CS, Palmisano WA. Aberrant CpG island methylation of the p16(INK4a) and estrogen receptor genes in rat lung tumors induced by particulate carcinogens. Carcinogenesis 2002; 23(2): 335-9.

[91]   Belinsky SA, Palmisano WA, Gilliland FD, *et al.* Aberrant promoter methylation in bronchial epithelium and sputum from current and former smokers. Cancer Res 2002; 62(8): 2370-7.

[92]   Liu H, Zhou Y, Boggs SE, Belinsky SA, Liu J. Cigarette smoke induces demethylation of prometastatic oncogene synuclein-gamma in lung cancer cells by downregulation of DNMT3B. Oncogene 2007; 26(40): 5900-10.

[93]   Pulling LC, Vuillemenot BR, Hutt JA, Devereux TR, Belinsky SA. Aberrant promoter hypermethylation of the death-associated protein kinase gene is early and frequent in murine lung tumors induced by cigarette smoke and tobacco carcinogens. Cancer Res 2004; 64(11): 3844-8.

[94]   Launay JM, Del Pino M, Chironi G, *et al.* Smoking induces long-lasting effects through a monoamine-oxidase epigenetic regulation. PloS one 2009; 4(11): e7959.

[95]   Breton CV, Byun HM, Wenten M, Pan F, Yang A, Gilliland FD. Prenatal tobacco smoke exposure affects global and gene-specific DNA methylation. Am J Respir Crit Care Med 2009; 180(5): 462-7.

[96]   Skinner MK, Manikkam M, Guerrero-Bosagna C. Epigenetic transgenerational actions of environmental factors in disease etiology. Trends Endocrinol Metab. 2010;21(4):214-22.

[97]   Rubin MM. Antenatal exposure to DES: lessons learned.future concerns. Obstet Gynecol Surv 2007; 62(8): 548-55.

[98]   Sato K, Fukata H, Kogo Y, Ohgane J, Shiota K, Mori C. Neonatal exposure to diethylstilbestrol alters the expression of DNA methyltransferases and methylation of genomic DNA in the epididymis of mice. Endocr J 2006; 53(3): 331-7.

[99]   Bromer JG, Zhou Y, Taylor MB, Doherty L, Taylor HS. Bisphenol-A exposure in utero leads to epigenetic alterations in the developmental programming of uterine estrogen response. FASEB J 2010; 24(7): 2273-80.

[100]   Dolinoy DC, Weidman JR, Waterland RA, Jirtle RL. Maternal genistein alters coat color and protects Avy mouse offspring from obesity by modifying the fetal epigenome. Environ Health Perspect 2006; 114(4): 567-72.

[101]   Day JK, Bauer AM, DesBordes C, *et al.* Genistein alters methylation patterns in mice. J Nutr 2002; 132(Suppl 8): 2419S-23S.

[102]   Anway MD, Cupp AS, Uzumcu M, Skinner MK. Epigenetic transgenerational actions of endocrine disruptors and male fertility. Science 2005; 308(5527): 1466-9.

[103]   Chang HS, Anway MD, Rekow SS, Skinner MK. Transgenerational epigenetic imprinting of the male germline by endocrine disruptor exposure during gonadal sex determination. Endocrinology 2006; 147(12): 5524-41.

[104]   Zama AM, Uzumcu M. Fetal and neonatal exposure to the endocrine disruptor methoxychlor causes epigenetic alterations in adult ovarian genes. Endocrinology 2009; 150(10): 4681-91.

[105]   Bowman RV, Wright CM, Davidson MR, Francis SM, Yang IA, Fong KM. Epigenomic targets for the treatment of respiratory disease. Expert Opin Ther Targets 2009; 13(6): 625-40.

[106]   Herceg Z. Epigenetics and cancer: towards an evaluation of the impact of environmental and dietary factors. Mutagenesis 2007; 22(2): 91-103.

[107]   Pilsner JR, Hu H, Ettinger A, *et al.* Influence of prenatal lead exposure on genomic methylation of cord blood DNA. Environ Health Perspect 2009; 117(9): 1466-71.

[108]   Desaulniers D, Xiao GH, Lian H, *et al.* Effects of mixtures of polychlorinated biphenyls, methylmercury, and organochlorine pesticides on hepatic DNA methylation in prepubertal female Sprague-Dawley rats. Int J Toxicol 2009; 28(4): 294-307.

[109]   Novikova SI, He F, Bai J, Cutrufello NJ, Lidow MS, Undieh AS. Maternal cocaine administration in mice alters DNA methylation and gene expression in hippocampal neurons of neonatal and prepubertal offspring. PloS one 2008; 3(4): e1919.

[110]   Zhu R, Li BZ, Li H, *et al.* Association of p16INK4A hypermethylation with hepatitis B virus X protein expression in the early stage of HBV-associated hepatocarcinogenesis. Pathology international 2007; 57(6): 328-36.

[111]   Graessmann A, Graessmann M. DNA methylation, chromatin structure and regulation of Herpes simplex virus tk gene expression. Gene 1988; 74(1): 135-7.

[112]   Kruger DH, Schroeder C, Santibanez-Koref M, Reuter M. Avoidance of DNA methylation. A virus-encoded methylase inhibitor and evidence for counterselection of methylase recognition sites in viral genomes. Cell Biophys 1989; 15(1-2): 87-95.

[113]   Nishida N. Impact of hepatitis virus and aging on DNA methylation in human hepatocarcinogenesis. Histol Histopathol 2010; 25(5): 647-54.

[114] Tao Q, Robertson KD. Stealth technology: how Epstein-Barr virus utilizes DNA methylation to cloak itself from immune detection. Clin Immunol 2003; 109(1): 53-63.

[115] Arbibe L, Kim DW, Batsche E, *et al.* An injected bacterial effector targets chromatin access for transcription factor NF-kappaB to alter transcription of host genes involved in immune responses. Nat Immunol 2007; 8(1): 47-56.

[116] Weidner-Glunde M, Ottinger M, Schulz TF. WHAT do viruses BET on? Front Biosci 2010; 15: 537-49.

[117] Evain-Brion D, Malassine A. Human placenta as an endocrine organ. Growth Horm IGF Res 2003; 13 (Suppl A): S34-7.

[118] Hemberger M. Epigenetic landscape required for placental development. Cell Mol Life Sci 2007; 64(18): 2422-36.

[119] Vlahovic M, Bulic-Jakus F, Juric-Lekic G, Fucic A, Maric S, Serman D. Changes in the placenta and in the rat embryo caused by the demethylating agent 5-azacytidine. The International journal of developmental biology 1999; 43(8): 843-6.

[120] Serman L, Vlahovic M, Sijan M, *et al.* The impact of 5-azacytidine on placental weight, glycoprotein pattern and proliferating cell nuclear antigen expression in rat placenta. Placenta 2007; 28(8-9): 803-11.

[121] Rahnama F, Shafiei F, Gluckman PD, Mitchell MD, Lobie PE. Epigenetic regulation of human trophoblastic cell migration and invasion. Endocrinology 2006; 147(11): 5275-83.

[122] Arima T, Hata K, Tanaka S, *et al.* Loss of the maternal imprint in Dnmt3Lmat-/-mice leads to a differentiation defect in the extraembryonic tissue. Developmental biology 2006; 297(2): 361-73.

[123] Li E, Bestor TH, Jaenisch R. Targeted mutation of the DNA methyltransferase gene results in embryonic lethality. Cell 1992; 69(6): 915-26.

[124] Chapman V, Forrester L, Sanford J, Hastie N, Rossant J. Cell lineage-specific undermethylation of mouse repetitive DNA. Nature 1984; 307(5948): 284-6.

[125] Gama-Sosa MA, Wang RY, Kuo KC, Gehrke CW, Ehrlich M. The 5-methylcytosine content of highly repeated sequences in human DNA. Nucleic Acids Res 1983; 11(10): 3087-95.

[126] Gama-Sosa MA, Midgett RM, Slagel VA, *et al.* Tissue-specific differences in DNA methylation in various mammals. Biochim Biophys Acta 1983; 740(2): 212-9.

[127] Gama-Sosa MA, Slagel VA, Trewyn RW, *et al.* The 5-methylcytosine content of DNA from human tumors. Nucleic Acids Res 1983; 11(19): 6883-94.

[128] Faulkner GJ, Kimura Y, Daub CO, *et al.* The regulated retrotransposon transcriptome of mammalian cells. Nature genetics 2009; 41(5): 563-71.

[129] Tsien F, Fiala ES, Youn B, *et al.* Prolonged culture of normal chorionic villus cells yields ICF syndrome-like chromatin decondensation and rearrangements. Cytogenet Genome Res 2002; 98(1): 13-21.

[130] Reiss D, Zhang Y, Mager DL. Widely variable endogenous retroviral methylation levels in human placenta. Nucleic Acids Res 2007; 35(14): 4743-54.

[131] Shen HM, Nakamura A, Sugimoto J, *et al.* Tissue specificity of methylation and expression of human genes coding for neuropeptides and their receptors, and of a human endogenous retrovirus K family. Journal of human genetics 2006; 51(5): 440-50.

[132] Cotton AM, Avila L, Penaherrera MS, Affleck JG, Robinson WP, Brown CJ. Inactive X chromosome-specific reduction in placental DNA methylation. Hum Mol Genet 2009; 18(19): 3544-52.

[133] Constancia M, Hemberger M, Hughes J, *et al.* Placental-specific IGF-II is a major modulator of placental and fetal growth. Nature 2002; 417(6892): 945-8.

[134] Tilghman SM. The sins of the fathers and mothers: genomic imprinting in mammalian development. Cell 1999; 96(2): 185-93.

[135] Renfree MB. Review: Marsupials: placental mammals with a difference. Placenta 2010; (Suppl 31): S21-6.

[136] Renfree MB, Hore TA, Shaw G, Graves JA, Pask AJ. Evolution of genomic imprinting: insights from marsupials and monotremes. Annual review of genomics and human genetics 2009; 10: 241-62.

[137] Reik W, Lewis A. Co-evolution of X-chromosome inactivation and imprinting in mammals. Nature reviews 2005; 6(5): 403-10.

[138] Tunster SJ, Tycko B, John RM. The imprinted Phlda2 gene regulates extraembryonic energy stores. Mol Cell Biol 2010; 30(1): 295-306.

[139] Burke W, Press N. Genetics as a tool to improve cancer outcomes: ethics and policy. Nat Rev Cancer 2006; 6(6): 476-82.

[140] Diplas AI, Lambertini L, Lee MJ, *et al.* Differential expression of imprinted genes in normal and IUGR human placentas. Epigenetics 2009; 4(4): 235-40.

[141] Guo L, Choufani S, Ferreira J, *et al*. Altered gene expression and methylation of the human chromosome 11 imprinted region in small for gestational age (SGA) placentae. Developmental biology 2008; 320(1): 79-91.

[142] Tabano S, Colapietro P, Cetin I, *et al*. Epigenetic modulation of the IGF2/H19 imprinted domain in human embryonic and extra-embryonic compartments and its possible role in fetal growth restriction. Epigenetics 2010; 5(4): 313-24.

[143] Mann MR, Lee SS, Doherty AS, *et al*. Selective loss of imprinting in the placenta following preimplantation development in culture. Development 2004; 131(15): 3727-35.

[144] Zechner U, Pliushch G, Schneider E, *et al*. Quantitative methylation analysis of developmentally important genes in human pregnancy losses after ART and spontaneous conception. Mol Hum Reprod 2010; 16(9): 704-13.

[145] Luo YM, Fang Q, Zhuang GL, Liang RC, Liu QL. [Characteristics of IGF-II gene imprinting in twin placentas] Zhonghua Yi Xue Yi Chuan Xue Za Zhi 2006; 23(5): 497-501.

[146] Rawn SM, Cross JC. The evolution, regulation, and function of placenta-specific genes. Annual review of cell and developmental biology 2008; 24: 159-81.

[147] Rakyan V, Down T, Thorne N, *et al*. An integrated resource for genome-wide identification and analysis of human tissue-specific differentially methylated regions (tDMRs). Genome research 2008; 18(9): 1518-29.

[148] Yuen RK, Avila L, Penaherrera MS, *et al*. Human placental-specific epipolymorphism and its association with adverse pregnancy outcomes. PloS one 2009; 4(10): e7389.

[149] Maccani MA, Marsit CJ. Epigenetics in the placenta. Am J Reprod Immunol 2009; 62(2): 78-89.

[150] Perry JK, Lins RJ, Lobie PE, Mitchell MD. Regulation of invasive growth: similar epigenetic mechanisms underpin tumour progression and implantation in human pregnancy. Clin Sci (Lond) 2010; 118(7): 451-7.

[151] Guilleret I, Osterheld MC, Braunschweig R, Gastineau V, Taillens S, Benhattar J. Imprinting of tumor-suppressor genes in human placenta. Epigenetics 2009; 4(1): 62-8.

[152] Novakovic B, Rakyan V, Ng HK, *et al*. Specific tumour-associated methylation in normal human term placenta and first-trimester cytotrophoblasts. Mol Hum Reprod 2008; 14(9): 547-54.

[153] Wong NC, Novakovic B, Weinrich B, *et al*. Methylation of the adenomatous polyposis coli (APC) gene in human placenta and hypermethylation in choriocarcinoma cells. Cancer letters 2008; 268(1): 56-62.

[154] Chiu RW, Chim SS, Wong IH, *et al*. Hypermethylation of RASSF1A in human and rhesus placentas. Am J Pathol 2007; 170(3): 941-50.

[155] Cohen CJ, Lock WM, Mager DL. Endogenous retroviral LTRs as promoters for human genes: a critical assessment. Gene 2009; 448(2): 105-14.

[156] Medstrand P, Landry JR, Mager DL. Long terminal repeats are used as alternative promoters for the endothelin B receptor and apolipoprotein C-I genes in humans. J Biol Chem 2001; 276(3): 1896-903.

[157] Redman CW, Sargent IL. Latest advances in understanding preeclampsia. Science 2005 10; 308(5728): 1592-4.

[158] Wallis AB, Saftlas AF, Hsia J, Atrash HK. Secular trends in the rates of preeclampsia, eclampsia, and gestational hypertension, United States, 1987-2004. Am J Hypertens 2008; 21(5): 521-6.

[159] Solomon CG, Seely EW. Preeclampsia--searching for the cause. N Engl J Med. 2004; 350(7): 641-2.

[160] Smith GC, Pell JP, Walsh D. Pregnancy complications and maternal risk of ischaemic heart disease: a retrospective cohort study of 129,290 births. Lancet 2001; 357(9273): 2002-6.

[161] Fisher SJ. The placental problem: linking abnormal cytotrophoblast differentiation to the maternal symptoms of preeclampsia. Reprod Biol Endocrinol. 2004; 5: 2-53.

[162] Barker DJ, Clark PM. Fetal undernutrition and disease in later life. Rev Reprod 1997; 2(2): 105-12.

[163] Huppertz B. Placental origins of preeclampsia: challenging the current hypothesis. Hypertension 2008; 51(4): 970-5.

[164] Jauniaux E, Poston L, Burton GJ. Placental-related diseases of pregnancy: Involvement of oxidative stress and implications in human evolution. Hum Reprod Update 2006; 12(6): 747-55.

[165] Robinson WP, McGillivray B, Lewis ME, Arbour L, Barrett I, Kalousek DK. Prenatally detected trisomy 20 mosaicism. Prenatal diagnosis 2005; 25(3): 239-44.

[166] Robinson WP, Penaherrera MS, Jiang R, *et al*. Assessing the role of placental trisomy in preeclampsia and intrauterine growth restriction. Prenatal diagnosis 2010; 30(1): 1-8.

[167] Yong PJ, Langlois S, von Dadelszen P, Robinson W. The association between preeclampsia and placental trisomy 16 mosaicism. Prenatal diagnosis 2006; 26(10): 956-61.

[168] Hung TH, Burton GJ. Hypoxia and reoxygenation: a possible mechanism for placental oxidative stress in preeclampsia. Taiwan J Obstet Gynecol 2006; 45(3): 189-200.

[169] Tsui DW, Chan KC, Chim SS, *et al*. Quantitative aberrations of hypermethylated RASSF1A gene sequences in maternal plasma in pre-eclampsia. Prenatal diagnosis 2007; 27(13): 1212-8.

[170] Yu L, Chen M, Zhao D, *et al.* The H19 gene imprinting in normal pregnancy and pre-eclampsia. Placenta 2009; 30(5): 443-7.

[171] Mutze S, Rudnik-Schoneborn S, Zerres K, Rath W. Genes and the preeclampsia syndrome. J Perinat Med 2008; 36(1): 38-58.

[172] GOPEC C. Disentangling fetal and maternal susceptibility for pre-eclampsia: a British multicenter candidate-gene study. Am J Hum Genet 2005; 77(1): 127-31.

[173] Sood R, Zehnder JL, Druzin ML, Brown PO. Gene expression patterns in human placenta. Proc Natl Acad Sci U S A 2006; 103(14): 5478-83.

[174] Farina A, Morano D, Arcelli D, *et al.* Gene expression in chorionic villous samples at 11 weeks of gestation in women who develop preeclampsia later in pregnancy: implications for screening. Prenatal diagnosis 2009; 29(11): 1038-44.

[175] Farina A, Sekizawa A, De Sanctis P, *et al.* Gene expression in chorionic villous samples at 11 weeks' gestation from women destined to develop preeclampsia. Prenatal diagnosis 2008; 28(10): 956-61.

[176] Founds SA, Conley YP, Lyons-Weiler JF, Jeyabalan A, Hogge WA, Conrad KP. Altered global gene expression in first trimester placentas of women destined to develop preeclampsia. Placenta 2009; 30(1): 15-24.

[177] Tycko B. Imprinted genes in placental growth and obstetric disorders. Cytogenetic and genome research 2006; 113(1-4): 271-8.

[178] Lambertini L, Diplas AI, Lee MJ, Sperling R, Chen J, Wetmur J. A sensitive functional assay reveals frequent loss of genomic imprinting in human placenta. Epigenetics 2008; 3(5): 261-9.

[179] Pozharny Y, Lambertini L, Ma Y, *et al.* Genomic loss of imprinting in first-trimester human placenta. Am J Obstet Gynecol 2010; 202(4): 391 e1-8.

[180] Bourque DK, Avila L, Penaherrera M, von Dadelszen P, Robinson WP. Decreased placental methylation at the H19/IGF2 imprinting control region is associated with normotensive intrauterine growth restriction but not preeclampsia. Placenta 2010; 31(3): 197-202.

[181] Yuen RK, Penaherrera MS, von Dadelszen P, McFadden DE, Robinson WP. DNA methylation profiling of human placentas reveals promoter hypomethylation of multiple genes in early-onset preeclampsia. Eur J Hum Genet 2010; 18(9): 1006-1012.

[182] Barker DJ. The intrauterine origins of cardiovascular disease. Acta Paediatr Suppl 1993; 82 (Suppl 391): 93-9; discussion 100.

[183] Barker DJ. Maternal nutrition and cardiovascular disease. Nutr Health. 1993;9(2):99-106.

[184] James WP. WHO recognition of the global obesity epidemic. Int J Obes (Lond) 2008; 32 (Suppl 7): S120-6.

[185] Catalano PM, Tyzbir ED, Roman NM, Amini SB, Sims EA. Longitudinal changes in insulin release and insulin resistance in nonobese pregnant women. American journal of obstetrics and gynecology 1991;165(6 Pt 1): 1667-72.

[186] Huda SS, Brodie LE, Sattar N. Obesity in pregnancy: prevalence and metabolic consequences. Seminars in fetal & neonatal medicine 2010; 15(2):70-6.

[187] Kerrigan AM, Kingdon C. Maternal obesity and pregnancy: a retrospective study. Midwifery 2010; 26(1): 138-46.

[188] Yogev Y, Visser GH. Obesity, gestational diabetes and pregnancy outcome. Seminars in fetal & neonatal medicine 2009; 14(2): 77-84.

[189] Chu SY, Callaghan WM, Kim SY, *et al.* Maternal obesity and risk of gestational diabetes mellitus. Diabetes Care 2007; 30(8): 2070-6.

[190] Budge H, Gnanalingham MG, Gardner DS, Mostyn A, Stephenson T, Symonds ME. Maternal nutritional programming of fetal adipose tissue development: long-term consequences for later obesity. Birth Defects Res C Embryo Today 2005; 75(3): 193-9.

[191] Oken E, Gillman MW. Fetal origins of obesity. Obes Res 2003; 11(4): 496-506.

[192] Kliegman RM, Gross T. Perinatal problems of the obese mother and her infant. Obstetrics and gynecology 1985; 66(3): 299-306.

[193] Ehrenberg HM, Durnwald CP, Catalano P, Mercer BM. The influence of obesity and diabetes on the risk of cesarean delivery. American journal of obstetrics and gynecology 2004; 191(3): 969-74.

[194] Whitaker RC. Predicting preschooler obesity at birth: the role of maternal obesity in early pregnancy. Pediatrics 2004; 114(1): e29-36.

[195] Whitaker RC, Pepe MS, Wright JA, Seidel KD, Dietz WH. Early adiposity rebound and the risk of adult obesity. Pediatrics 1998; 101(3): E5.

[196] Sorensen HT, Sabroe S, Rothman KJ, Gillman M, Fischer P, Sorensen TI. Relation between weight and length at birth and body mass index in young adulthood: cohort study. BMJ 1997; 315(7116): 1137.

[197] Boney CM, Verma A, Tucker R, Vohr BR. Metabolic syndrome in childhood: association with birth weight, maternal obesity, and gestational diabetes mellitus. Pediatrics 2005; 115(3): e290-6.

[198] Fall CH, Stein CE, Kumaran K, *et al.* Size at birth, maternal weight, and type 2 diabetes in South India. Diabet Med 1998; 15(3): 220-7.

[199] Forsen T, Eriksson JG, Tuomilehto J, Teramo K, Osmond C, Barker DJ. Mother's weight in pregnancy and coronary heart disease in a cohort of Finnish men: follow up study. BMJ 1997; 315(7112): 837-40.

[200] Rich-Edwards JW, Stampfer MJ, Manson JE, *et al.* Birth weight and risk of cardiovascular disease in a cohort of women followed up since 1976. BMJ 1997; 315(7105): 396-400.

[201] Samuelsson AM, Matthews PA, Argenton M, *et al.* Diet-induced obesity in female mice leads to offspring hyperphagia, adiposity, hypertension, and insulin resistance: a novel murine model of developmental programming. Hypertension 2008; 51(2): 383-92.

[202] Gabbe SG. Definition, detection, and management of gestational diabetes. Obstetrics and gynecology 1986; 67(1): 121-5.

[203] Gabbe SG. Gestational diabetes mellitus. N Engl J Med 1986; 315(16): 1025-6.

[204] Linne Y, Barkeling B, Rossner S. Natural course of gestational diabetes mellitus: long term follow up of women in the SPAWN study. BJOG 2002; 109(11): 1227-31.

[205] Leikin E, Jenkins JH, Graves WL. Prophylactic insulin in gestational diabetes. Obstetrics and gynecology1987; 70(4): 587-92.

[206] Surkan PJ, Hsieh CC, Johansson AL, Dickman PW, Cnattingius S. Reasons for increasing trends in large for gestational age births. Obstetrics and gynecology 2004; 104(4): 720-6.

[207] Heerwagen MJ, Miller MR, Barbour LA, Friedman JE. Maternal Obesity and Fetal Metabolic Programming: A Fertile Epigenetic Soil. Am J Physiol Regul Integr Comp Physiol 2010; 299(3): R711-22.

[208] Bar-Zohar D, Azem F, Klausner J, Abu-Abeid S. Pregnancy after laparoscopic adjustable gastric banding: perinatal outcome is favorable also for women with relatively high gestational weight gain. Surg Endosc 2006; 20(10): 1580-3.

[209] Dixon JB, Dixon ME, O'Brien PE. Pregnancy after Lap-Band surgery: management of the band to achieve healthy weight outcomes. Obes Surg 2001; 11(1): 59-65.

[210] Maggard MA, Yermilov I, Li Z, *et al.* Pregnancy and fertility following bariatric surgery: a systematic review. JAMA 2008; 300(19): 2286-96.

[211] Skull AJ, Slater GH, Duncombe JE, Fielding GA. Laparoscopic adjustable banding in pregnancy: safety, patient tolerance and effect on obesity-related pregnancy outcomes. Obes Surg 2004; 14(2): 230-5.

[212] Allison DB, Paultre F, Heymsfield SB, Pi-Sunyer FX. Is the intra-uterine period really a critical period for the development of adiposity? Int J Obes Relat Metab Disord 1995; 19(6): 397-402.

[213] Poulsen P, Vaag AA, Kyvik KO, Moller Jensen D, Beck-Nielsen H. Low birth weight is associated with NIDDM in discordant monozygotic and dizygotic twin pairs. Diabetologia 1997; 40(4): 439-46.

[214] Loos RJ, Beunen G, Fagard R, Derom C, Vlietinck R. Birth weight and body composition in young adult men--a prospective twin study. Int J Obes Relat Metab Disord 2001; 25(10): 1537-45.

[215] Loos RJ, Fagard R, Beunen G, Derom C, Vlietinck R. Birth weight and blood pressure in young adults: a prospective twin study. Circulation 2001; 104(14): 1633-8.

[216] Dabelea D, Hanson RL, Lindsay RS, *et al.* Intrauterine exposure to diabetes conveys risks for type 2 diabetes and obesity: a study of discordant sibships. Diabetes 2000; 49(12): 2208-11.

[217] Aagaard-Tillery KM, Grove K, Bishop J, *et al.* Developmental origins of disease and determinants of chromatin structure: maternal diet modifies the primate fetal epigenome. Journal of molecular endocrinology 2008; 41(2): 91-102.

[218] Zhang J, Zhang F, Didelot X, *et al.* Maternal high fat diet during pregnancy and lactation alters hepatic expression of insulin like growth factor-2 and key microRNAs in the adult offspring. BMC genomics 2009; 10: 478.

[219] Plagemann A, Roepke K, Harder T, *et al.* Epigenetic malprogramming of the insulin receptor promoter due to developmental overfeeding. J Perinat Med 2010; 38(4): 393-400.

[220] Shao WJ, Tao LY, Gao C, Xie JY, Zhao RQ. Alterations in methylation and expression levels of imprinted genes H19 and Igf2 in the fetuses of diabetic mice. Comp Med 2008; 58(4): 341-6.

[221] Mujezinovic F, Alfirevic Z. Procedure-related complications of amniocentesis and chorionic villous sampling: a systematic review. Obstetrics and gynecology 2007; 110(3): 687-94.

[222] Papageorgiou EA, Fiegler H, Rakyan V, *et al.* Sites of differential DNA methylation between placenta and peripheral blood: molecular markers for noninvasive prenatal diagnosis of aneuploidies. Am J Pathol 2009; 174(5): 1609-18.

[223] Chu T, Burke B, Bunce K, Surti U, Allen Hogge W, Peters DG. A microarray-based approach for the identification of epigenetic biomarkers for the noninvasive diagnosis of fetal disease. Prenat Diagn 2009; 29(11): 1020-30.

[224] Papageorgiou EA, Karagrigoriou A, Tsaliki E, Velissariou V, Carter NP, Patsalis PC. Fetal-specific DNA methylation ratio permits noninvasive prenatal diagnosis of trisomy 21. Nat Med 2011; 17(4): 510-3.

[225] Tong YK, Jin S, Chiu RW, et al. Noninvasive prenatal detection of trisomy 21 by an epigenetic-genetic chromosome-dosage approach. Clinical chemistry 2010; 56(1): 90-8.

[226] Brown L, Brown G, Vacek P, Brown S. Aneuploidy detection in mixed DNA samples by methylation-sensitive amplification and microarray analysis. Clinical chemistry 2010; 56(5): 805-13.

[227] Litton C, Stone J, Eddleman K, Lee MJ. Noninvasive Prenatal Diagnosis: Past, Present, and Future. The Mount Sinai journal of medicine, New York 2009; 76(6): 521-8.

[228] Poon LC, Nekrasova E, Anastassopoulos P, Livanos P, Nicolaides KH. First-trimester maternal serum matrix metalloproteinase-9 (MMP-9) and adverse pregnancy outcome. Prenatal diagnosis 2009; 29(6): 553-9.

[229] Poon LC, Kametas NA, Maiz N, Akolekar R, Nicolaides KH. First-trimester prediction of hypertensive disorders in pregnancy. Hypertension 2009; 53(5): 812-8.

[230] Than NG, Romero R, Hillermann R, Cozzi V, Nie G, Huppertz B. Prediction of preeclampsia-a workshop report. Placenta 2008; 29(Suppl A): S83-5.

[231] Smith GC, Crossley JA, Aitken DA, et al. Circulating angiogenic factors in early pregnancy and the risk of preeclampsia, intrauterine growth restriction, spontaneous preterm birth, and stillbirth. Obstetrics and gynecology 2007; 109(6): 1316-24.

[232] Spencer CA, Allen VM, Flowerdew G, Dooley K, Dodds L. Low levels of maternal serum PAPP-A in early pregnancy and the risk of adverse outcomes. Prenatal diagnosis 2008; 28(11): 1029-36.

[233] Bellido ML, Radpour R, Lapaire O, et al. MALDI-TOF mass array analysis of RASSF1A and SERPINB5 methylation patterns in human placenta and plasma. Biol Reprod 2010; 82(4): 745-50.

[234] Chelbi ST, Mondon F, Jammes H, et al. Expressional and epigenetic alterations of placental serine protease inhibitors: SERPINA3 is a potential marker of preeclampsia. Hypertension 2007; 49(1): 76-83.

Subject Index

Oocytes; 21-22, 25, 28

Oxidative stress; 61, 35, 80, 90-92, 100, 103-106, 109-110

Oxygen tension; 101-103

Parathyroid hormone related protein (PTHr); 98

Peroxisome proliferator-activated receptors (PPARs); 41-42, 138

Placental epigenetics; 134-136

Placental inhibitor growth factor (PIGF); 43, 62-63

Placental growth hormone (pGH); 40-41, 47, 49-50

Placental lactogen, human(hPL); 40, 47-49, 90

Placentation; 35-51, 64, 68, 83, 98, 100-103, 112

Platelet-derived growth factor (PDGF); 43, 107

Preeclampsia (PE); 20, 27, 29, 35, 38, 49, 58-59, 61-62, 67, 74, 76-77, 81, 83, 97-113

Pregnancy associated plasma protein-A (PAPP-A); 26, 41-42, 61-62, 64-66

Prenatal screening of chromosomal abnormalities; 26, 63-64

Preterm birth (PTB); 20, 26-29, 58, 60, 62, 64, 83,

Primordial germ; 131

Progesterone; 3-6, 9, 11, 40, 47, 50-51, 64, 77-78, 83

Progesterone receptor (PR); 5

Prostacyclins; 6, 7, 108-109

Prostaglandins; 6-7, 40-41, 61, 79, 108

Proteinuria; 58-59, 62, 80, 97-100, 103, 107, 110-112, 136

Reactive oxygen species (ROS); 92, 103-106

Renin-angiotensin system (RAS); 98

Retinoic acid receptors (RARs); 41

Selectins; 8, 64-66, 107

Singleton pregnancy; 20, 24, 26-27, 29, 92

Small for gestational age (SGA); 20, 27, 29, 62, 65, 112, 136

Smoking; 60, 62, 132-314

Soluble fms-like tyrosine kinase-1 (s-Fit-1); 61-64, 77-78, 82-83, 104, 106-107

Spontaneous abortion; 20, 24-25, 74, 77-78, 119

SR-B1; 47, 51

Steroids; 3, 5-6, 40-41, 49-51, 90

Stress; 50, 60-61, 63, 90, 100, 103, 105-107, 131-133, 138

Syncytin (HERV); 38-40, 135-136

Syncytiotrophoblast; 4, 35-40, 42, 45-51, 63-65, 89-90, 100-101, 103-106, 112, 134

T cell receptors (TCR); 74-84

T cells; 74-84, 103

T helper (Th); 74-84

Thromboxane; 61, 108-109

Thyroid hormone receptor (THR); 41

Toll-like receptors (TLRs); 74, 76, 83

Transforming growth factor (TGF); 11-12, 40-41, 49, 61, 63-64, 75, 77-80, 82-83, 102, 106

Trisomy; 38, 48, 50, 63, 139

Trophoblast; 3-6, 8-9, 11-12, 35-51, 61-62, 64, 74-78, 80-82, 89, 97, 100-103, 105-106, 112, 136

Twin; 24-25, 50, 138

Vaginal bleeding; 20, 25

Vascular cell adhesion molecule (VCAM); 61-62, 65, 107

Vascular epidermal growth factor (VEGF); 43, 49, 61-64, 76-78, 80, 82-83, 106

Very low birth weight (VLBW); 24, 27

Very low-density lipoproteins(VLDL); 46-47, 49, 51, 89-90

Villous trophoblast; 35, 37, 39- 40, 43, 81, 102, 105-106, 112

Villous trophoblast differentiation; 39

Vitamin C; 109-110

Vitamin D; 110

www.ingramcontent.com/pod-product-compliance
Lightning Source LLC
Chambersburg PA
CBHW041709210326
41598CB00007B/589